T0259337

Dangerous Fever in the Emergency Department

Editors

EMILIE J.B. CALVELLO
CHRISTIAN THEODOSIS

EMERGENCY MEDICINE CLINICS OF NORTH AMERICA

www.emed.theclinics.com

Consulting Editor
AMAL MATTU

November 2013 • Volume 31 • Number 4

ELSEVIER

1600 John F. Kennedy Boulevard • Suite 1800 • Philadelphia, Pennsylvania, 19103-2899

http://www.theclinics.com

EMERGENCY MEDICINE CLINICS OF NORTH AMERICA Volume 31, Number 4
November 2013 ISSN 0733-8627, ISBN-13: 978-0-323-24219-6

Editor: Patrick Manley
Developmental Editor: Donald Mumford

Emergency Medicine Clinics of North America (ISSN 0733-8627) is published quarterly by Elsevier Inc., 360 Park Avenue South, New York, NY, 10010-1710. Months of issue are February, May, August, and November. Business and Editorial Offices: 1600 John F. Kennedy Boulevard, Suite 1800, Philadelphia, PA 19103-2899. Customer Service Office: 6277 Sea Harbor Drive, Orlando, FL 32887-4800. Periodicals postage paid at New York, NY, and additional mailing offices. Subscription prices are $149.00 per year (US students), $298.00 per year (US individuals), $507.00 per year (US institutions), $211.00 per year (international students), $428.00 per year (international individuals), $609.00 per year (international institutions), $211.00 per year (Canadian students), $368.00 per year (Canadian individuals), and $609.00 per year (Canadian institutions). International air speed delivery is included in all *Clinics'* subscription prices. All prices are subject to change without notice. **POSTMASTER:** Send address changes to *Emergency Medicine Clinics of North America*, Elsevier Periodicals Customer Service, 11830 Westline Industrial Drive, St. Louis, MO 63146. Customer Service (orders, claims, online, change of address): Elsevier Periodicals Customer Service, 11830 Westline Industrial Drive, St. Louis, MO 63146. Tel: 1-800-654-2452 (U.S. and Canada); 314-453-7041 (outside U.S. and Canada). Fax: 314-453-5170. E-mail: journalscustomerservice-usa@elsevier.com (for print support); journalsonline support-usa@elsevier.com (for online support).

Reprints. For copies of 100 or more of articles in this publication, please contact the Commercial Reprints Department, Elsevier Inc., 360 Park Avenue South, New York, NY 10010-1710. Tel.: 212-633-3874; Fax: 212-633-3820; E-mail: reprints@elsevier.com.

Emergency Medicine Clinics of North America is covered in *MEDLINE/PubMed (Index Medicus), Current Contents/Clinical Medicine, EMBASE/Excerpta Medica, BIOSIS, SciSearch, CINAHL, ISI/BIOMED,* and *Research Alert.*

Printed and bound by CPI Group (UK) Ltd, Croydon, CR0 4YY

Transferred to digital print 2012

Contributors

CONSULTING EDITOR

AMAL MATTU, MD
Professor and Vice Chair, Department of Emergency Medicine, University of Maryland
School of Medicine, Baltimore, Maryland

EDITORS

EMILIE J.B. CALVELLO, MD, MPH
Assistant Professor, Department of Emergency Medicine, University of Maryland School
of Medicine, Baltimore, Maryland

CHRISTIAN THEODOSIS, MD, MPH
Assistant Professor, Department of Emergency Medicine, University of Maryland,
Baltimore, Maryland

AUTHORS

WALTER F. ATHA, MD, FACEP
Director, Department of Emergency Medicine, Howard County General Hospital;
Instructor, Department of Emergency Medicine, Johns Hopkins School of Medicine,
Columbia, Maryland

FERMIN BARRUETO Jr, MD
Clinical Associate Professor, Department of Emergency Medicine, University of Maryland
School of Medicine, Baltimore; Chairman, Department of Emergency Medicine, Upper
Chesapeake Health Systems, Bel Air, Maryland

JANAÉ E.P. DARK, MD, MPH
Department of Emergency Medicine, George Washington University School of Medicine,
Washington, DC

MAYA R. DOR, DO
Pediatric Resident, Department of Pediatrics, University of Massachusetts Medical
School, Worcester, Massachusetts

LUCY FRANJIC, MD
Resident Physician, Division of Emergency Medicine, Washington University School of
Medicine, St Louis, Missouri

S. ELIZA HALCOMB, MD
Section Chief, Medical Toxicology, Assistant Professor, Division of Emergency Medicine,
Washington University School of Medicine, St Louis, Missouri

KARIN M. HALVORSON, MD
Pulmonary Critical Care Fellow, Department of Pulmonary and Critical Care, Brown
University, Providence, Rhode Island

RAQUEL F. HARRISON, MD
Resident Physician, Department of Emergency Medicine, New York-Presbyterian Hospital, The University Hospitals of Columbia and Cornell, New York, New York

BRYAN D. HAYES, PharmD
Clinical Assistant Professor, Department of Emergency Medicine, University of Maryland School of Medicine; Clinical Pharmacist of Emergency Medicine and Toxicology, Department of Pharmacy, University of Maryland Medical Center, Baltimore, Maryland

SIMON KOTLYAR, MD, MSc
Assistant Professor, Division of Global Health, Department of Emergency Medicine, Yale University School of Medicine, New Haven, Connecticut

AISHA T. LIFERIDGE, MD, MPH
Assistant Professor, Department of Emergency Medicine, George Washington University School of Medicine, Washington, DC

JOSEPH P. MARTINEZ, MD
Assistant Professor, Department of Emergency Medicine, University of Maryland School of Medicine, Baltimore, Maryland

PATRICIA A. MCQUILKIN, MD
Department of Pediatrics, University of Massachusetts Medical School, Worcester, Massachusetts

SANDRA P. MEDINILLA, MD, MPH
Assistant Professor of Trauma Surgery and Critical Care, Department of Surgery, Christiana Care Health Services, Newark, Delaware

MAYUR NARAYAN, MD, MPH, MBA, FACS
Assistant Professor, Department of Surgery; Program in Trauma, Director, Center for Injury Prevention and Policy, Associate Director, Division of Medical Education, R Adams Cowley Shock Trauma Center, University of Maryland School of Medicine, Baltimore, Maryland

HELEN OUYANG, MD, MPH
Associate Director, International Emergency Medicine Fellowship; Assistant Professor, Department of Emergency Medicine, Columbia University Medical Center, New York, New York

MARY S. PADEN, MD
Resident Physician, Division of Emergency Medicine, Washington University School of Medicine, St Louis, Missouri

DEVANG M. PATEL, MD
Assistant Professor, Division of Infectious Disease, Department of Medicine, Institute of Human Virology, University of Maryland School of Medicine, Baltimore, Maryland

JENNIFER M. REIFEL SALTZBERG, MD, MPH
Assistant Professor, Department of Emergency Medicine, University of Maryland School of Medicine, Baltimore, Maryland

BRIAN T. RICE, MDCM
Clinical Instructor, Division of Global Health, Department of Emergency Medicine, Yale University School of Medicine, New Haven, Connecticut

DAVID J. RIEDEL, MD
Assistant Professor, Division of Infectious Disease, Department of Medicine, Institute of Human Virology, University of Maryland School of Medicine, Baltimore, Maryland

ANDREA G. TENNER, MD, MPH
Assistant Professor, Department of Emergency Medicine, University of Maryland, Baltimore, Maryland

ROBYN WING, MD
Pediatric Chief Resident, Department of Pediatrics, University of Massachusetts Medical School, Worcester, Massachusetts

Contents

A common cause of fever with signs of shock is sepsis. Sepsis describes the spectrum of illness caused by severe infection. The incidence of sepsis is increasing and mortality can be high. Diagnosing the disease and implementing treatment early can decrease mortality. Early treatment includes empirical antibiotics and resuscitation. The diverse physiology present in sepsis can make the resuscitation complex; many different types of hemodynamic monitoring may be necessary. Even with this complexity, an organized approach can improve patient outcomes.

Fever in ill travelers returning home from developing nations is common. Most travelers present with undifferentiated febrile syndromes. Regional proportionate morbidity rates and patients' travel histories are essential in narrowing the differential diagnosis. Most patients in whom a diagnosis is confirmed have malaria, dengue fever, enteric fever, or rickettsial disease. Empiric treatment based on the clinical presentation is required in many cases, because acquisition of confirmatory laboratory data is often delayed. The focus of this article is travel-related illness that falls within the spectrum of the acute febrile syndrome.

Any patient presenting to the emergency department (ED) with fever triggers consideration of the administration of an antimicrobial. Empiric antimicrobial therapy has become a cornerstone of treatment. Frequently, the decision to initiate empiric treatment needs to be made before the definitive diagnosis is known. In such cases, an organized approach is helpful. This article aims to provide a systems-based approach to prescribing antimicrobials to patients presenting to the ED with fever, while understanding the risk associated with overutilization. An understanding of the key considerations is needed to ensure that decisions are made well and appropriate treatment begins promptly.

EMERGENCY MEDICINE CLINICS OF NORTH AMERICA

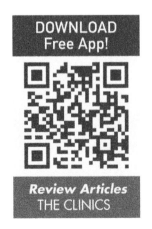

PROGRAM OBJECTIVE
The goal of *Emergency Medicine Clinics of North America* is to keep practicing emergency medicine physicians and emergency medicine residents up to date with current clinical practice in emergency medicine by providing timely articles reviewing the state of the art in patient care.

TARGET AUDIENCE
All practicing physicians and healthcare professionals who provide patient care utilizing findings from *Emergency Medicine Clinics of North America*.

LEARNING OBJECTIVES
Upon completion of this activity, participants will be able to:
1. Identify heat-related illness.
2. Discuss fever in the returning traveler, immunocompromised host, pediatric patient, and the postoperative patient.
3. Determine the rational use of antimicrobials for the treatment of fevers in the emergency department.

ACCREDITATION
The Elsevier Office of Continuing Medical Education (EOCME) is accredited by the Accreditation Council for Continuing Medical Education (ACCME) to provide continuing medical education for physicians.

The EOCME designates this enduringmaterial for a maximum of 15 *AMA PRA Category 1 Credit*(s)™. Physicians should claim only the credit commensurate with the extent of their participation in the activity.

All other health care professionals requesting continuing education credit for this enduring material will be issued a certificate of participation.

DISCLOSURE OF CONFLICTS OF INTEREST
The EOCME assesses conflict of interest with its instructors, faculty, planners, and other individuals who are in a position to control the content of CME activities. All relevant conflicts of interest that are identified are thoroughly vetted by EOCME for fair balance, scientific objectivity, and patient care recommendations. EOCME is committed to providing its learners with CME activities that promote improvements or quality in healthcare and not a specific proprietary business or a commercial interest.

The planning committee, staff, authors and editors listed below have identified no financial relationships or relationships to products or devices they or their spouse/life partner have with commercial interest related to the content of this CME activity:
Walter Atha, MD, FACEP; Fermin Barrueto, Jr, MD; Emilie Calvello, MD, MPH; Janae E. Dark, MD, MPH; Maya R. Dor, DO; Lucy Franjic, MD; Eliza Halcomb, MD; Karin Halvorson, MD; Raquel F. Harrison, MD; Bryan Hayes, PharmD; Kristen Helm; Brynne Hunter; Simon Kotlyar, MD, MSc, DTM&H; Indu Kumari; Sandy Lavery; Aisha Liferidge, BS, MD, MPH; Patrick Manley; Joseph P. Martinez, MD; Amal Mattu, MD; Jill McNair; Patricia McQuilkin, MD; Sandra Medinilla, MD, MPH; Mayur Narayan; Helen Ouyang, MD, MPH; Mary Paden, MD; Nagarajan Paramasivam; Devang Patel, MD, MS; Jenny Reifel Saltzberg, MD, MPH; Brian Travis Wilcox Rice, MDCM; David J. Riedel, MD; Andrea Tenner, MD, MPH; Christian Theodosis, MD, MPH; Robyn Wing, MD.

The planning committee, staff, authors and editors listed below have identified financial relationships or relationships to products or devices they or their spouse/life partner have with commercial interest related to the content of this CME activity:

UNAPPROVED/OFF-LABEL USE DISCLOSURE
The EOCME requires CME faculty to disclose to the participants:
1. When products or procedures being discussed are off-label, unlabelled, experimental, and/or investigational (not US Food and Drug Administration (FDA) approved); and
2. Any limitations on the information presented, such as data that are preliminary or that represent ongoing research, interim analyses, and/or unsupported opinions. Faculty may discuss information about pharmaceutical agents that is outside of FDA-approved labelling. This information is intended solely for CME and is not intended to promote off-label use of these medications. If you have any questions, contact the medical affairs department of the manufacturer for the most recent prescribing information.

TO ENROLL
To enroll in the *Emergency Medicine Clinics* Continuing Medical Education program, call customer service at 1-800-654-2452 or sign up online at http://www.theclinics.com/home/cme. The CME program is available to subscribers for an additional annual fee of $212 USD.

METHOD OF PARTICIPATION

In order to claim credit, participants must complete the following:

1. Complete enrolment as indicated above.
2. Read the activity.
3. Complete the CME Test and Evaluation. Participants must achieve a score of 70% on the test. All CME Tests and Evaluations must be completed online.

CME INQUIRIES/SPECIAL NEEDS

For all CME inquiries or special needs, please contact elsevierCME@elsevier.com.

Foreword

Dangerous Fever in the Emergency Department

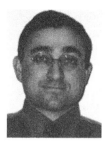

Amal Mattu, MD
Consulting Editor

I used to love "fever." As a chief complaint, I generally thought "fever" was easy: check urine and a chest X-ray, listen for a murmur, tap on the spine, and check for a stiff neck. It was even easier if the patient also complained of a focal area of pain: check the throat, check the skin, do a pelvic exam, and so on. Look for an infection wherever there's pain. If the patient looked really sick, then pan-culture, check a lactate, and initiate the latest broad-spectrum "gorrilacillins." And no matter how vague the related complaints were, if we found an infection, we could usually treat it and end the workup. "Fever" was pretty much a piece of cake, as emergency department (ED) workups go.

During a shift last week, I received a firm reminder that nothing is truly easy in the ED for long. A 45-year-old woman was brought to the ED by friends for a chief complaint of "fever." She was not only febrile but also tachycardic and confused. This would normally be far from a diagnostic dilemma and would elicit a reflexive order set of labs, blood cultures, head computerized tomogram, and intravenous ceftriaxone followed by lumbar puncture. However, we soon discovered from her friends that the patient had just returned from a trip to Nepal and had been taking some "prophylactic medications" along with a medicine for a recently diagnosed thyroid problem. At that point, I'm not sure if it was my jaw or my confidence that caused the loud "thud" on the floor. Yes, the patient had a fever...but was this truly an infection or was it a toxicologic or endocrine etiology? Was there an antidote? Did she need β-blockers and iodine? Even if it were an infection, was the choice of antibiotics appropriate? Did she have some unusual type of bacteria or a parasite or the latest form of Asian flu that we were missing? Did I need to contact the local Health Department and quarantine her close contacts? I decided at that point that I *hate* "fever."

Maybe "hate" is an overstatement, but that case certainly taught me to *respect* fever. Although fever is common and usually somewhat mundane, I was reminded of the broad differential diagnosis associated with this vital sign abnormality. Many of these

Emerg Med Clin N Am 31 (2013) xiii–xiv
http://dx.doi.org/10.1016/j.emc.2013.09.007
emed.theclinics.com

etiologies are easily forgotten because of the frequency with which we see fevers associated with simple infections, yet they are nevertheless deadly if not diagnosed and treated quickly. The astute health care provider must always consider these less common conditions or they will easily be missed.

In this issue of *Emergency Medicine Clinics of North America*, Drs Emilie Calvello and Christian Theodosis provide us with an outstanding reference that covers the gamut of potential ED conditions that can present with fever. They address not only "typical" infections and sepsis but also less common lethal infections from atypical organisms. Especially important is their article that addresses a growing ED presentation: fever in the returning traveler. Fevers caused by medications are addressed, as well as fevers caused by endocrine and environmental conditions. Three special patient populations are addressed with individual articles: the pediatric patient, the postprocedure patient, and the immunocompromised patient. Finally, important reminders are provided regarding the rational use of antibiotics in ED practice.

The guest editors and authors are to be commended for providing us with a practical and important reference for everyday use in the ED. I suppose if I had had this issue of *Emergency Medicine Clinics of North America* last week, my shift would have been much smoother...and my patient's thyroid storm would have been diagnosed with far less stress. Drs Calvello and Theodosis may help me love "fever" once again.

Amal Mattu, MD
Department of Emergency Medicine
University of Maryland School of Medicine
Baltimore, MD 21201, USA

E-mail address:
amattu@smail.umaryland.edu

Preface

Dangerous Fever in the Emergency Department

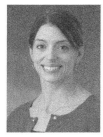 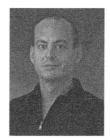

Emilie J.B. Calvello, MD, MPH   Christian Theodosis, MD, MPH
Editors

The importance and significance of fever as a sign or symptom of severe illness or severe infection have been known for thousands of years. Long before any type of standardized measuring device was crafted to report temperature objectively, people knew the experience of "fever." Fever is among the commonest causes of concern among patients seeking health services and is associated with many health emergencies. Here we describe several deadly conditions commonly associated with fever. Topics have been selected for their clinical and educational significance. The material is presented in conventional terms, whereby "diseases" are understood in terms of interaction between hosts, vectors, and the environment.

"Fever" is selected as a prime organizing unit for discussion with foreknowledge of its broad scope. When fever is associated with infection, it is because the architecture of the common disease model connects the concepts of host, pathogen, and environment to the possibilities of susceptible host, vector of contagion, and permissive environment. Likewise, noninfectious causes of pyrexia are markedly influenced by vulnerability—otherwise understood as host-specific attributes. With limited expansion, "vectors of disease" can include both endogenous (eg, hypermetabolic states due to endocrine derangements) and exogenous causes of disease (eg, toxins, poisons, drugs). The environment itself can be more or less permissive to the development of several noninfectious disease states. Indeed, hosts can be killed outright by the environment. They can also be injured by identified specific risks that are external to themselves but confined by the environment.

This issue of *Emergency Medicine Clinics of North America* updates the emergency physician on recent advances in the diagnosis and management of sentinel syndromes associated with fever. The content of this issue is organized around pathogenicity, vulnerability, and environmental exposure. Sepsis, the classical dangerous fever,

Emerg Med Clin N Am 31 (2013) xv–xvi
http://dx.doi.org/10.1016/j.emc.2013.09.006
0733-8627/13/$ – see front matter © 2013 Elsevier Inc. All rights reserved.
emed.theclinics.com

and its management are reviewed in the first article. The broad and mostly infectious differential of fever in the returned traveler is covered in the second article, followed by the rational application of antimicrobials to fever caused by infectious organisms. The next two articles represent fever within the intricate architecture of their physiological causes and effects. The following two articles untangle cases of fever caused mostly by toxic, exogenic, and iatrogenic events. The next three articles are devoted to fevers that cause particular concern among specific groups of people—the immunocompromised, the pediatric patient, and those with recent surgery. Finally, in the last article we cover dangerous fever caused by the exposure of the host to environmental extremes.

It is our intent that the content of this issue will be a guide and resource to the emergency physician faced with the conundrum of the complicated patient with undifferentiated pyrexia. We wish to thank the authors who dedicated much time and effort to this project. We also acknowledge with much gratitude the support of Dr Amal Mattu and Patrick Manley throughout the creation of this issue.

Emilie J.B. Calvello, MD, MPH
Department of Emergency Medicine
University of Maryland School of Medicine
6th Floor, Suite 200
110 South Paca Street
Baltimore, MD 21201, USA

Christian Theodosis, MD, MPH
Department of Emergency Medicine
University of Maryland School of Medicine
6th Floor, Suite 200
110 South Paca Street
Baltimore, MD 21201, USA

E-mail addresses:
emiliejbc@gmail.com (E.J.B. Calvello)
christian.theodosis@gmail.com (C. Theodosis)

Fever and Signs of Shock
The Essential Dangerous Fever

Jennifer M. Reifel Saltzberg, MD, MPH

KEYWORDS

- Sepsis • Septic shock • Severe sepsis • Early goal-directed therapy • Resuscitation
- Sepsis bundles

KEY POINTS

- Sepsis is a complex disease process, with an incidence that is increasing globally.
- Early resuscitation reduces mortality substantially.
- Administration of empirical antibiotics within an hour reduces mortality.
- Resuscitation needs to address the multiple possible clinical manifestations of sepsis.

Fever with signs of shock is a common presentation in the emergency department and requires prompt evaluation and treatment. When the underlying cause is infectious, the patient is diagnosed with sepsis, specifically septic shock. Sepsis is the systemic response to infection that manifests as a continuum of illness from mild vital sign abnormalities to cardiovascular collapse. The disease is widespread, and the incidence is growing.[1–3] In the past 12 years, effective therapy for sepsis has been developed and has reduced mortality, hospital length of stay, and treatment costs when implemented in a timely manner.[4–7]

Other causes of fever with signs of shock include pulmonary embolus; toxidromes such as salicylate toxicity and neuroleptic malignant syndrome; and endocrine emergencies such as adrenal crisis, pheochromocytoma, or diabetic ketoacidosis. These other possible diagnoses require specific interventions, but treatment of sepsis should not be delayed because it is time dependent and does not worsen most other possible illnesses. Sepsis care can begin while the diagnosis is being confirmed. The importance of this early diagnosis and treatment means that the emergency department plays a fundamental role in reducing the mortality associated with sepsis.

EPIDEMIOLOGY

Severe sepsis and septic shock are common clinical scenarios. In the United States, the incidence is 3 cases per 1000, or 751,000 cases annually.[1] Many of these cases

Disclosures: None.
Department of Emergency Medicine, University of Maryland School of Medicine, 110 South Paca Street, 6th Floor, Suite 200, Baltimore, MD 21201, USA
E-mail address: jreifelsaltzberg@umem.org

Emerg Med Clin N Am 31 (2013) 907–926
http://dx.doi.org/10.1016/j.emc.2013.07.009
0733-8627/13/$ – see front matter © 2013 Elsevier Inc. All rights reserved.

present to an emergency department first. Severe sepsis accounts for more than 500,000 emergency department visits each year.[1,8] Despite improvements in antibiotic therapy and expansion of preventive measures such as vaccines, the incidence of sepsis has been increasing[1,8] as much as 8.7% per year.[9]

The sepsis-related mortality in the United States is an estimated 215,000 deaths per year, with 9.3% of all deaths attributed to sepsis.[1] This mortality is not uniform across the country and ranges from 41 to 88 deaths per 100,000, depending on the state.[10] The geographic variability of sepsis mortality is also shown between countries even when matched for relative level of available resources. A study in Australia[11] showed that patients admitted to an intensive care unit (ICU) with sepsis had a mortality of 24.7%. In Spain, a similar population had a mortality of 37.5%.[12] Internationally the most common infectious source of sepsis is respiratory, accounting for 44% of cases.[1,9] There is some geographic variability in the source; intra-abdominal infections are more common in Mexico, accounting for 47% of ICU sepsis admissions.[13]

PATHOPHYSIOLOGY

An infection stimulates an inflammatory response, which, under some circumstances, becomes systemic and causes sepsis. Early triggers of sepsis are inflammatory mediators such as tumor necrosis factor α and interleukin-1.[14] The activity of these cytokines decreases later in sepsis, when other mediators of an antiinflammatory response, including interleukin-4 and interleukin-10, become more prevalent.[14] This downregulation of the inflammatory system has been shown histologically with a decrease in B cells, dendritic cells, and CD4 T cells in spleens of septic patients.[14] A patient's location along this continuum of inflammation and antiinflammatory response is influenced by host characteristics and comorbidities as well as the infectious agent.

The inflammatory pathways that are activated in sepsis interact with the blood hemostasis pathways. When an infection and its response are localized, the two systems slow local blood flow through the microcirculation and increase endothelial permeability, allowing the immune system to clear the pathogen.[15] When the response is generalized, as in sepsis, the actions of the inflammatory and blood hemostasis pathways decrease blood flow through the microcirculation systemically and limit oxygen delivery.[16] Nitric oxide (NO) is also produced, but the amount changes with time like the other inflammatory mediators. Initially, NO causes vasodilation, but then its production decreases and vasoconstriction occurs. These processes contribute to arteriovenous shunting and blood pressure abnormalities.[16]

Microcirculatory changes might be difficult to measure at the onset of illness, but as the disease progresses, these changes contribute to the overall clinical picture. Decreased systemic vascular resistance and capillary leak caused by endothelial dysfunction[15] combine with insensible fluid losses from fever, tachypnea, and poor oral intake to cause hypovolemia and distributive shock. Some patients have cardiogenic dysfunction caused by an interaction of multiple secondary mediators acting on the cardiac tissue.[17] These diverse influences cause variability of the clinical presentation: some patients have hypotension and high cardiac output, others show hypovolemia and low cardiac output, and others have no hypotension but show evidence of microcirculatory deficits and tissue hypoperfusion.

The treatment of sepsis is based on optimizing the cardiovascular system to improve oxygen delivery in the microcirculation. Therapies targeting secondary mediators are not generalizable and are still under investigation.[14,18] The diagnosis of sepsis must consider the disease in its various clinical presentations, and treatment must adapt to changes in the patient's hemodynamics as the disease progresses.

CASE DEFINITION

The last 2 decades have witnessed significant progress toward a better definition of sepsis. A set of criteria is now used to define cases and facilitate early detection (**Fig. 1**). The severity of illness is also important to categorize, because it is explicitly connected to intervention, treatment targets, and outcome. Sepsis is stratified by inflammation, end-organ involvement, and tissue hypoperfusion. Even patients with uncomplicated sepsis are important to identify early. Glickman and colleagues[19]

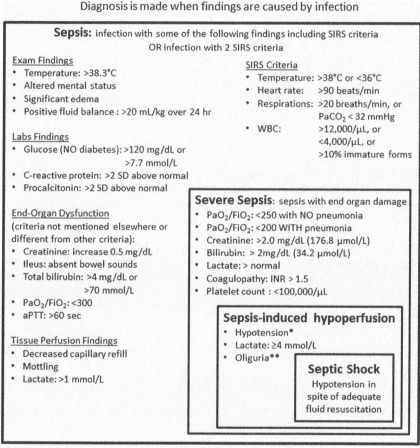

Diagnosis is made when findings are caused by infection

Sepsis: infection with some of the following findings including SIRS criteria OR infection with 2 SIRS criteria

Exam Findings
• Temperature: >38.3°C
• Altered mental status
• Significant edema
• Positive fluid balance : >20 mL/kg over 24 hr

Labs Findings
• Glucose (NO diabetes): >120 mg/dL or >7.7 mmol/L
• C-reactive protein: >2 SD above normal
• Procalcitonin: >2 SD above normal

End-Organ Dysfunction
(criteria not mentioned elsewhere or different from other criteria):
• Creatinine: increase 0.5 mg/dL
• Ileus: absent bowel sounds
• Total bilirubin: >4 mg/dL or >70 mmol/L
• PaO_2/FiO_2: <300
• aPTT: >60 sec

Tissue Perfusion Findings
• Decreased capillary refill
• Mottling
• Lactate: >1 mmol/L

SIRS Criteria
• Temperature: >38°C or <36°C
• Heart rate: >90 beats/min
• Respirations: >20 breaths/min, or $PaCO_2 < 32$ mmHg
• WBC: >12,000/μL, or <4,000/μL, or >10% immature forms

Severe Sepsis: sepsis with end organ damage
• PaO_2/FiO_2: <250 with NO pneumonia
• PaO_2/FiO_2: <200 WITH pneumonia
• Creatinine: >2.0 mg/dL (176.8 μmol/L)
• Bilirubin: > 2mg/dL (34.2 μmol/L)
• Lactate: > normal
• Coagulopathy: INR > 1.5
• Platelet count : <100,000/μL

Sepsis-induced hypoperfusion
• Hypotension*
• Lactate: ≥4 mmol/L
• Oliguria**

Septic Shock
Hypotension in spite of adequate fluid resuscitation

*HYPOTENSION: SYSTOLIC BLOOD PRESSURE (SBP) < 90 MM HG
MEAN ARTERIAL PRESSURE (MAP) < 70 MM HG
SBP DECREASE > 40 MM HG
≤ 2 SD BELOW NORMAL FOR AGE
**OLIGURIA: < 0.5 ML/KG/HR FOR MORE THAN 2 HR DESPITE ADEQUATE FLUID RESUSCITATION

Fig. 1. Definition of sepsis, based on past definitions conferences[20,21] and the SSC guidelines.[7] Note the discrepancy in the criteria with some values to diagnose sepsis different from those to diagnose severe sepsis. When there is a question if a patient has severe sepsis or sepsis, clinical judgment is important for discerning where the patient is on the spectrum of disease. aPTT, activated thromboplastin time; Fio_2, fraction of inspried oxyge; INR, international normalized ratio; $Paco_2$, partial pressure of arterial carbon dioxide; Pao_2, partial pressure of arterial oxygen; SD, standard deviation; SIRS, systemic inflammatory response syndrome; WBC, white blood cells.

documented that uncomplicated sepsis progressed to more serious stages of illness in 22.7% of patients within 72 hours. A plan for management and reevaluation is important at all levels of disease.

Patients could have signs of inflammation due to causes other than infection. Systemic inflammatory response syndrome (SIRS) can be caused by infection, trauma, thermal injury, pancreatitis, or pulmonary embolism (**Fig. 2**). SIRS is diagnosed when 2 of the following criteria are present: body temperature greater than 38°C or less than 36°C; heart rate greater than 90 beats per minute; respiratory rate greater than 20 breaths per minute or $Paco_2$ less than 32 mm Hg; and a white blood cell count greater than 12,000/mm^3, less than 4000/mm^3, or with more than 10% immature forms.[20] Sepsis is diagnosed when SIRS is caused by a suspected infection. These criteria simplify the diagnosis and are useful, but they do not replace clinical judgment.[21] Some patients have SIRS but no infection; others have sepsis but show a blunted SIRS response. Elderly patients do not always have fever,[22] and immunocompromised patients might not have leukocytosis. Patients taking β-blockers or calcium channel blockers might not have tachycardia. Although they are helpful, SIRS criteria do not have ideal sensitivity or specificity for diagnosis.

In 2001, the diagnostic criteria were revisited and expanded.[21] The expanded definition does not rely exclusively on SIRS criteria and allows clinicians to incorporate other aspects of the bedside examination. The additional signs and laboratory values include a higher body temperature of 38.3°C or greater, altered mental status, significant edema, hyperglycemia, increased C-reactive protein level, increased procalcitonin level, increased lactate concentration, ileus, and markers of end-organ dysfunction and hypovolemia (see **Fig. 1**). This expanded definition allows the identification of sepsis throughout the continuum of disease, because it includes markers used to identify patients with a more serious clinical status. These expanded criteria allow clinicians to identify sepsis based on the bedside examination, whereas SIRS criteria identify septic patients based on vital sign abnormalities and a blood test. Once sepsis is recognized, illness severity should be assessed to identify patients who need a higher level of care. Both diagnostic methods have value,[21] and the most appropriate criteria may vary with clinical setting.

Severe sepsis is defined as sepsis with end-organ damage.[21] Patients with this condition are not in shock but are at high risk for hypoperfusion. This can be a difficult

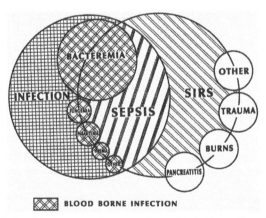

Fig. 2. The interrelationship between SIRS, sepsis, and infection. (*From* Bone RC, Balk RA, Cerra FB, et al. Definitions for sepsis and organ failure and guidelines for the use of innovative therapies in sepsis. Chest 1992;101:1645; with permission.)

diagnosis to make because these patients do not always have marked vital sign abnormalities, and the diagnosis usually depends on laboratory values. The specific thresholds for organ dysfunction vary slightly, depending on the criteria being used. Some definitions are adapted from the expanded criteria to make the sepsis definition reflect findings from the clinical examination.[21] Some diagnostic thresholds are adapted from these criteria as well as clinical severity scores.[7,21,23] Just as with the expanded definition for sepsis, the criteria for end-organ dysfunction and severe sepsis also include defining symptoms for patients who have more serious clinical presentations and require a higher level of care.[7] This strategy helps ensure that patients with more serious illness receive the time-dependent treatments for severe sepsis as well those for more serious presentations. Patients with severe sepsis can be difficult to distinguish from those with uncomplicated sepsis, but it is important to make this diagnosis and begin appropriate treatment because severe sepsis is associated with a higher mortality.[2,24,25]

Sepsis-induced tissue hypoperfusion is defined as sepsis with hypotension, an increased blood lactate concentration of 4 mmol/L or greater, or oliguria less than 0.5 mL/kg/h for 2 hours.[7] Some clinicians use a lower threshold for lactate, but this practice has not been rigorously evaluated, so no recommendation can be made.[7] Septic shock is defined as hypotension despite adequate fluid resuscitation.[21] The recommended treatment of these patient groups is the same,[7] and the terms are used interchangeably in this document. Hypoperfusion can occur with no hypotension.[26–28] Patients with an increased lactate level but no hypotension (ie, cryptic shock) have a similar mortality to patients with hypotension[26,27] and respond to the same measures that improve septic shock.[26,27]

TREATMENT

As the epidemiology and pathophysiology suggest, patients with sepsis are a heterogeneous group. The condition can be caused by different infectious agents, and the disease progresses over time to involve different organ systems. Two patients with similar infections can have a different course; the same patient can have a change in physiology. Sepsis treatment needs to address the diverse and evolving physiology of a patient with sepsis as well as treat the infection causing hemodynamic instability (**Fig. 3**). The goals of interventions can be summarized succinctly as follows:

1. Control the infectious source.
2. Restore end-organ perfusion.

An international effort, the Surviving Sepsis Campaign (SSC), developed multiple tools to help implement these therapies, with the goal of reducing mortality. The SSC developed guidelines that emphasize the timing of interventions and help to standardize treatment by recommending a series of best practices.[7] To encourage standardization of therapy, recommendations are grouped into bundles, with the important interventions highlighted as bundle elements. The most recent guidelines were adapted to improve care by focusing on the time-dependent aspects of sepsis care. Treatment is divided into 3-hour and 6-hour bundles (**Box 1**). The recommendations not incorporated into the bundles are still important but are not time dependent. The SSC guidelines are a collection of best practices and should not replace clinical decision making. They were written as recommendations and do not represent a standard of care.

The guidelines for pediatric patients are different from those for adults with sepsis.[7,29] Sepsis in the pediatric population has a lower mortality, and the physiologic

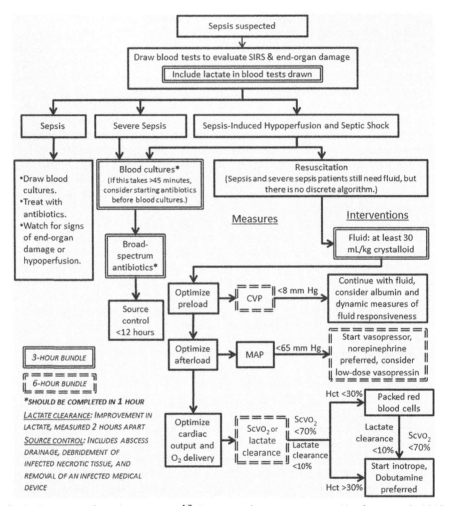

Fig. 3. Summary of sepsis treatment.[4,7] CVP, central venous pressure; Hct, hematocrit; MAP, mean arterial blood pressure; Scvo$_2$, central venous oxygen saturation; SIRS, systemic inflammatory response syndrome.

response to severe infection changes with age, which means that different medications are useful for resuscitation. The basic principles associated with sepsis treatment still apply. Early resuscitation and timely antibiotics should be administered to patients in shock, followed by best practices regarding supportive therapy.[7,29]

Case Management: Controlling the Infectious Source

Blood cultures

Patients should be started on broad-spectrum antibiotics, but that treatment should be de-escalated as soon as possible. To facilitate de-escalation, samples of blood and other possibly infected body fluids should be collected for culture before antibiotics are started. To improve the likelihood of culturing the pathogenic agent, blood samples should be collected for 2 sets of aerobic and anaerobic blood cultures, with at least 1 set drawn percutaneously. The recommended volume of blood for

---

Box 1
Surviving Sepsis Campaign bundles

To be completed within 3 hours:

1. Measure lactate level

2. Obtain blood cultures before administration of antibiotics

3. Administer broad-spectrum antibiotics

4. Administer 30 mL/kg crystalloid for hypotension or lactate 4 mmol/L or greater

To be completed within 6 hours:

5. Apply vasopressors (for hypotension that does not respond to initial fluid resuscitation) to maintain an MAP of 65 mm Hg or greater

6. In the event of persistent arterial hypotension despite volume resuscitation (septic shock) or initial lactate ≥4 mmol/L (36 mg/dL):

   a. Measure central venous pressure (CVP)[a]

   b. Measure central venous oxygen saturation ($Scvo_2$).[a]

7. Remeasure lactate if initial lactate was increased.[a]

[a] Targets for quantitative resuscitation included in the guidelines are CVP 8 mm Hg or greater, $Scvo_2$ 70% or greater, and normalization of lactate.
From Dellinger RP, Levy MM, Rhodes A, et al. Surviving sepsis campaign: international guidelines for management of severe sepsis and septic shock: 2012. Crit Care Med 2013;41:580–637; with permission.

---

culture is 10 mL or greater per culture tube.[7] If the patient has an indwelling vascular device that was placed more than 48 hours before sepsis developed, 1 set of samples should be drawn from that device. Other body fluids, (eg, urine, sputum, wound drainage, or cerebrospinal fluid) should be collected for culture if they are suspected of being infected. When samples cannot be processed immediately, they may be refrigerated or frozen until they can be analyzed. If the collection of a sample delays the administration of antibiotics by more than 45 minutes, priority should be given to antibiotic administration, because the antibiotics are more important than cultures for reducing the mortality.[7]

β-*D*-Glucan assay and mannan and antimannan antibody assays may be helpful in identifying fungal causes of sepsis.[1,3,7] Many empirical antibiotic regimens do not treat fungal infections, and fungal infection is often diagnosed by blood culture, long after treatment has started. These assays could be helpful in reducing the time to diagnosis and appropriate treatment. These tests are recommended for directing antibiotics only in centers that are familiar with them. The recommendation is not universal, because these assays individually do not have the sensitivity to identify all invasive fungal infections.[30,31] They are more useful when combined[30] or paired with a clinical prediction tool for fungal infection.[31] They should be used by clinicians who are familiar with the tests and can interpret the results appropriately.[7]

Biomarkers
Pierrakos and Vincent[18] determined that 178 biomarkers have been studied in sepsis but only a few of them have the sensitivity and specificity necessary to facilitate diagnosis. Procalcitonin is increased in bacterial infections but does not have the specificity and sensitivity to identify sepsis; however, it has shown usefulness in de-escalating antibiotics.[32–34] There are questions about the most useful algorithm[32]

and the safety of using procalcitonin levels to guide therapy,[34] so it should be used only in centers experienced at interpreting the results.[7] If procalcitonin is followed, the patient can be evaluated for withdrawal of antibiotics when the level decreases to normal or by 80%.[7,32,33] Clinicians experienced with other biomarkers may use them at their own discretion.[7]

Antibiotics

Appropriate early antibiotics significantly reduce the mortality from sepsis. Kumar and colleagues[6] showed that, for every hour that antibiotics are delayed after hypotension, mortality increases 7.6% (**Fig. 4**). A protocol for resuscitation that included antibiotics reduced the time to administration,[35] and antibiotics should be included in any treatment protocol for patients with sepsis. The antimicrobials must be active against the infectious agent. Ineffective antibiotics increase mortality.[36,37] If the wrong antimicrobial is administered first, several hours might pass until an effective one is given. In Kumar and colleagues' study,[6] only 32% of patients who received ineffective antibiotics before the onset of hypotension received effective antibiotics within 3 hours after the onset of hypotension. Many patients who receive ineffective therapy meet the criteria for a nosocomial infection.[38] A protocol for antibiotic selection in these patients may be helpful.

Given the importance of administering effective antibiotics, broad-spectrum antibiotics that are active against all the possible infective agents should be administered as early as possible in the patient's treatment. This recommendation extends to antivirals if the infectious cause is viral (eg, influenza, varicella, or herpes simplex).[7] Empiric antibiotic choice varies regionally depending on prevalence of bacteria and resistance patterns. Some areas also need to address the possibility of infections such as malaria, tuberculosis, and tropical diseases such as melioidosis or dengue.[39] Even in these situations, empiric antibiotics should be given, because delays quickly increase mortality. Combination antibiotic therapy should be administered to certain patients, eg, neutropenic patients with severe sepsis, patients with multidrug-resistant

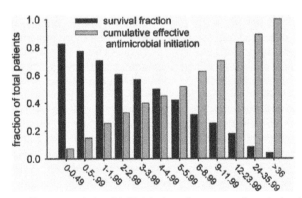

Fig. 4. Cumulative effective antimicrobial initiation after onset of septic shock–associated hypotension and associated survival. The x-axis represents time (in hours) after first documentation of septic shock–associated hypotension. The *black bars* represent the fraction of patients surviving to hospital discharge for effective therapy initiated within the given time interval. The *gray bars* represent the cumulative fraction of patients having received effective antimicrobials at any given time point. (*From* Kumar A, Roberts D, Wood K, et al. Duration of hypotension prior to initiation of effective antimicrobial therapy is the critical determinant of survival in human septic shock. Crit Care Med 2006;34:1592; with permission.)

pathogens such as *Acinetobacter* and *Pseudomonas* spp, and patients with septic shock and respiratory failure. The recommended combination is an extended-spectrum β-lactam and either an aminoglycoside or a fluoroquinolone.[7] Patients with septic shock caused by *Streptococcus pneumoniae* should receive a β-lactam and a macrolide.[7]

After the infectious agent is identified, the antibiotic regimen can be targeted to that organism.[7,38] The patient should be assessed daily for de-escalation of antibiotics, and broad-spectrum antibiotics should be narrowed in 3 to 5 days.[7] Most antibiotics are needed for a total of 7 to 10 days, unless the clinical situation requires a longer course. If a patient's symptoms of sepsis are attributed to a noninfectious cause, all antibiotics can be stopped. This does not mean that antibiotics should be stopped if cultures are negative, because 50% of sepsis cases have no obvious source identified.[7] However, when another diagnosis is made, there is no need to continue the antibiotics.

Given that rapid antibiotic administration can improve mortality, clinical guidelines recommend collection of blood samples for culture and initiating antibiotic treatment within 1 hour of diagnosis of severe sepsis or septic shock. SSC guidelines discuss strategies to facilitate achieving these goals, such as increasing the number of vascular access sites and storing antibiotics in the locations where they are administered, not in the pharmacy. It is acknowledged that the goal of 1 hour might not be feasible for every patient.[7] To emphasize the importance of the timing of these interventions, obtaining blood for culture and administering antibiotics are part of the 3-hour bundle.

Source control

The source of the infection should be treated within 12 hours after diagnosis. An abscess should be drained, and infected necrotic tissue should be debrided. If possible, these procedures should be conducted in a way that causes the least amount of stress on the patient, for example, percutaneous drainage of an abscess instead of abdominal surgery. If an infected medical device is suspected, it should be removed and replaced as soon as possible.[7] The recommendation for early source control must be interpreted within the clinical context. Occasionally, delayed intervention is recommended, such as in patients with peripancreatic necrosis.[7]

Case Management: Restore End-Organ Perfusion

Treatment of a patient with hypoperfusion requires a comprehensive approach, with goals for time to intervention and hemodynamic measures. Septic shock is usually a combination of vasodilation and hypovolemia. Some patients also have a component of cardiogenic shock. This heterogeneity of patients with sepsis is one of the factors complicating resuscitation. Early goal-directed therapy (EGDT) introduced a protocol-based approach to treating septic shock and addressed its heterogeneity by optimizing certain hemodynamic parameters.[4] The protocol aims to improve oxygen delivery by optimizing preload, afterload, cardiac output, and oxygen-carrying capacity. This goal is achieved in a step-wise approach, because actions to improve afterload and cardiac output are not effective until preload is optimized, and treating preload can improve the other measures. Many of the interventions that are part of EGDT have also been incorporated into the SSC's guidelines[7] and represent key elements of the 3-hour and 6-hour bundles. Some studies and past SSC guidelines recommend EGDT for severe sepsis as well as septic shock. Current guidelines recommend EGDT interventions for sepsis-induced tissue hypoperfusion and septic shock.

Preload

Preload is assessed using a central line to measure central venous pressure (CVP), with the recommendation to resuscitate with fluid until the pressure normalizes at 8 to 12 mm Hg. The goal for intubated patients is higher, at 12 to 15 mm Hg. Although CVP is an imperfect measure of intravascular volume status,[40] "it is the most readily obtainable target" when evaluating preload[7] and, when low, it suggests a positive response to fluids. The initial bolus should be a minimum of 30 mL/kg of crystalloid or equivalent of colloid.[7,40] This quantity is recommended only for patients with sepsis-induced tissue hypoperfusion or septic shock, and it should be given as quickly as possible, with the goal of completing the administration within 3 hours of diagnosis. Patients with uncomplicated sepsis and severe sepsis may also need fluid, but no specific quantity is recommended.

The SSC guidelines state that preload should be measured via CVP within 6 hours, which means that treatment can start before the end point is known. In patients with hypovolemia and septic shock, the initial fluid resuscitation is the suggested minimum intervention, and patients may need more volume than the initial bolus. These recommendations allow the treatment of hypovolemia while arranging for central access.

The initial fluid should be 0.9% normal saline, lactated Ringer solution, or albumin. Hydroxyethyl starches should not be the first choice for fluid resuscitation because the safety evidence has been mixed.[7,41–43] Resuscitation with albumin might be just as effective as crystalloid and may even reduce mortality.[44] Albumin use was associated with a slight improvement in mortality in a meta-analysis that compared albumin with crystalloid.[44] More specific information about albumin use in sepsis will be known after 3 current studies are completed.[44] Given the cost differential between crystalloid and albumin solutions, the small suggested mortality benefit, and the lack of definitive evidence, current recommendations are to use albumin only after substantial crystalloid has been infused.[7] The interpretation of how much fluid is substantial is left to clinical judgment.

Fluids should be administered even to patients with comorbidities such as heart failure and end-stage renal disease, in which pulmonary edema is a common complication. These patients need fluid because they become intravascularly depleted when septic. There are no specific published alterations of recommendations for these patients, and they have not been excluded from experimental protocols or guidelines.[4,7,45] Close monitoring of respiratory status and hemodynamic measures may be necessary when treating these patients, but some amount of fluid resuscitation is necessary.

CVP is an imperfect measure of fluid responsiveness, because it does not reflect the interaction between contractility and preload on stroke volume and subsequent oxygen delivery.[46] Several dynamic measures of fluid responsiveness can evaluate whether continuing to increase preload will improve cardiac output. These measures can be categorized as those that measure pressure variations in either the venous or arterial system in response to respirations and those that evaluate the hemodynamic response to a fluid challenge.[46] All methods require ultrasonography evaluation, invasive monitoring, or the use of proprietary devices. Methods that use pulse pressure variations have been validated only in controlled situations (ie, in intubated, heavily sedated patients with no spontaneous breaths and a regular heart rhythm). Few patients in septic shock meet these criteria. A fluid challenge is better suited to the septic patient, because it can be used when a heart arrhythmia is present, and in patients who are breathing spontaneously. The fluid challenge can be a small fluid bolus of 250 to 500 mL or a passive leg raise, in which the patient is lying flat or recumbent and the legs are raised at least 45°.[46,47] To assess fluid responsiveness, cardiac output, stroke volume, or pulse pressure is measured immediately before and after the challenge. This measurement requires invasive monitoring, proprietary devices, or ultrasonographic evaluation. The dynamic measures of fluid responsiveness can provide a more accurate understanding of a patient's hemodynamic status, but specialized monitoring must be used.

Afterload

When hypotension persists after adequate fluid is given to correct preload, vasoactive agents may be useful. The goal for afterload optimization is a mean arterial pressure (MAP) greater than 65 mm Hg.[4,7] Norepinephrine is the preferred vasopressor in adults.[7] Epinephrine is a reasonable alternative, but clinicians should be aware that it could increase lactate production.[7] Dopamine is not recommended, because it is associated with more adverse events caused by arrhythmias and has higher associated mortality.[48,49] It should be used only in a select group of patients in whom the clinical scenario suggests a low risk for tachyarrhythmia and a need for chronotropy in addition to increased systemic vascular resistance, such as a patient with hypotension caused by bradycardia.[7] Treatment of hypotension and optimizing MAP above the threshold of 65 mm Hg is part of the 6-hour bundle.

Vasopressin can be a beneficial second agent when added as a low-dose infusion of 0.03 units/min, with the goal of achieving the desired MAP and weaning vasopressors.[50] Vasopressin is released early in the course of septic shock, and the endogenous stores become depleted. The introduction of low-dose vasopressin has been shown to reduce the dose of norepinephrine and decrease the length of time it is needed. Even patients who require a lower dose of norepinephrine might benefit from vasopressin. Russell and colleagues[51] found that patients with a norepinephrine requirement of less than 15 μg/min had lower mortality with low-dose vasopressin administration compared with those who received only norepinephrine. Vasopressin should not be used as a single agent.[7] It can cause complications from vasoconstriction, such as mesenteric ischemia, cardiac ischemia, and skin necrosis when used in high doses.[50] When administered as a low-dose infusion, it has shown no increase in 28-day mortality.[51]

Cardiac output and oxygen delivery

Poor cardiac output occurs in septic patients with a history of heart failure as well as those with no history of cardiac disease. As many as 60% of patients with septic shock have a reduced ejection fraction.[52] This dysfunction can be corrected with inotropic support[52] and usually resolves in 7 to 10 days. The high rate of cardiac dysfunction has been associated with 14 different intracellular and extracellular processes.[17] No specific cause is present in all instances of cardiac dysfunction; and an interaction of pathologic processes is the likely cause.[17] Cardiac involvement cannot be reliably predicted by patient characteristics. Comprehensive care of septic patients and their appropriate resuscitation includes monitoring cardiac function.

One measure of cardiac function, cardiac index, correlates with oxygen consumption and with pulmonary artery (PA) measures of mixed venous oxygen saturation (Svo_2).[53,54] A low Svo_2 (<65%) usually represents decreased cardiac function or anemia.[54] Measurement of venous oxygen saturation from a central line ($Scvo_2$) is the recommended end point in EGDT, because it is less invasive and corresponds with Svo_2.[55] $Scvo_2$ does not always accurately represent Svo_2 and can change with left-to-right shunt or position of the catheter tip. When the catheter terminates in the right atrium, a more accurate representation of Svo_2 is provided.[54] Ideally, $Scvo_2$ is measured continuously, but if that is not possible, it can be measured intermittently.[7]

If the $Scvo_2$ is low (<70%) and preload and afterload are optimized, treatments are targeted to correct the 2 possible causes: low cardiac output or anemia. If the hematocrit level is less than 30%, transfusion is recommended. If preload, afterload, and hematocrit are optimized but the $Scvo_2$ is still low, then inotropic agents are recommended to maximize oxygen delivery.[4] Dobutamine is the recommended inotrope for a patient who has already been fluid resuscitated.[7]

Svo_2 and $Scvo_2$ are less helpful when increased. Occasionally, certain sedation agents and hypothermia can cause low oxygen consumption, leading to an unusual situation in which the cardiac output is low but the $Scvo_2$ is high.[55] Usually, supranormal values of $Scvo_2$ accurately represent cardiac function and oxygen extraction, but this might not represent an improved physiologic state. Sepsis can cause a maldistribution of blood flow and arteriovenous shunting due to endothelial dysfunction. This situation leads to diminished oxygen delivery and extraction, which causes a high $Scvo_2$. This situation may represent disease progression, because a $Scvo_2$ greater than 80% corresponds with increased mortality.[56,57] There is no specific threshold for a $Scvo_2$ value that is too high, so it must be judged based on the clinical scenario.

Lactate has been proposed as an alternative end point to $Scvo_2$. Lactate is an independent predictor of mortality, and lactate clearance is an important prognostic indicator.[26,28,45,58] Jones and colleagues[59] showed, in a randomized trial, that poor lactate clearance can be used just as successfully as $Scvo_2$ to identify patients who might benefit from blood transfusion or inotropic therapy. The goal for lactate clearance is a 10% improvement after 2 hours. One disadvantage to using lactate to titrate medications is that it can only be measured with a blood test and cannot provide immediate feedback when processing times are long. There are several devices that can measure lactate concentration at the bedside,[60,61] which may be a reasonable alternative if efficient laboratory testing is not available.[62] Measuring $Scvo_2$ and lactate clearance is part of the 6-hour bundle. The first lactate measurement should be completed as part of the 3-hour bundle, and it should be measured again as part of the 6-hour bundle if the first value is elevated.[7] However, it is reasonable to assess lactate a second time when the first measure is normal if the patient has other evidence of hypoperfusion.[59]

Although lactate is important in the treatment of septic shock, it does not measure the same thing that $Scvo_2$ measures.[63] Lactate is produced when an insufficient amount of oxygen is supplied to mitochondria, inducing anaerobic metabolism. $Scvo_2$ can be low when oxygen supply does not meet oxygen demand. Factors other than oxygen delivery influence $Scvo_2$ and lactate levels, and those influences do not apply to the 2 markers equally. The lactate level is increased by certain vasopressors[7] and overdoses.[64] Its level can also be influenced by organ failure and excretion. $Scvo_2$ can be influenced by arteriovenous shunting and poor microvascular perfusion. Although both markers are vital to resuscitation, it is important to recognize that both are falsely reassuring in certain classes of patients.[45,56] As stated earlier, patients with sepsis are a heterogeneous group. When $Scvo_2$ and lactate both suggest decreased cardiac output, it is clear how to proceed with treatment. Patients with discordant $Scvo_2$ and lactate measurements have a more complex physiologic state and may need other measures to determine the best plan of care.

EGDT has been the subject of much criticism since its introduction.[65] However, some concepts of EGDT are not debated. The importance of early optimization of hemodynamic parameters is recognized universally. The resuscitation process should start as soon as a patient arrives in the emergency department. EGDT has been good at standardizing resuscitation. It provides clear indications for beginning and ending therapies. This data-driven approach to resuscitation can be useful when patient care is being transferred from one area to another or from one provider to another. Having a protocol that delineates expected therapy is helpful to the many providers caring for the patient as they prioritize interventions.

Ultrasonography use during resuscitation

Point-of-care ultrasonography has been proposed as a noninvasive method of measuring many of the end points targeted by EGDT and the SSC guidelines.[66] It can evaluate preload and fluid responsiveness as well as identify patients with impaired cardiac function, who may benefit from inotropy. The information gathered by an ultrasonographic examination to assess preload and cardiac output has been shown to guide treatment plans and increase provider confidence in the chosen treatment.[67] Performing point-of-care ultrasonography requires specific education, and this training is feasible.[68] The major limitation of using ultrasonography instead of invasive monitoring is that it represents 1 point in time, so multiple assessments are needed if ultrasonography is to guide therapy as medication is titrated. However, in settings with no capacity for invasive monitoring, ultrasonography is an excellent clinical adjunct.[66] Ultrasonographic evaluation is particularly useful if resources are limited. After the initial investment, it is a tool that can be used multiple times and can provide information about end points that could not otherwise be obtained without invasive monitors.[66]

Case Management: Supportive Therapy and Other Interventions

Other recommended therapies are not as time sensitive as antibiotic therapy and resuscitation. Some of these other recommendations made by the SSC guidelines are specific to patients with sepsis, but most are therapies that apply to many critically ill patients.

Steroids

Septic shock can have a component of adrenal dysfunction, and the use of steroids can increase the survival rate.[69] However, it is difficult to identify patients who will benefit from steroids. The cosyntropin stimulation test does not reliably identify sepsis-induced adrenal dysfunction. Consequently, the decision to start steroids is based on the clinical scenario. The current SSC guidelines recommend low-dose steroids for patients with hypotension that responds poorly to fluid and vasopressors. Hydrocortisone should be started at 200 mg per day as divided doses or a continuous infusion.[7,69] A continuous infusion results in fewer incidents of hyperglycemia.[69] There is no specific recommendation regarding the duration of therapy, but it should continue while the patient is hypotensive and be tapered when the hypotension resolves.

It is important to accurately identify patients for whom this therapy is appropriate given the associated risks of superinfection and myopathy. Adverse reactions and the difficulty identifying sepsis-induced adrenal insufficiency have produced studies with conflicting results. Some trials have shown no mortality benefit after administration of steroids but did find an increase in the occurrence of adverse events.[70] A large meta-analysis showed that low-dose steroids reduce 28-day mortality.[69] Given these mixed results, steroids are recommended only for patients who do not respond to other interventions in the resuscitation bundle to improve blood pressure.[7]

Activated protein C

The interaction between the immune system and blood hemostasis has been investigated extensively in sepsis.[14] The serum concentration of protein C was observed to be decreased in sepsis. Attempts were made to treat sepsis by replacing the protein.[71] After the US Food and Drug Administration approved the use of recombinant human-activated protein C, drotrecogin α (activated), it became part of sepsis care.[72] However, the European Medicines Agency required monitoring after its initial approval and doubts were raised about its effectiveness. A second large study showed no mortality benefit,[73] so the manufacturer, Eli Lily, removed drotrecogin α (activated) from the marketplace in 2012.

Ventilation support

Sepsis is the most common cause of acute lung injury (ALI) and acute respiratory distress syndrome (ARDS). Forty-six percent of patients with ALI have sepsis with a pulmonary cause and 33% have sepsis with no pulmonary source.[74] Clinicians caring for septic patients should be prepared to manage ALI and ARDS. The ventilator management recommendations are based on a lung-protective strategy. To keep plateau pressures 30 cm H_2O or lower, permissive hypercapnia and low-volume ventilation with a tidal volume of 6 mL/kg can be used.[7] Other recommendations for patients with ALI include positive end-expiratory pressure to prevent alveolar collapse, raising the head of the bed, and the regular use of spontaneous breathing trials. Prone position, as feasible, can also be helpful. A short course of neuromuscular blockade lasting less than 48 hours may be considered early in patients with sepsis-induced ARDS and a Pao_2/Fio_2 less than 150 mm Hg. PA catheters and large amounts of fluid are not helpful if the patient is no longer volume depleted. For patients with ARDS, a conservative approach to fluid administration is advised if tissue hypoperfusion has resolved. β_2-agonists should be used only in patients with bronchospasm.[7]

Glucose control

Glucose control reduces the morbidity and mortality of patients admitted to the ICU. The target glucose level and ideal insulin protocol are still not well understood. The initial benefit of glucose control in ICU patients was shown using a glucose goal of 80 to 110 mg/dL.[75] Subsequent studies have shown that a slightly higher glucose goal has fewer complications related to hypoglycemia.[76] In light of these findings, an ideal glucose goal has not been universally accepted. The safest recommendation is to target a moderate glucose goal of 180 mg/dL or less.[7]

Other therapies for sepsis care

The guidelines have many other recommendations that are beneficial for most critically ill patients.[7] Some recommendations are for intubated patients and most apply only to hemodynamically stable patients.

- Sedation protocols for intubated patients should be used with planned daily interruptions or decreases in sedation to allow titration of the sedation agents.
- Neuromuscular blockade should be used in intubated patients only when appropriate sedation cannot be achieved with other medications. Train-of-4 monitoring should be used to monitor neuromuscular blockade and titrate the medication.
- Oral chlorhexadine gluconate can be used to decontaminate the mouths of intubated patients to decrease the incidence of ventilator-associated pneumonia.
- Selective oral and digestive decontamination can be used to decrease the incidence of ventilator-associated pneumonia in settings in which this has been shown to be effective.
- Packed red blood cells should be transfused when the hemoglobin level decreases lower than 7 g/dL. This goal is different from the resuscitation goal and applies when the patient is hemodynamically stable.

- Erythropoietin is not useful unless there is an indication for its administration other than sepsis, such as chronic renal failure with anemia.
- Fresh frozen plasma has no benefit unless a procedure is planned or the patient has active bleeding.
- Platelets should be transfused if the patient is thrombocytopenic with a platelet count 10,000/mm^3 or less. If the patient is at risk of bleeding, platelets can be transfused when the count is 20,000/mm^3 or less. If the patient is actively bleeding or an invasive procedure is planned, platelets should be transfused to a count of greater than 50,000/mm^3.
- Renal replacement should be used when necessary for renal failure, but one modality is not recommended over another.
- Measures should be taken to prevent deep vein thrombosis. A combination of intermittent pneumatic compression devices and heparin is recommended in most patients. If patients have a contraindication to heparin, mechanical prophylactic devices should be used.
- Feeding should be started as tolerated in the first 48 hours. Enteral feeding is preferred, but if this route is not possible, parenteral feeding can be started.
- Patients with risk factors for gastrointestinal (GI) bleeding should be started on histamine 2 blockers or proton pump inhibitors. Proton pump inhibitors are preferred. Certain risk factors for GI bleeding are common in patients with sepsis and include coagulopathy and intubation for more than 48 hours. This therapy should be used only in patients with risk factors.
- Bicarbonate should not be given routinely for acidosis. It can be considered if the pH is less than 7.15.
- The prognosis and expected outcome of patients with sepsis should be discussed with the patient's decision makers to allow less aggressive therapy or withdrawal of care when appropriate.

Standardizing Care

Ideally, patients receive all elements in a bundle instead of the therapies that are easiest or most convenient to perform. When all pieces of the bundles are performed, mortality decreases.[45] Some of the recommended interventions require many resources, are time consuming, and can be difficult or impractical to implement.[77,78] Compliance rates with bundle recommendations range from 11% to 67%.[11,45,79,80] These compliance rates were measured in settings with no resource limitations and with providers well trained in sepsis care. Interventions designed to increase bundle compliance, such as quality improvement techniques[79] and sepsis response teams, were used.[80] The low compliance rates show the difficulty in achieving all bundle elements for all patients. The recent guidelines changed the bundles to emphasize the time-dependent interventions and improve compliance. Included in the guidelines are recommendations for quality improvement techniques and screening tools to improve treatment of the patients who need it.

SUMMARY

The most important step in treating a patient with fever and signs of shock is recognizing the need for early and comprehensive resuscitation. Septic patients are a heterogeneous group, and many aspects of their physiology must be assessed as the disease progresses. Understanding the possible physiologic states in sepsis and the capacity and limitations of monitors and biomarkers is essential for sepsis care. These patients have a high mortality, but early intervention can reduce that mortality.

REFERENCES

1. Angus DC, Linde-Zwirble WT, Lidicker J, et al. Epidemiology of severe sepsis in the United States: analysis of incidence, outcome, and associated costs of care. Crit Care Med 2001;29:1303–10.
2. Brun-Buisson C, Meshaka P, Pinton P, The EPISEPSIS Study Group. EPISEPSIS: a reappraisal of the epidemiology and outcome of severe sepsis in French intensive care units. Intensive Care Med 2004;30:580–8.
3. Martin GS, Mannino DM, Eaton S, et al. The epidemiology of sepsis in the United States from 1979 through 2000. N Engl J Med 2003;348:1546–54.
4. Rivers E, Nguyen B, Havstad S, et al. Early goal-directed therapy in the treatment of severe sepsis and septic shock. N Engl J Med 2001;345:1368–77.
5. Shorr AF, Micek ST, Jackson WL, et al. Economic implications of an evidence-based sepsis protocol: can we improve outcomes and lower costs? Crit Care Med 2007;35:1257–62.
6. Kumar A, Roberts D, Wood K, et al. Duration of hypotension prior to initiation of effective antimicrobial therapy is the critical determinant of survival in human septic shock. Crit Care Med 2006;34:1589–96.
7. Dellinger RP, Levy MM, Rhodes A, et al. Surviving sepsis campaign: international guidelines for management of severe sepsis and septic shock: 2012. Crit Care Med 2013;41:580–637.
8. Wang HE, Shapiro NI, Angus DC, et al. National estimates of severe sepsis in United States emergency departments. Crit Care Med 2007;35:1928–36.
9. Levy MM, Dellinger RP, Townsend SR, et al. The surviving sepsis campaign: results of an international guideline-based performance improvement program targeting severe sepsis. Intensive Care Med 2010;36:222–31.
10. Wang HE, Devereaux RS, Yealy DM, et al. National variation in United States sepsis mortality: a descriptive study. Int J Health Geogr 2010;9:9.
11. Peake SL, Bailey M, Bellomo R, et al. Australasian resuscitation of sepsis evaluation (ARISE): a multi-centre, prospective, inception cohort study. Resuscitation 2009;80:811–8.
12. Castellanos-Ortega A, Suberviola B, García-Astudillo LA, et al. Impact of the surviving sepsis campaign protocols on hospital length of stay and mortality in septic shock patients: results of a three-year follow-up quasi-experimental study. Crit Care Med 2010;38:1036–43.
13. Carrillo-Esper R, Carrillo-Córdova JR, Carrillo-Córdova LD. Epidemiological study of sepsis in Mexican intensive care units. Cir Cir 2009;77:301–8 [in English, Spanish].
14. Hotchkiss RS, Karl IE. The pathophysiology and treatment of sepsis. N Engl J Med 2003;348:138–50.
15. Ait-Oufella H, Maury E, Lehoux S, et al. The endothelium: physiological functions and role in microcirculatory failure during severe sepsis. Intensive Care Med 2010;36:1286–98.
16. Spronk PE, Zandstra DF, Ince C. Bench-to-bedside review: sepsis is a disease of the microcirculation. Crit Care 2004;8:462–8.
17. Romero-Bermejo FJ, Ruiz-Bailen M, Gil-Cebrian J, et al. Sepsis-induced cardiomyopathy. Curr Cardiol Rev 2011;7:163–83.
18. Pierrakos C, Vincent JL. Sepsis biomarkers: a review. Crit Care 2010;14:R15.
19. Glickman SW, Cairns CB, Otero RM, et al. Disease progression in hemodynamically stable patients presenting to the emergency department with sepsis. Acad Emerg Med 2010;17:383–90.

20. Bone RC, Balk RA, Cerra FB, et al. Definitions for sepsis and organ failure and guidelines for the use of innovative therapies in sepsis. The ACCP/SCCM Consensus Conference Committee. American College of Chest Physicians/Society of Critical Care Medicine. Chest 1992;101:1644–55.

21. Levy MM, Fink MP, Marshall JC, et al, SCCM/ESICM/ACCP/ATS/SIS. 2001 SCCM/ESICM/ACCP/ATS/SIS International Sepsis Definitions Conference. Crit Care Med 2003;31:1250–6.

22. Girard TD, Opal SM, Ely EW. Insights into severe sepsis in older patients: from epidemiology to evidence-based management. Clin Infect Dis 2005;40:719–27.

23. Ferreira FL, Bota DP, Bross A, et al. Serial evaluation of the SOFA score to predict outcome in critically ill patients. JAMA 2001;286:1754–8.

24. Cardoso T, Henriques Carneiro A, Ribeiro O, et al. Reducing mortality in severe sepsis with the implementation of a core 6-hour bundle: results from the Portuguese community-acquired sepsis study (SACiUCI study). Crit Care 2010;14: R83.

25. Silva E, Pedro MA, Sogayar AC, et al. Brazilian sepsis epidemiological study (BASES study). Crit Care 2004;8:R251–60.

26. Mikkelsen ME, Miltiades AN, Gaieski DF, et al. Serum lactate is associated with mortality in severe sepsis independent of organ failure and shock. Crit Care Med 2009;37:1670–7.

27. Puskarich MA, Trzeciak S, Shapiro NI, et al, Emergency Medicine Shock Research Network (EMSHOCKNET). Outcomes of patients undergoing early sepsis resuscitation for cryptic shock compared with overt shock. Resuscitation 2011;82:1289–93.

28. Howell MD, Donnino M, Clardy P, et al. Occult hypoperfusion and mortality in patients with suspected infection. Intensive Care Med 2007;33:1892–9.

29. Carcillo JA, Fields AI. Clinical practice parameters for hemodynamic support of pediatric and neonatal patients in septic shock. Crit Care Med 2002;30: 1365–78.

30. Alam FF, Mustafa AS, Khan ZU. Comparative evaluation of (1, 3)-beta-D-glucan, mannan and anti-mannan antibodies, and *Candida* species-specific snPCR in patients with candidemia. BMC Infect Dis 2007;7:103.

31. Pemán J, Zaragoza R. Current diagnostic approaches to invasive candidiasis in critical care settings. Mycoses 2009;53:424–33.

32. Schuetz P, Chiappa V, Briel M, et al. Procalcitonin algorithms for antibiotic therapy decisions: a systematic review of randomized controlled trials and recommendations for clinical algorithms. Arch Intern Med 2011;171:1322–31.

33. Nobre V, Harbarth S, Graf JD, et al. Use of procalcitonin to shorten antibiotic treatment duration in septic patients: a randomized trial. Am J Respir Crit Care Med 2008;177:498–505.

34. Heyland DK, Johnson AP, Reynolds SC, et al. Procalcitonin for reduced antibiotic exposure in the critical care setting: a systematic review and an economic evaluation. Crit Care Med 2011;39:1792–9.

35. Francis M, Rich T, Williamson T, et al. Effect of an emergency department sepsis protocol on time to antibiotics in severe sepsis. CJEM 2010;12:303–10.

36. Kollef MH, Sherman G, Ward S, et al. Inadequate antimicrobial treatment of infections: a risk factor for hospital mortality among critically ill patients. Chest 1999;115:462–74.

37. Vallés J, Rello J, Ochagavía A, et al. Community-acquired bloodstream infection in critically ill adult patients: impact of shock and inappropriate antibiotic therapy on survival. Chest 2003;123:1615–24.

38. Capp R, Chang Y, Brown DF. Effective antibiotic treatment prescribed by emergency physicians in patients admitted to the intensive care unit with severe sepsis or septic shock: where is the gap? J Emerg Med 2011;41:573–80.

39. Cheng AC, West TE, Limmathurotsakul D, et al. Strategies to reduce mortality from bacterial sepsis in adults in developing countries. PLoS Med 2008;5: e175.

40. Marik PE. Surviving sepsis: going beyond the guidelines. Ann Intensive Care 2011;1:17.

41. Perner A, Haase N, Guttormsen AB, et al, Scandinavian Critical Care Trials Group. Hydroxyethyl starch 130/0.42 versus Ringer's acetate in severe sepsis. N Engl J Med 2012;367:124–34.

42. Guidet B, Martinet O, Boulain T, et al. Assessment of hemodynamic efficacy and safety of 6% hydroxyethylstarch 130/0.4 vs. 0.9% NaCl fluid replacement in patients with severe sepsis: the CRYSTMAS study. Crit Care 2012;16:R94.

43. Myburgh JA, Finfer S, Bellomo R, et al. Hydroxyethyl starch or saline for fluid resuscitation in intensive care. N Engl J Med 2012;367:1901–11.

44. Delaney AP, Dan A, McCaffrey J, et al. The role of albumin as a resuscitation fluid for patients with sepsis: a systematic review and meta-analysis. Crit Care Med 2011;39:386–91.

45. Cannon CM, Holthaus CV, Zubrow MT, et al. The GENESIS Project (GENeralized Early Sepsis Intervention Strategies): a multicenter quality improvement collaborative. J Intensive Care Med 2012. http://dx.doi.org/10.1177/0885066612453025.

46. Shujaat A, Bajwa AA. Optimization of preload in severe sepsis and septic shock. Crit Care Res Pract 2012;2012:761051.

47. Cavallaro F, Sandroni C, Marano C, et al. Diagnostic accuracy of passive leg raising for prediction of fluid responsiveness in adults: systematic review and meta-analysis of clinical studies. Intensive Care Med 2010;36:1475–83.

48. Vasu TS, Cavallazzi R, Hirani A, et al. Norepinephrine or dopamine for septic shock: systematic review of randomized clinical trials. J Intensive Care Med 2012;27:172–8.

49. De Backer D, Aldecoa C, Njimi H, et al. Dopamine versus norepinephrine in the treatment of septic shock: a meta-analysis. Crit Care Med 2012;40:725–30.

50. Russell JA. Bench-to-bedside review: vasopressin in the management of septic shock. Crit Care 2011;15:226.

51. Russell JA, Walley KR, Singer J, et al, VASST Investigators. Vasopressin versus norepinephrine infusion in patients with septic shock. N Engl J Med 2008;358: 877–87.

52. Vieillard-Baron A, Caille V, Charron C, et al. Actual incidence of global left ventricular hypokinesia in adult septic shock. Crit Care Med 2008;36:1701–6.

53. Gattinoni L, Brazzi L, Pelosi P, et al. A trial of goal-oriented hemodynamic therapy in critically ill patients. N Engl J Med 1995;333:1025–32.

54. Vincent JL, Rhodes A, Perel A, et al. Clinical review: update on hemodynamic monitoring–a consensus of 16. Crit Care 2011;15:229.

55. Reinhart K, Rudolph T, Bredle DL, et al. Comparison of central-venous to mixed-venous oxygen saturation during changes in oxygen supply/demand. Chest 1989;95:1216–21.

56. Pope JV, Jones AE, Gaieski DF, et al, Emergency Medicine Shock Research Network (EMShock Net) Investigators. Multicenter study of central venous oxygen saturation (ScvO2) as a predictor of mortality in patients with sepsis. Ann Emerg Med 2010;55:40–6.

57. Textoris J, Fouché L, Wiramus S, et al. High central venous oxygen saturation in the latter stages of septic shock is associated with increased mortality. Crit Care 2011;15:R176.
58. Shapiro NI, Howell MD, Talmor D, et al. Serum lactate as a predictor of mortality in emergency department patients with infection. Ann Emerg Med 2005;455: 524–8.
59. Jones AE, Shapiro NI, Trzeciak S, et al. Clinical trial as goals of early sepsis therapy: a randomized lactate clearance vs central venous oxygen saturation. JAMA 2010;303:739–46.
60. Karon BC, Scott R, Burritt MF, et al. Comparison of lactate values between point-of-care and central laboratory analyzers. Am J Clin Pathol 2007;128:168–71.
61. Tanner RK, Fuller KL, Ross ML. Evaluation of three portable blood lactate analysers: lactate pro, lactate scout and lactate plus. Eur J Appl Physiol 2010;109:551–9.
62. Moyo S, Bussmann H, Mangwendeza P, et al. Validation of a point-of-care lactate device for screening at-risk adults receiving combination antiretroviral therapy in Botswana. J Antivir Antiretrovir 2011;3:45–8.
63. Puskarich MA, Trzeciak S, Shapiro NI, et al. Prognostic value and agreement of achieving lactate clearance or central venous oxygen saturation goals during early sepsis resuscitation. Acad Emerg Med 2012;19:252–8.
64. Dell'Aglio DM, Perino LJ, Kazzi Z, et al. Acute metformin overdose: examining serum pH, lactate level, and metformin concentrations in survivors versus non-survivors: a systematic review of the literature. Ann Emerg Med 2009;54:818–23.
65. Perel A. Bench-to-bedside review: the initial hemodynamic resuscitation of the septic patient according to Surviving Sepsis Campaign guidelines–does one size fit all? Crit Care 2008;12:223.
66. Via G, Storti E, Spreafico A, et al. Point of care ultrasound for sepsis management in resource-limited settings: time for a new paradigm for global health care. Intensive Care Med 2012;38:1405–7.
67. Haydar SA, Moore ET, Higgins GL, et al. Effect of bedside ultrasonography on the certainty of physician clinical decisionmaking for septic patients in the emergency department. Ann Emerg Med 2012;60:346–58.
68. Shah S, Noble VE, Umulisa I, et al. Development of an ultrasound training curriculum in a limited resource international setting: successes and challenges of ultrasound training in rural Rwanda. Int J Emerg Med 2008;1(3):193–6.
69. Annane D, Bellissant E, Bollaert PE, et al. Corticosteroids in the treatment of severe sepsis and septic shock in adults: a systematic review. JAMA 2009;301: 2362–75.
70. Sprung CL, Annane D, Keh D, et al. Hydrocortisone therapy for patients with septic shock. N Engl J Med 2008;358:111–24.
71. Bernard GR, Vincent JL, Laterre PF, et al, Recombinant Human Protein C Worldwide Evaluation in Severe Sepsis (PROWESS) Study Group. Efficacy and safety of recombinant human activated protein C for severe sepsis. N Engl J Med 2001;344:699–709.
72. Dellinger RP, Levy MM, Carlet JM, et al, for the International Surviving Sepsis Campaign Guidelines Committee. Surviving sepsis campaign: international guidelines for management of severe sepsis and septic shock. Crit Care Med 2008;36:296–327.
73. Ranieri VM, Thompson BT, Barie PS, et al, PROWESS-SHOCK Study Group. Drotrecogin alfa (activated) in adults with septic shock. N Engl J Med 2012; 366:2055–64.

74. Rubenfeld GD, Caldwell E, Peabody E, et al. Incidence and outcomes of acute lung injury. N Engl J Med 2005;353:1685–93.
75. Van den Berghe G, Wouters P, Weekers F, et al. Intensive insulin therapy in critically ill patients. N Engl J Med 2001;345:1359–67.
76. The NICE-SUGAR Study Investigators, Finfer S, Liu B, et al. Hypoglycemia and risk of death in critically ill patients. N Engl J Med 2012;367:1108–18.
77. Jones AE, Shapiro NI, Roshon M. Implementing early goal-directed therapy in the emergency setting: the challenges and experiences of translating research innovations into clinical reality in academic and community settings. Acad Emerg Med 2007;14:1072–8.
78. Nguyen HB, Lynch EL, Mou JA, et al. The utility of a quality improvement bundle in bridging the gap between research and standard care in the management of severe sepsis and septic shock in the emergency department. Acad Emerg Med 2007;14:1079–86.
79. Nguyen HB, Corbett SW, Steele R, et al. Implementation of a bundle of quality indicators for the early management of severe sepsis and septic shock is associated with decreased mortality. Crit Care Med 2007;35:1105–12.
80. Casserly B, Baram M, Walsh P, et al. Implementing a collaborative protocol in a sepsis intervention program: lessons learned. Lung 2011;189:11–9.

Fever in the Returning Traveler

Simon Kotlyar, MD, MSc*, Brian T. Rice, MDCM

KEYWORDS

- Fever • International travel • Imported infectious disease • Tropical disease

KEY POINTS

- Fever in ill travelers returning home from developing nations is common.
- Most travelers present with undifferentiated febrile syndromes. Regional proportionate morbidity rates and the patient's travel history are essential in narrowing the differential diagnosis.
- Most patients in whom a diagnosis is confirmed have malaria, dengue, enteric fever, or rickettsial disease.
- Empiric treatment based on the clinical presentation is required in many cases because acquisition of confirmatory laboratory data is often delayed.

INTRODUCTION

Worldwide, more than 940 million international journeys were undertaken in 2010.[1] Global travel on such a scale exposes individuals to a range of health risks and poses a challenge to clinicians caring for patients who return home ill from international travel. Of the more than 80 million people who travel from industrialized to developing nations, between 20% and 70% report some illness associated with their travel.[2–4] A small proportion, between 5% and 19%, of those who develop a travel-associated illness seek medical attention either during or immediately after travel.[3–7] Mortality in this population is low (1 per 100,000) but the associated morbidity is significant, with high rates of hospitalization and missed work for what is largely a preventable spectrum of disease.

Much of the current epidemiologic understanding of travel-associated illness in developed nations is based on data acquired through surveillance systems such as GeoSentinel (a system of the International Society of Travel Medicine and the Centers for Disease Control and Prevention [CDC]) and TropNet Europe (the European

Disclosures: No financial disclosures.

Conflicts of Interest: None.

Division of Global Health, Department of Emergency Medicine, Yale University School of Medicine, 464 Congress Avenue, Suite 260, New Haven, CT 06519, USA

* Corresponding author.

E-mail address: simonkotlyar@mac.com

Emerg Med Clin N Am 31 (2013) 927–944

http://dx.doi.org/10.1016/j.emc.2013.07.001

0733-8627/13/$ – see front matter

Network on Imported Infectious Disease Surveillance). GeoSentinel sites are located on 6 continents and collect clinician-based surveillance data on travel-associated disease from more than 30 locations. TropNet Europe has 68 member sites, which contribute surveillance data for travel-associated illness in Europe. A case definition for travel-associated illness is a patient has who crossed an international border within the past 10 years and presents for a presumed travel-related illness.[5] This definition encompasses a very broad set of clinical conditions, including dermatologic disease, injury, tuberculosis, and chronic diarrhea. The focus of this article is on travel-related illness that falls within the spectrum of the acute febrile syndrome.

Fever was the chief complaint of 6957 (28%) of the 24,920 ill travelers who were treated in GeoSentinel sites between 1997 and 2006.[8] These patients visited clinics in Europe (53%), North America (25%), Israel (9%), Australia/New Zealand (8%), Asia (5%), and other sites (1%), and one-fourth of them were hospitalized.[8] Their characteristics are summarized in **Table 1**. Most patients in this group were middle-aged men, and most people in the study group had traveled for tourism, on business, or to visit friends and relatives. These individuals (those visiting friends and relatives) constitute a high-risk group because they are much less likely than tourist travelers to receive prophylaxis, and tend to use fewer preventive measures. Consequently they are almost 9 times more likely than other groups to require inpatient treatment when they return with febrile complications of travel.[9] Most individuals with fever after travel present within 1 to 3 weeks after returning home. These presentations, considered

Table 1 Characteristics of returned ill travelers with fever: GeoSentinel Surveillance Network	
Characteristic	Number (%)
Age (y)	
<20	429 (6)
20–64	6230 (89)
≥65	244 (4)
Sex	
Male	3995 (57)
Female	2891 (43)
Reason for Travel	
Tourism	3802 (55)
Business	1036 (15)
Research/education	283 (4)
Missionary/volunteer	384 (6)
Visiting friends and relatives	1431 (21)
Duration of Travel (d)	
≤30	4134 (59)
≥31	2597 (41)
Interval from Travel to Presentation (wk)	
<1	2789 (40)
1–6	2437 (36)
>6	1551 (22)
Total	6957

Data from Wilson ME, Weld LH, Boggild A, et al. Fever in returned travelers: results from the GeoSentinel Surveillance Network. Clin Infect Dis 2007;44(12):1560–8.

acute and subacute, are within the direct purview of the emergency medicine specialist. Among those in whom a definitive diagnosis is reached the majority have malaria, acute diarrheal disease, acute respiratory tract infections, or dengue fever (**Fig. 1**).[8] More than 35% of patients presenting with a febrile syndrome after travel do not receive a definitive diagnosis, even in the hands of trained experts, which highlights the importance of a structured diagnostic approach.

One of the key principles in approaching the presentation of fever in the returning traveler is a thorough understanding of epidemiology as it applies to the individual's circumstances. Most patients present with undifferentiated and nonlocalizing systemic febrile syndromes, so the clinical decision-making process and the diagnostic algorithm should reflect the likelihood of acquiring a specific disease based on regional morbidity, host-pathogen interaction, and the clinical assessment. Accordingly, the following 3 key areas are discussed in the next section of this review:

1. Destination-specific variations in proportionate morbidity. What are the most common/likely infections that someone can bring home from a given region?
2. Assessment of travel history, with emphasis on exposure, incubation period, and vaccination/chemoprophylaxis. What did the patient do/not do that might put him or her at risk for a certain infection? Does the course of illness fit with the expected incubation period for that infection?
3. Clinical presentation. What patterns of the fever and other signs/symptoms point toward or rule out a diagnosis?

DESTINATION-SPECIFIC VARIATIONS IN PROPORTIONATE MORBIDITY

Arguably the most important feature to consider in the initial assessment is the region of travel. Several diagnoses, and their empiric therapies, can be guided by an understanding of regional risk.[10] GeoSentinel data, collected from 17,353 patients who traveled to 230 countries between June 1996 and August 2004, demonstrate significant regional differences in proportionate morbidity for 16 of 21 broad syndromic categories, including systemic febrile syndrome.[5] In the context of systemic febrile illness, destination-specific variations in proportionate morbidity are stark (**Fig. 2**). Proportionate morbidity rates for malaria and enteric fever are regionally disparate, whereas

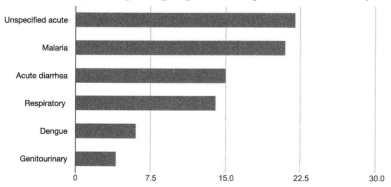

Summary of diagnosis groups in febrile patients after travel (n = 6,957)

Fig. 1. Summary of diagnosis groups in returned ill travelers with fever (N = 6957). GeoSentinel Surveillance Network. (*Data from* Wilson ME, Weld LH, Boggild A, et al. Fever in returned travelers: results from the GeoSentinel Surveillance Network. Clin Infect Dis 2007;44(12):1560–8.)

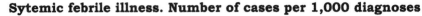

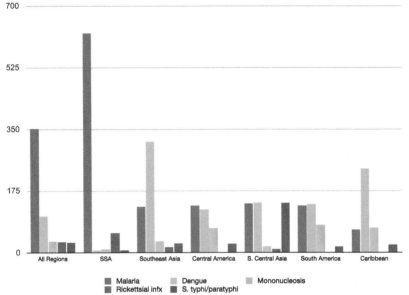

Fig. 2. Infectious cases of malaria, dengue, mononucleosis, rickettsial disease, and enteric fever per 1000 diagnoses by region. GeoSentinel Surveillance Network. SSA, sub-Saharan Africa. (*Adapted from* Freedman DO, Weld LH, Kozarsky PE, et al. Spectrum of disease and relation to place of exposure among ill returned travelers. N Engl J Med 2006;354(2):119–30; with permission.)

dengue fever has a fairly broad global distribution. EuroTravelNet data from 17,228 patients show similar patterns of distribution (**Fig. 3**).[11] Data from 1842 febrile returned travelers in Belgium demonstrated that 91% of all imported malaria cases were from sub-Saharan Africa, all cases of enteric fever were from Asia, and dengue was nearly evenly split between Asia and the Americas.[12] Data from Australia found 6-fold higher rates of malaria in itineraries that included Africa, 13-fold increases in dengue for itineraries that included Asia, and high rates of malaria among visitors to Oceania.[13,14] Although a thorough understanding of destination-specific proportionate morbidity rates is important, other considerations must be incorporated into the assessment process. Generally speaking, geographic trends correlate with the diagnosis in roughly one-third of febrile patients returning from developing nations; the other two-thirds have undifferentiated fever and other diagnoses.

ASSESSMENT OF TRAVEL HISTORY

The importance of obtaining a detailed travel history cannot be overstated in the evaluation of the febrile traveler. Determination of possible infectious exposures and their associated incubation periods can be particularly helpful in ruling out causes of fever. For example, a fever that began more than 3 weeks after a traveler returned home is very unlikely to be caused by dengue, rickettsial disease, or viral hemorrhagic fever; it is much more likely to be caused by malaria (particularly the forms caused by *Plasmodium vivax* or *Plasmodium ovale*) if the infection was acquired abroad. Careful attention to the exposure history, immunization status, and use of malarial chemoprophylaxis can be very helpful in establishing a diagnosis. In a series of 2071 fever

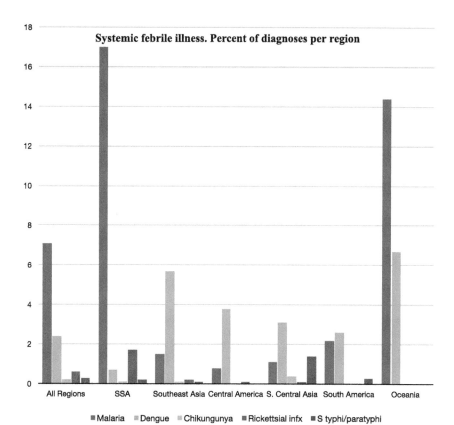

Fig. 3. Infectious cases of malaria, dengue, Chikungunya, rickettsial disease, and enteric fever percentage per region. EuroTravelNet. SSA, sub-Saharan Africa. (*Adapted from* Gautret P, Schlagenhauf P, Gaudart J, et al. Multicenter EuroTravNet/GeoSentinel study of travel-related infectious diseases in Europe. Emerg Infect Dis 2009;15(11):1783–90.)

episodes from 1962 patients in Europe, the majority (78%) presented within 1 month after return from travel.[15] GeoSentinel data for 6957 patients presenting with fever found that after malaria, the most common specific infections causing systemic febrile illness were dengue, enteric fever, and rickettsioses, all of which have short to medium incubation periods (<21 days).[8] Incubation periods for common infectious agents are presented in **Table 2**. Whereas most infections in travelers have incubation periods of less than 21 days, several can manifest more than 30 days after return (eg, malaria, tuberculosis, hepatitis, filariasis). Furthermore, patients might spend several weeks to months overseas and then present within a short time after returning home with infections that were acquired months earlier. The most common infection presenting more than 30 days after exposure is *P vivax* malaria (25% of patients with this infection in the United States present after 30 days).[16]

The emergency physician who is evaluating a traveler with a febrile illness should inquire about the following topics:

- Details of itinerary/travel dates/seasonality
- Countries and destinations (rural/urban locations) visited
- Exposure to bites/vectors/animals

Table 2
Incubation periods for common and severe infections acquired during travel

Short (<10 d)	Medium (11–21 d)	Long (>30 d)
Typhoid	Malaria	Reactivation malaria
Dengue	Typhoid	Tuberculosis
Rickettsial	Hepatitis A	Leishmaniasis
Meningitis/encephalitis	Schistosomiasis	Filariasis
Chikungunya	Amebic liver abscess	Schistosomiasis
Salmonellosis	Leptospirosis	Rabies
Shigellosis	Q-fever	African trypanosomiasis
VHF	African trypanosomiasis	Enteric protozoal
Influenza	Brucellosis	Enteric helminthic
Legionella	VHF	
Mononucleosis	Rickettsial	
	HIV Seroconversion	

Abbreviations: HIV, human immunodeficiency virus; VHF, viral hemorrhagic fever.

- Types of food and water that were consumed
- Vaccination and chemoprophylaxis history
- Unprotected intercourse and partners
- Timing and sequence of illness/symptoms

Once an appropriate travel history is obtained, this information, in conjunction with a destination-specific assessment of risk, can be used to formulate a fairly narrow differential diagnosis, which can then be applied to the clinical presentation. Of importance is that although exotic infectious agents are often the focus of interest, nonexotic infectious processes, such as pneumonia, urinary tract infection, and unspecified viral syndromes, are more common than exotic ones and must remain high on the differential diagnosis.[17]

CLINICAL PRESENTATION

Because the vast majority (close to 80%) of travelers with fever seeks medical care within 1 month after return, this discussion focuses primarily on presentations that are likely to be seen within this time frame.[15] In nearly 20% of patients fever is the only symptom, and more than 50% of patients have noncontributory findings on physical examination.[15] When associated symptoms are present, they are often nonlocalizing and tend to represent manifestations of systemic disease (eg, headache, fatigue, myalgia). Fever associated with genitourinary, respiratory, and gastrointestinal symptoms should focus on the diagnostic pathway; these combinations rarely pose a major diagnostic challenge. The following sections focus on recognizable fever with concomitant complexes of signs and symptoms, and their associated diagnostic considerations, in patients returning from the tropics.

Fever and Rash

Fever and rash should prompt an urgent and cautionary assessment, as several rare but potentially life-threatening diagnoses are possible. Patients with this combination should undergo respiratory and droplet-isolation precautions until a diagnosis is confirmed. A list of rash characteristics and their associated diagnoses are presented in

Table 3. This list is by no means comprehensive, but does highlight the more common and relevant syndromes presenting with fever and rash in returned travelers. Several nonemergent tropical infections can present with dermatologic manifestations; the absence of an associated acute systemic febrile syndrome usually suggests an indolent process. The majority of patients with fever and rash after travel to the tropics should be admitted to hospital for observation and confirmatory diagnosis of causes, which often take time to isolate via culture or serology.

Fever and Jaundice

The association of the systemic febrile syndrome and jaundice is rare after travel. Its presentation should prompt a cautious investigation that targets common domestic causes such as cholangitis, hepatitis, and severe sepsis. In the context of pathogens that could have been acquired abroad, the viral hepatitides (A–E) rarely present concurrently with fever and jaundice.[10]

Common infectious causes of fever and jaundice acquired abroad are malaria with hemolysis, leptospirosis (Weil disease), the hemolytic-uremic syndrome (associated with *Escherichia coli*), enteric fever, and the viral hemorrhagic fevers. Close attention to regional risk and the incubation period is essential, and can help to rule out several of the aforementioned conditions. Patients with fever and jaundice should be admitted to hospital with appropriate contact precautions, pending diagnostic confirmation, for observation and appropriate therapy.

Fever and Central Nervous System Involvement

Neurologic presentations are seen in 15 of 1000 ill travelers. When they are associated with a febrile syndrome, urgent treatment and diagnosis are necessary.[5] The most common treatable causes are malaria and meningitis, and these must be ruled out or treated promptly in most cases. All common domestic causes of meningitis should be considered, and treatment should be initiated before confirmatory diagnosis if there is a high index of suspicion for cerebral malaria or bacterial meningitis. Patients

Table 3	
Infectious causes of fever and rash based on rash type	
Rash	**Infection**
Purpuric	Dengue hemorrhagic syndrome
	Meningococcal infection
	Viral hemorrhagic fever
	Rickettsial infection, severe
	Leptospirosis
Maculopapular	Arboviral infection
	Rickettsial infection
	VHF
	HIV seroconversion
	Typhoid
	Dengue fever
	Leptospirosis
	Brucellosis
Vesicular	Herpes simplex virus
	Varicella
Ulcerative	Chancre: trypanosomiasis
	Eschar: anthrax, African tick typhus
	Ulcer: leishmaniasis, syphilis, tropical ulcer

traveling within the meningitis belt and pilgrims traveling with the Hajj to Mecca should be treated promptly for meningococcal disease, which carries a 5% to 10% case-fatality rate, even with antibiotic treatment.[18] Nonbacterial encephalitis has a broad differential diagnosis, which includes common arboviral infections native to the Americas and Asia, and often requires reference laboratory analysis for confirmation. Other considerations include tuberculosis, opportunistic disease associated with human immunodeficiency virus (HIV) infection, leptospirosis, rabies, and alcohol withdrawal. Lastly, there have been several reports of tourists who acquired trypanosomal infections (African sleeping sickness) transmitted through bites of the tsetse fly in game parks in east and central Africa.[19,20] Central nervous system (CNS) disease is a late presentation of these infections, although fulminant cases of rapidly progressive *Trypanosoma gambiense* have been described. Suspected trypanosomal disease should prompt expert consultation for diagnosis and treatment.

Fever and Eosinophilia

Peripheral eosinophilia is generally a result of acute allergic reaction, malignancy, or parasitic infection.[21] In the context of fever and eosinophilia in the returned traveler, a high index of suspicion for helminthic infections, in which worms migrate or dwell in tissues, should be considered. Whereas mild elevation in the peripheral eosinophil count (351–1500 cells/mL) can be nonspecific, moderate (1500–5000 cells/mL) to severe (>5000 cells/mL) elevations in individuals traveling to nonindustrialized regions are highly suggestive of invasive helminthic infection.[21] Diagnoses to be considered in febrile travelers with eosinophilia include the following:

- Schistosomiasis (Katayama fever)
- *Strongyloides* hyperinfestation
- Lymphatic filariasis
- Invasive hookworm disease
- Migratory *Ascaris lumbricoides*

Initial workup should include stool analysis for ova and parasites, serology for strongyloidiasis, and examination of blood smears and skin snips to detect microfilariae, depending on the clinical picture and the area of travel.[22,23]

Undifferentiated Fever

Febrile patients without localizing symptoms, presenting after travel to nonindustrialized nations, accounted for 23% to 35% of GeoSentinel cases, with similar proportions reported in smaller European and Australian series.[5,8,15,24,25] In returning travelers with undifferentiated fever, malaria (all species) was the cause of disease in 14% to 35% of patients, accounting for the largest proportion of diagnoses.[5,12,13,15,24,26–28] When destination-specific morbidity is considered, the proportion of undifferentiated fever diagnosed as malaria in travelers returning from sub-Saharan Africa is 32% to 62%. Therefore, all patients with fever after returning from the tropics, particularly sub-Saharan Africa, should be considered as having malaria until proven otherwise.[5,8,12,13,15] Following malaria, the most common imported communicable diseases causing undifferentiated fever are dengue, enteric fever, and rickettsial disease.

Dengue virus infection is confirmed serologically in 3% to 10% of travelers with undifferentiated fever on return from the tropics.[5,8,12,13,15,24,26] In patients returning from Central or South America, dengue virus is the causative agent in 8% to 14%, and in those returning from southeast Asia dengue is responsible for 13% to 32% of cases of undifferentiated fever.[5,8,13] For enteric fever, pooled data demonstrate *Salmonella typhi/paratyphi* in 1% to 4% of cases of undifferentiated fever.[5,8,12,13,15,24,26] Enteric fever should be considered strongly in travelers returning from south Asia, particularly the Indian subcontinent; travel to pockets of sub-Saharan Africa can also pose a risk. When the diagnosis of malaria has been excluded or if the patient has a rash, a heightened index of suspicion for rickettsial infection should be maintained, particularly in patients returning from sub-Saharan Africa. In this group, up to 5% of patients with undifferentiated fever have been found to harbor rickettsial infection (namely, African tick typhus).[15]

Although the evaluation and workup of patients with undifferentiated fever after travel can be complex and intimidating, there is room for simplification and an evidence-based approach. Because a large proportion of diagnoses will remain in the scope of "cosmopolitan infections," a practical approach to the workup of patients with imported disease is warranted. Initial assessment should include evaluation for common local causes of fever. Given that no source will be identified in one-third of patients and that a cosmopolitan cause will be identified also in about one-third of patients, it is the remaining third that is the focus of the imported disease workup. The vast majority of patients (>95%) in whom a causative agent is identified will have malaria, dengue, enteric fever, or rickettsial disease.[5,8,12,15,17] Therefore, a detailed clinical discussion focuses on these 4 essential disease entities and their recognition, diagnosis, and treatment.

PEDIATRIC CONSIDERATIONS

Most travel-related morbidity data for children stem from limited single-center studies.[29,30] Analysis of data from 1849 pediatric patients from GeoSentinel surveillance found that children can be grouped into 4 general categories of illness after travel: diarrheal syndrome (28%), dermatologic disorders (25%), systemic febrile illness (23%), and respiratory disorders (11%).[31] Children were more likely to require hospitalization, were less likely to receive pretravel advice, and generally presented earlier than adults.[31] Of those children with systemic febrile syndromes, the majority (35%) was diagnosed with malaria; the remaining diagnoses were viral syndrome (28%), dengue fever (7%), enteric fever (6%), and unspecified febrile illness (24%).[31] For children presenting with undifferentiated fever after travel, a high index of suspicion should be maintained for both cosmopolitan and imported causes. The same geographic considerations as for adults hold true. All evaluations for fever in children returning from the tropics should include consideration of malaria, dengue, and enteric fever. A low threshold for admitting pediatric patients with undifferentiated fever after travel should be maintained.

MALARIA

In 2010, the CDC received notification of 1691 cases of malaria, 1688 (99.8%) of which were classified as imported, representing a 14% increase from the 1484 recorded in 2009.[32] *P falciparum* and *P vivax* represented the majority of infections and were identified in 74% and 18% of cases, respectively.[32] These infections occurred primarily in United States nationals (75%), and probably underestimate the total disease burden. Of the 828 patients (76%) who reported a purpose for their travel, the largest proportion (71%) were visiting friends or relatives. At least 56% of all patients were hospitalized and 9 of them died (all cases of severe *P falciparum*).[32] Imported cases of malaria in Europe and the United Kingdom number close to 11,000 per annum, making this one of the principal imported tropical infections.[33]

In patients returning from travel to malaria-endemic regions, the diagnosis must be excluded in those with a history of fever, regardless of travel duration or use of chemoprophylaxis. Of the several species of *Plasmodium* that cause disease in humans, 4 are of clinical relevance: *P falciparum, P vivax, P ovale*, and *P malariae*. Of these, *P falciparum* poses the highest risk for severe disease and complications while *P vivax* constitutes the bulk of chronic and recrudescent disease. Transmission occurs through the bite of the female *Anopheles* mosquito, with multiple species responsible for transmission. Life cycles involve both hepatic and hematologic stages; the intraerythrocytic stages account for the clinical spectrum of disease. The minimum incubation period for *P falciparum* is 6 days, with most clinical symptoms developing between 9 and 14 days after exposure (median 12) days.[34] Incubation periods for *P vivax* and *P ovale* are significantly longer, ranging from 8 days to several months. The majority of cases of *P vivax* infection present within 2 months after exposure; however, cases of *P vivax* and *P ovale* have presented several years after exposure, which likely constitutes disease recrudescence.

No specific signs and symptoms are pathognomonic for malaria. Most patients present with a constellation of fever, myalgia, arthralgia, and headache. Patients present occasionally with concomitant abdominal pain, diarrhea, cough, and dyspnea. Rash and lymphadenopathy are rarely present and are clues to an alternative diagnosis. Roughly 10% to 40% of patients with malaria are afebrile on presentation, and, although textbooks frequently describe tertian and quaternary cyclical fevers, they are rarely seen in practice.[35,36] Adults with severe cases of *P falciparum* infection may present with renal failure, jaundice, and respiratory failure, including acute respiratory distress syndrome. Children with severe disease typically present with severe anemia, acidosis, and respiratory distress. Both adults and children with severe disease can present with CNS involvement, which carries a 15% to 20% mortality rate and can lead to neurologic sequelae in survivors.[34] Patients who present with fever and neurologic findings after returning from the tropics should be evaluated for malaria and meningitis, and treated promptly as warranted.

Laboratory diagnosis of malaria is classically made by examination of Giemsa-stained blood films. Thick peripheral blood films have an advantage of allowing more red blood cells to be examined per high-powered field, and therefore have increased sensitivity in comparison with thin films, which are used primarily for parasite speciation. The sensitivity of individual thick smears is variable, and depends on smear preparation and the technical experience of laboratory personnel. In recent years, malarial rapid diagnostic tests (RDTs) have been introduced into clinical practice for antigen detection. Similar to other point-of-care tests, RDTs are fairly simple to use and numerous brands are available worldwide. In the United States, only one RDT has been approved by the US Food and Drug Administration, namely the BinaxNOW Malaria Test kit, which is 97% sensitive for all species of malaria and 100% sensitive for *P falciparum*.[37] Many laboratories find this test to be superior to microscopic diagnosis, particularly when smears are performed infrequently. Other rarely used diagnostic strategies include the quantitative buffy coat technique, which allows centrifugation and separation of parasitized from unparasitized cells to facilitate parasite detection, and polymerase chain reaction (PCR) tests to detect parasite DNA. Regardless of the diagnostic strategy used, it is important that diagnosis should never supersede empiric treatment when severe *P falciparum* infection is suspected.

Two major classes of drugs are available for the parenteral treatment of severe malaria: the cinchona alkaloids (quinine and quinidine) and the artemisinin derivatives (artesunate and artemether). A meta-analysis of randomized controlled trials that compared mortality rates among patients with severe malaria treated with parenteral

artesunate or quinine demonstrated a clear advantage for artemisinin-based compounds (odds ratio [OR] for death, 0.69; 95% confidence interval [CI] 0.57–0.84;
P<.00001) in favor of artesunate, with no significant increase in adverse effects.[38,39]
Artemisinin derivatives also clear parasitemia more rapidly and are effective against a
broader range of parasite stages.[40] Despite these advantages, no parenteral formulations of artemisinin-based compounds are available in the United States, and only
one oral artemisinin-based combination (artemether/lumefantrine) is approved but is
not widely available. As it stands, the CDC recommends parenteral quinidine for
severe malaria. Quinidine remains available and effective, and should be considered
first-line until parenteral artemisinin therapy is made available.[41] Therapy with quinidine should be combined with doxycycline or clindamycin, and a 7-day course
should be completed. For cases of uncomplicated malaria, 3 options exist in the
United States. Most patients with uncomplicated disease should receive either
atovaquone-proguanil (Malarone), artemether-lumefantrine (Coartem) or oral quinidine plus doxycycline. The CDC maintains a 24-hour hotline and updated online
treatment guidelines, which should be referenced when treating patients with
imported malaria. All nonimmune patients with P falciparum should be admitted to
hospital, and infectious disease consultation should be obtained.

DENGUE FEVER

Dengue fever is caused by a family of 4 arboviruses that are endemic in most tropical
and subtropical regions and represent the most common causes of arboviral disease.[42] The viruses are transmitted primarily by the *Aedes aegypti* mosquito, which
is day-biting and has an affinity for small containers and pools of water in urban environments. Approximately one-third of the world's population lives in dengue-endemic
countries, with the highest prevalence in Southeast Asia, Oceania, the Caribbean, and
Latin America.[43,44] Close to 100 million cases of dengue fever occur per annum,
including 250,000 cases of dengue hemorrhagic fever (DHF), accounting for 25,000
deaths per year.[45] The proportion of febrile illness attributed to dengue in returning
travelers has increased greatly, from 2% in the 1990s to 16% in 2005. Dengue is
currently more than twice as common as malaria in febrile travelers returning from
Southeast Asia.[46] For United States travelers, the number of confirmed or probable
cases rose from 33.5 cases per year in 1990 to 2005 to 244 cases per year in 2006
to 2008.[47] At present, no effective vaccine exists for the virus.

Dengue virus has an incubation period of 4 to 8 days. Classic dengue fever is characterized by a clinical syndrome of fever (typically lasting 5–7 days), retro-orbital pain,
myalgia, arthralgia ("break-bone fever"), and rash. The rash often begins with an eryth-
rodermic pattern and progresses to a petechial appearance, with desquamation in the
convalescent phase. The petechiae are usually seen during the early febrile phase and
appear as discrete fine purpura on the face, soft palate, extremities, and axilla.

Dengue infection presents in a spectrum of disease ranging from mild febrile illness
(dengue fever) to DHF and dengue shock syndrome (DSS). The more severe syndromes were thought to be rare in returning travelers, as they are associated with
repeated infection; however, up to 16% of cases reported to the CDC between
2006 and 2008 were classified as DHF/DSS.[47]

Progression to the more serious spectrum of DHF/DSS is marked by coagulopathy
and increased vascular permeability.[48] Hemorrhagic manifestations include easy
bruising, bleeding at venipuncture sites, and a positive tourniquet test. On the third
to seventh day of illness, often as the fever subsides, changes in vascular permeability
may lead to edema, effusions, and the circulatory collapse that marks DSS. Risk

factors for developing more severe disease are poorly understood; however, individuals with a history of dengue infection are more likely to develop DHF/DSS (OR 5.1, 95% CI 1.4–17.7).[49] Low platelet counts correlate with increased bleeding (OR 3.1, 95% CI 0.95–10.7), and an elevated aminotransferase concentration is associated with progression to DHF (OR 3.5, 95% CI 1.2–10.0).[50]

The initial diagnosis of dengue fever is clinical, typified by fever and constitutional symptoms in individuals returning from endemic areas. Laboratory features suggestive of dengue infection include thrombocytopenia, leukopenia, and elevated levels of liver enzymes. DHF (mortality rate 10%–20%) is defined as the triad of:

- Thrombocytopenia (<100,000 platelets)
- Hemorrhagic manifestations
- Objective evidence of plasma leakage (hematocrit increase >20%, hypoproteinemia, or evidence of effusions)

DSS (with a mortality rate of up to 40%) is characterized by hypotension (systolic blood pressure <90%) or a narrow pulse pressure (<20 mm Hg). Patients with DHF/DSS warrant admission to a high level of care, as profound hemodynamic shock may rapidly ensue. Leukopenia (<5000 cells/mL) coupled with thrombocytopenia also warrants admission of patients with suspected dengue infection. Serologic diagnosis relies on acute and convalescent serum titers, with convalescent samples drawn 3 weeks after infection. During the acute stage of early infection, a PCR can be used identify dengue viremia.

Mild or classic dengue fever can be treated conservatively with antipyretics, oral fluids, and bed rest. Outpatients should be followed with daily monitoring of the complete blood count for 7 days.[50] The day of defervescence (usually between days 4 and 7 of illness) is a common period when capillary leakage and more severe disease can develop. If DHF/DSS is suspected, aggressive fluid replacement with normal saline or lactated Ringer solution is appropriate, and has been shown to decrease the mortality rate.[51] In patients with DHF/DSS the hypotension is often profound, although the clinical course is short. Patients with DSS typically either recover rapidly after fluid administration or die within 12 to 24 hours, with an overall mortality rate of 40%.[45]

ENTERIC FEVER (TYPHOID AND PARATYPHOID)

Typhoid fever is caused by 2 serotypes of the gram-negative bacillus *Salmonella enterica*: serovar typhi and serovar paratyphi. When these disseminate to cause systemic illness, they are collectively called enteric fever. Infection typically occurs via an oral-fecal route and comes from contaminated food and water, most commonly where standards of personal and environmental hygiene are low. In 2000, enteric fever affected 21.6 million people and claimed 216,500 lives.[52] The burden of disease is highest in south central Asia, Southeast Asia, and sub-Saharan Africa (>100 cases/100,000 people per year), and moderately high in the rest of Asia, Africa, Latin America, and Oceania (10–100 cases/100,000 people per year).[53] Enteric fever accounts for 2.9% of diagnosed causes of fever in returned travelers, and 14.1% among travelers returning from the Indian subcontinent.[5] Two typhoid vaccines are available: the single-dose Vi vaccine (55%–72% effective) and the 3-dose Ty21a vaccine (33%–96% effective).[53]

Typhoid fever has an incubation period of 7 to 18 days. Affected individuals invariably present with fever. The bacteria initially invade the intestinal mucosa and then pass from the lymphatics to the bloodstream, where they replicate and cause systemic illness. The fever often starts as low grade and then proceeds "stepwise" to become persistent and high grade by the second week. Headache (typically dull and frontal), abdominal pain, constipation or diarrhea, and cough are common symptoms, and can be confused with malaria. Classically, "rose spots" (2–3-mm blanching, pink-red macules) appear early in the course of the disease, but they appear only briefly and are often difficult to detect except in light-skinned persons.[17] The Faget sign (relative bradycardia during high fever) has been described in association with typhoid fever, but is rarely seen in clinical practice.

Complications such as disseminated intravascular coagulation, intestinal perforation, gastrointestinal bleeding, and meningitis/encephalitis occur in 10% to 15% of patients, most commonly as delayed manifestations. Peyer patches within the intestinal mucosa are the focus for gastrointestinal hemorrhage and perforation. Intestinal perforation occurs in 1% to 3% of patients and is associated with male sex (OR 4.39, 95% CI 1.37–14.09), leukopenia (OR 3.88, 95% CI 1.46–10.33), and delayed treatment (OR 4.58, 95% CI 1.14–18.35).[54] The case-fatality rate for typhoid is less than 1% in the setting of adequate antibiotic treatment and supportive therapy, but can approach 30% to 50% among patients with severe illness in low-resource settings.

The gold standard for diagnosis of enteric fever is blood culture, although stool cultures, urine cultures, bone marrow biopsy, and serology can play a role. During the first week of illness blood cultures have their highest yield, but their diagnostic sensitivity is only 40% to 80%, which underscores the importance of serial cultures.[55,56] Bone marrow biopsies, though rarely indicated, can have a higher yield.[57] Serologic testing using the Widal test is not recommended because of its poor sensitivity (47%–77%) and specificity (50%–92%). Newer serologic tests (Typhidot-M, Tubex) are available and may have some utility.[57] Because culture data and serology take time to be obtained, presumptive diagnosis and empiric treatment based on clinical diagnosis are required in suspected cases.

Prompt diagnosis coupled with early administration of appropriate antibiotics, supportive care, and correction of fluid losses should be the primary goals of care. Patients suspected of having enteric fever (S typhi or S paratyphi bacteremia) warrant admission for diagnostic and therapeutic considerations. Previous guidelines recommended treatment with fluoroquinolones; however, recent data have demonstrated up to 70% resistance of strains acquired by United Kingdom travelers in Asia.[58] Because fluoroquinolone-resistant strains are all sensitive to ceftriaxone, third-generation cephalosporins are considered first-line therapy. In patients with abdominal tenderness, a low index of suspicion should be maintained for complications, including gastrointestinal bleeding and perforation. Imaging and early surgical consultation are warranted in patients with peritonitis.

RICKETTSIAL INFECTION

Rickettsial diseases are a host of zoonotic infections caused by obligate intracellular, gram-negative bacteria of the order Rickettsiales. The vectors are typically arthropods, encompassing ticks, fleas, lice, and mites. More than 280 diagnoses of rickettsial disease were reported in GeoSentinel Surveillance data from 1996 to 2008, with the majority (82.5%) being spotted fever rickettsiosis.[59] Surveillance data from returned travelers with undifferentiated fever show rickettsial disease to account for almost 2% of all fevers and 5.6% of fevers in travelers returning from sub-Saharan Africa, making it the second most common identifiable cause of imported fever in that region behind malaria.[5]

Rickettsial diseases typically have an incubation period of 1 to 2 weeks following a bite from an infected arthropod vector. Although myriad bacteria, vectors, and hosts are intermixed in complex pathways, all rickettsial diseases share clinical features, diagnostic challenges, and treatment recommendations.

Classic rickettsial disease features short (5–7-day) incubation periods, primary lesions (eschars) at the bite site, fever lasting for a few days up to 2 weeks, lymphadenitis, and a maculopapular rash that develops 3 to 5 days after onset of symptoms.[60] Of note, less than 50% of patients exhibit the classic triad of eschar, lymphadenitis, and rash.[61] In addition to these symptoms, patients often experience headache, myalgia, arthralgia, and malaise, with up to one-third experiencing diarrhea.[17] On physical examination, an eschar at the site of a tick or louse bite, which the patient describes as lasting for 1 or 2 weeks, is found more than 80% of the time, but its absence does not rule out the disease. Less than 20% of patients remember the culprit bite.[60] Lymphadenitis is the next most common examination finding. Of note, the clinical presentation of rickettsial disease is similar to that of other diagnoses presenting with undifferentiated fever after travel.

Definitive microbiological diagnosis is available via PCR, culture, and serologic analysis. PCR is sensitive, specific, and rapid. Serologic studies are used more commonly but offer only retrospective diagnosis.

Because this diagnosis is difficult to make and is frequently delayed, clinical suspicion and presumptive diagnosis are required to initiate prompt and appropriate treatment in the absence of confirmatory data. Tetracyclines remain the mainstay of treatment, with doxycycline (100 mg twice daily for 3–14 days, depending on the clinical scenario) being the preferred regimen. Patients should improve within the first 48 hours. Failure to do so should prompt the treating physician to revisit the original diagnosis. Mediterranean spotted fever and murine typhus carry higher mortality rates, and scrub typhus, if left untreated, carries significant morbidity.[62,63] Nonetheless, complications are exceedingly rare and prognosis is usually good, with outpatient treatment being appropriate.

PROTECTION OF CONTACTS AND STAFF

Until potentially hazardous diseases are excluded, routine infectious precautions, with source isolation and respiratory/droplet confinement, should be implemented for all patients with undifferentiated fever after travel to the tropics. Local hospital guidelines should be followed. The following suspected or confirmed infections require special consideration[10]: anthrax, diphtheria, encephalitis, enteric fever, hepatitis (acute), novel influenza, measles, meningitis, mumps, pertussis, plague, poliomyelitis, rabies, and tuberculosis; travelers with respiratory illness and rash, varicella and herpes zoster, and viral hemorrhagic fever.

Several infections pose a risk of infection to laboratory staff from improper sample handling and processing. Laboratory staff should therefore be informed if any of the following infections are being considered: enteric fever, brucellosis, Q-fever, melioidosis, and, in particular, the viral hemorrhagic fevers.

The CDC maintains statutory requirements for notification of certain infectious diseases via the National Notifiable Disease Surveillance System. Current guidelines and case definitions can be accessed online at wwwn.cdc.gov/nndss/document/2012_Case%20Definitions.pdf.

Notifiable infections include suspected or confirmed cases of the following: anthrax, arboviral disease, babesiosis, botulism, brucellosis, chancroid, *Chlamydia trachomatis*, cholera, coccidioidomycosis, cryptosporidiosis, cyclosporiasis, dengue fever, diphtheria, ehrlichiosis, giardiasis, gonorrhea, *Haemophilus influenzae*, Hansen disease, hantavirus, hemolytic-uremic syndrome, hepatitis, HIV, legionellosis, listeriosis,

Lyme disease, malaria, measles, meningococcal disease, mumps, novel influenza, pertussis, plague, polio, psittacosis, Q-fever, rabies, rubella, salmonellosis, severe acute respiratory syndrome, Shiga toxigenic *E coli*, shigellosis, smallpox, spotted fever, streptococcal toxic shock, syphilis, tetanus, trichinellosis, tularemia, typhoid, vibriosis, viral hemorrhagic fever, and yellow fever.

The most important facet of public health surveillance begins at local, state, and regional levels. Each state has laws that mandate reporting of certain diseases. Clinicians working with patients who return ill from travel should be familiar with state and national requirements as they relate to these infections. Reporting and surveillance are within the scope of practice for health care providers, and are essential for proper surveillance and disease control.

SUMMARY

Fever in ill travelers returning home from developing nations is common. Most travelers present with undifferentiated febrile syndromes. Regional proportionate morbidity rates and the patient's travel history are essential in narrowing the differential diagnosis. Most patients in whom a diagnosis is confirmed have malaria, dengue, enteric fever, or rickettsial disease. Emergency clinicians should have a high index of suspicion for these diagnoses. Empiric treatment based on the clinical presentation is required in many cases because acquisition of confirmatory laboratory data is often delayed.

REFERENCES

1. World Health Organization. International travel and health. 2012. Available at: www.who.int/ith/en. Accessed March 6, 2013.
2. Ryan ET, Kain KC. Health advice and immunizations for travelers. N Engl J Med 2000;342(23):1716–25.
3. Steffen R, deBernardis C, Banos A. Travel epidemiology—a global perspective. Int J Antimicrob Agents 2003;21(2):89–95.
4. Steffen R, Rickenbach M, Wilhelm U, et al. Health problems after travel to developing countries. J Infect Dis 1987;156(1):84–91.
5. Freedman DO, Weld LH, Kozarsky PE, et al. Spectrum of disease and relation to place of exposure among ill returned travelers. N Engl J Med 2006;354(2): 119–30.
6. Bruni M, Steffen R. Impact of travel-related health impairments. J Travel Med 1997;4(2):61–4.
7. Hill DR. Health problems in a large cohort of Americans traveling to developing countries. J Travel Med 2000;7(5):259–66.
8. Wilson ME, Weld LH, Boggild A, et al. Fever in returned travelers: results from the GeoSentinel Surveillance Network. Clin Infect Dis 2007;44(12):1560–8.
9. Leder K, Tong S, Weld L, et al. Illness in travelers visiting friends and relatives: a review of the GeoSentinel Surveillance Network. Clin Infect Dis 2006;43(9): 1185–93.
10. Johnston V, Stockley JM, Dockrell D, et al. Fever in returned travellers presenting in the United Kingdom: recommendations for investigation and initial management. J Infect 2009;59(1):1–18.
11. Gautret P, Schlagenhauf P, Gaudart J, et al. Multicenter EuroTravNet/GeoSentinel study of travel-related infectious diseases in Europe. Emerg Infect Dis 2009; 15(11):1783–90.

12. Bottieau E, Clerinx J, Schrooten W, et al. Etiology and outcome of fever after a stay in the tropics. Arch Intern Med 2006;166(15):1642–8.

13. O'Brien D, Tobin S, Brown GV, et al. Fever in returned travelers: review of hospital admissions for a 3-year period. Clin Infect Dis 2001;33(5):603–9.

14. O'Brien DP, Leder K, Matchett E, et al. Illness in returned travelers and immigrants/refugees: the 6-year experience of two Australian infectious diseases units. J Travel Med 2006;13(3):145–52.

15. Bottieau E, Clerinx J, Van den Enden E, et al. Fever after a stay in the tropics: diagnostic predictors of the leading tropical conditions. Medicine (Baltimore) 2007;86(1):18–25.

16. Mali S, Tan KR, Arguin PM. Malaria surveillance—United States, 2009. MMWR Surveill Summ 2011;60(3):1–15.

17. Spira AM. Assessment of travellers who return home ill. Lancet 2003;361(9367):1459–69.

18. Memish ZA. Meningococcal disease and travel. Clin Infect Dis 2002;34(1):84–90.

19. Jelinek T, Bisoffi Z, Bonazzi L, et al. Cluster of African trypanosomiasis in travelers to Tanzanian national parks. Emerg Infect Dis 2002;8(6):634–5.

20. Moore AC, Ryan ET, Waldron MA. Case records of the Massachusetts General Hospital. Weekly clinicopathological exercises. Case 20-2002. A 37-year-old man with fever, hepatosplenomegaly, and a cutaneous foot lesion after a trip to Africa. N Engl J Med 2002;346(26):2069–76.

21. Rothenberg ME. Eosinophilia. N Engl J Med 1998;338(22):1592–600.

22. Doherty JF, Moody AH, Wright SG. Katayama fever: an acute manifestation of schistosomiasis. BMJ 1996;313(7064):1071–2.

23. Schulte C, Krebs B, Jelinek T, et al. Diagnostic significance of blood eosinophilia in returning travelers. Clin Infect Dis 2002;34(3):407–11.

24. Antinori S, Galimberti L, Gianelli E, et al. Prospective observational study of fever in hospitalized returning travelers and migrants from tropical areas, 1997-2001. J Travel Med 2004;11(3):135–42.

25. Parola P, Soula G, Gazin P, et al. Fever in travelers returning from tropical areas: prospective observational study of 613 cases hospitalised in Marseilles, France, 1999-2003. Travel Med Infect Dis 2006;4(2):61–70.

26. Ansart S, Perez L, Vergely O, et al. Illnesses in travelers returning from the tropics: a prospective study of 622 patients. J Travel Med 2005;12(6):312–8.

27. Casalino E, Le Bras J, Chaussin F, et al. Predictive factors of malaria in travelers to areas where malaria is endemic. Arch Intern Med 2002;162(14):1625–30.

28. West NS, Riordan FA. Fever in returned travellers: a prospective review of hospital admissions for a 2(1/2) year period. Arch Dis Child 2003;88(5):432–4.

29. Herbinger KH, Drerup L, Alberer M, et al. Spectrum of imported infectious diseases among children and adolescents returning from the tropics and subtropics. J Travel Med 2012;19(3):150–7.

30. Naudin J, Blonde R, Alberti C, et al. Aetiology and epidemiology of fever in children presenting to the emergency department of a French paediatric tertiary care centre after international travel. Arch Dis Child 2012;97(2):107–11.

31. Hagmann S, Neugebauer R, Schwartz E, et al. Illness in children after international travel: analysis from the GeoSentinel Surveillance Network. Pediatrics 2010;125(5):e1072–80.

32. Mali S, Kachur SP, Arguin PM. Malaria surveillance—United States, 2010. MMWR Surveill Summ 2012;61(2):1–17.

33. Smith AD, Bradley DJ, Smith V, et al. Imported malaria and high risk groups: observational study using UK surveillance data 1987-2006. BMJ 2008;337: a120.
34. Severe falciparum malaria. World Health Organization, communicable diseases cluster. Trans R Soc Trop Med Hyg 2000;94(Suppl 1):S1–90.
35. Dorsey G, Gandhi M, Oyugi JH, et al. Difficulties in the prevention, diagnosis, and treatment of imported malaria. Arch Intern Med 2000;160(16):2505–10.
36. Nic Fhogartaigh C, Hughes H, Armstrong M, et al. Falciparum malaria as a cause of fever in adult travellers returning to the United Kingdom: observational study of risk by geographical area. QJM 2008;101(8):649–56.
37. Stauffer WM, Cartwright CP, Olson DA, et al. Diagnostic performance of rapid diagnostic tests versus blood smears for malaria in US clinical practice. Clin Infect Dis 2009;49(6):908–13.
38. Dondorp A, Nosten F, Stepniewska K, et al. Artesunate versus quinine for treatment of severe falciparum malaria: a randomised trial. Lancet 2005;366(9487): 717–25.
39. Dondorp AM, Fanello CI, Hendriksen IC, et al. Artesunate versus quinine in the treatment of severe falciparum malaria in African children (AQUAMAT): an open-label, randomised trial. Lancet 2010;376(9753):1647–57.
40. Rosenthal PJ. Artesunate for the treatment of severe falciparum malaria. N Engl J Med 2008;358(17):1829–36.
41. Treatment with quinidine gluconate of persons with severe *Plasmodium falciparum* infection: discontinuation of parenteral quinine from CDC Drug Service. MMWR Recomm Rep 1991;40(RR-4):21–3.
42. Wilder-Smith A, Schwartz E. Dengue in travelers. N Engl J Med 2005;353(9): 924–32.
43. Gubler DJ, Clark GG. Dengue/dengue hemorrhagic fever: the emergence of a global health problem. Emerg Infect Dis 1995;1(2):55–7.
44. Mohammed HP, Ramos MM, Rivera A, et al. Travel-associated dengue infections in the United States, 1996 to 2005. J Travel Med 2010;17(1):8–14.
45. Gibbons RV, Vaughn DW. Dengue: an escalating problem. BMJ 2002; 324(7353):1563–6.
46. Wilder-Smith A, Renhorn KE, Tissera H, et al. DengueTools: innovative tools and strategies for the surveillance and control of dengue. Glob Health Action 2012;5: 17274.
47. Centers for Disease Control and Prevention (CDC). Travel-associated Dengue surveillance—United States, 2006-2008. MMWR Morb Mortal Wkly Rep 2010; 59(23):715–9.
48. Halstead SB. Dengue. Lancet 2007;370(9599):1644–52.
49. Guzman MG, Kouri G. Dengue: an update. Lancet Infect Dis 2002;2(1):33–42.
50. Wichmann O, Gascon J, Schunk M, et al. Severe dengue virus infection in travelers: risk factors and laboratory indicators. J Infect Dis 2007;195(8):1089–96.
51. Dung NM, Day NP, Tam DT, et al. Fluid replacement in dengue shock syndrome: a randomized, double-blind comparison of four intravenous-fluid regimens. Clin Infect Dis 1999;29(4):787–94.
52. Crump JA, Luby SP, Mintz ED. The global burden of typhoid fever. Bull World Health Organ 2004;82(5):346–53.
53. Bhan MK, Bahl R, Bhatnagar S. Typhoid and paratyphoid fever. Lancet 2005; 366(9487):749–62.
54. Hosoglu S, Aldemir M, Akalin S, et al. Risk factors for enteric perforation in patients with typhoid Fever. Am J Epidemiol 2004;160(1):46–50.

55. Vallenas C, Hernandez H, Kay B, et al. Efficacy of bone marrow, blood, stool and duodenal contents cultures for bacteriologic confirmation of typhoid fever in children. Pediatr Infect Dis 1985;4(5):496–8.
56. World Health Organization. Background document: the diagnosis, treatment and prevention of typhoid fever. Geneva (Switzerland): World Health Organization; 2003.
57. Bhutta ZA. Current concepts in the diagnosis and treatment of typhoid fever. BMJ 2006;333(7558):78–82.
58. Threlfall EJ, de Pinna E, Day M, et al. Alternatives to ciprofloxacin use for enteric fever, United kingdom. Emerg Infect Dis 2008;14(5):860–1.
59. Jensenius M, Davis X, von Sonnenburg F, et al. Multicenter GeoSentinel analysis of rickettsial diseases in international travelers, 1996-2008. Emerg Infect Dis 2009;15(11):1791–8.
60. Jelinek T, Loscher T. Clinical features and epidemiology of tick typhus in travelers. J Travel Med 2001;8(2):57–9.
61. Jensenius M, Fournier PE, Vene S, et al. African tick bite fever in travelers to rural sub-Equatorial Africa. Clin Infect Dis 2003;36(11):1411–7.
62. Raoult D, Zuchelli P, Weiller PJ, et al. Incidence, clinical observations and risk factors in the severe form of Mediterranean spotted fever among patients admitted to hospital in Marseilles 1983-1984. J Infect 1986;12(2):111–6.
63. Dumler JS, Taylor JP, Walker DH. Clinical and laboratory features of murine typhus in south Texas, 1980 through 1987. JAMA 1991;266(10):1365–70.

Fever and the Rational Use of Antimicrobials in the Emergency Department

Raquel F. Harrison, MD[a], Helen Ouyang, MD, MPH[b],*

KEYWORDS

- Fever • Antibiotics • Antivirals • Antifungals • Antimicrobial resistance
- Hospital-acquired infections

KEY POINTS

- Emergency physicians must balance public health concerns about increasing antimicrobial resistance with the need for early antimicrobial therapy in febrile, ill patients.
- Institutional antibiograms should help guide antibiotic choices.
- Antimicrobial choices are affected by factors such as cost, dosing frequency, side effects, administration route, and infusion properties.
- Empiric antimicrobial therapy is challenging and ever-changing; it is the responsibility of the emergency physician to remain up to date.

INTRODUCTION

According to the 2009 National Hospital Ambulatory Medical Survey, 5.6% of patients who sought treatment in emergency departments (EDs) were febrile at the time of presentation. Second only to abdominal pain and cramps, fever was the second most common chief complaint for patients who came to EDs that year, and the most common chief complaint of patients younger than 15 years. The presence of fever prompts the question of whether antimicrobials should be administered empirically. The survey data also indicate that antimicrobials were the most prescribed drug category, second only to analgesics.[1] In EDs around the United States, 7% to 8% of visits involve the administration of at least 1 antimicrobial.[2]

Antimicrobials are ordered in the ED every day. Sometimes the indication is straightforward and the choices are simple; at other times the decisions are more

The authors have no conflicts of interest to disclose.
[a] Department of Emergency Medicine, New York-Presbyterian Hospital, The University Hospitals of Columbia and Cornell, New York, NY, USA; [b] Department of Emergency Medicine, Columbia University Medical Center, New York, NY, USA
* Corresponding author. Department of Emergency Medicine, New York-Presbyterian Hospital/Columbia, PH 1-137, 622 West 168th Street, New York, NY 10032.
E-mail address: houyang@post.harvard.edu

difficult. Any patient presenting with fever triggers consideration of the administration of an antimicrobial. Frequently, the decision to initiate empiric treatment needs to be made before the definitive diagnosis is known. In such cases, an organized approach is helpful.[3–5]

Determining the cause of a fever and subsequently treating it appropriately depend on multiple factors. Ideally each patient enters the ED with a clear history, and classic physical examination findings and the results of diagnostic tests mark an obvious path. However, a thorough history and physical examination can be hindered by uncontrollable elements, such as altered mental status. Results of diagnostic tests can be equivocal or even false. Therefore, empiric antimicrobial therapy has become a cornerstone of treatment. How does the emergency physician balance responsible stewardship of health resources with the need to provide effective treatment promptly?

The goal of this review is to provide a systems-based approach to prescribing antimicrobials to patients presenting to the ED with fever, while understanding the risk associated with overutilization. It seeks to provide an understanding of the key considerations needed to ensure that decisions are made well and appropriate treatment begins promptly.

GENERAL CONSIDERATIONS
When Should Antimicrobials be Used Empirically?

Not uncommonly, a physician decides that antimicrobials are needed even though a definitive infectious diagnosis has not yet been established. In these cases, "empiric therapy" is initiated, targeting potential sources of infection deemed likely and serious.[6] The spectrum of coverage is guided by a preliminary impression of probable infectious site based on the history and physical examination, relevant demographic information, medical history, laboratory data, and results of diagnostic imaging. Therefore, a good understanding of the surrounding epidemiology is particularly important. Many hospitals routinely gather culture results and sensitivity data for analysis and construction of a hospital antibiogram that provides antibiotic recommendations linked to specific clinical scenarios. This information is particularly useful for emergency service providers and others who see patients early in the course of illness, before cases have been definitively differentiated.

The need to administer antibiotics early and empirically is particularly pressing in the setting of severe infectious illnesses, including sepsis, pneumonia, and meningitis. Although some controversies remain, it is well established that antibiotics need to be administered empirically and early in selected cases, based on clinical judgment.[2] A particularly well-known illustration is found in the work of Emanuel Rivers and others, in which the strategy known as early goal-directed therapy[5] showed a significant positive impact on outcomes among patients with septic shock.[6] The 2012 Surviving Sepsis Guidelines emphasize administration of effective antimicrobials within the first hour after recognition of severe sepsis or septic shock.[7]

Assessing Vulnerability of the Patient

Comorbid conditions
The decision to prescribe antimicrobials can be informed by a thorough assessment of variables related to the host.[8] Some patients are unable to tolerate certain treatments because of hypersensitivity reactions. Patients might report a history of "allergy" in the past, even though no true allergy exists. It is important to investigate whether a history of intolerance is based on a true allergy or a less serious problem; for example, a

patient might have experienced gastrointestinal distress after taking a macrolide in the past, and therefore refuses to take it despite not having a true hypersensitivity reaction to the antibiotic.[9]

Patients with acute or chronic organ dysfunction might require antibiotic strategies that deviate from routine standard approaches. A particularly common example is renal dysfunction. Renal failure (whether acute or chronic) can affect elimination of antibiotics, which should be considered when establishing the appropriate dose and timing interval of antibiotics that are cleared by the kidneys. In addition, some antibiotics can directly cause renal or hepatic toxicity, and should be avoided in patients with underlying disease.

Immunocompromised patients raise particularly important issues. Such patients are exposed to all of the same common pathogens that infect otherwise healthy individuals and, at the same time, are particularly susceptible to atypical infections, including fungal infections and infections with resistant or particularly virulent organisms (eg, *Pseudomonas*) to which immunocompetent patients are less vulnerable. Understanding the host's response to the infection can have a significant impact on treatment choices and timing. Immunocompromised hosts can present atypically; they may not mount a fever and may not show classic signs of severity until late in the disease course. This situation could lead to delayed administration of antibiotics and failure to manage the patient aggressively on initial presentation.[2]

Drug interactions and side effects
Drug interactions can heighten patients' vulnerability to certain complications. For example, patients on warfarin for anticoagulation therapy may need to avoid fluoroquinolones to prevent coagulopathy. When quinolones must be used (or have been used inadvertently), it is essential to check the international normalized ratio to monitor coagulation status. Similarly, patients who are receiving metronidazole should be advised to avoid alcohol, because of the associated disulfiram-like reaction of nausea, vomiting, flushing of the skin, and tachycardia.

Socioeconomic status
Although not a comorbid medical condition per se, socioeconomic variables can render patients more vulnerable to infection and less able to access appropriate treatment. When financial barriers are significant, the cost of medicines needs to be considered in relation to patients' capacity to comply with recommendations. When patients are discharged with recommended outpatient follow-up, the cost of an antimicrobial and its dosing schedule become significant drivers of adherence. Generic brands that can be found in the formularies of large pharmacies are typically more affordable. Medicines that require frequent dosing are more difficult to take correctly and, as a result, compliance with therapy might be suboptimal.

Useful Clues to Support Targeting of Empiric Antibiotics

Identifying probable site(s) of infection
The history and physical examination, coupled with laboratory tests and imaging, should help identify the site of possible infection in a patient presenting with fever to the ED. Some sites of infection are difficult to penetrate with antibiotics, given the anatomy of the blood flow, and therefore limit the concentration of the antibiotic that can reach that organ. Areas that suffer significantly from lower concentrations of antibiotic include the cerebrospinal fluid (CSF), the prostate, the pancreas, the skin, soft tissue in patients with poorly controlled diabetes or peripheral vascular disease, and the vitreous humor of the eye.[9]

Which pathogens are most likely?

If multiple antibiotics are to be administered, consider first giving the antibiotic that is most likely to attack the offending organism, with guidance from the systems-based review that follows. For example, in a diabetic nursing-home patient at risk for *Pseudomonas aeruginosa*, the most likely cause of pneumonia remains a gram-positive coccus; therefore, *Streptococcus pneumoniae* should be targeted first, after which the need to also cover *P aeruginosa* should be addressed.

Using Antimicrobials Wisely and Strategically

Timing and sequence of administration

When choosing empiric antimicrobials, it is important to consider the pharmacokinetic and practical features of the options under consideration. For example, the combination of pipericillin-tazobactam and vancomycin is commonly used to provide broad-spectrum coverage when the prescribing physician judges that both methicillin-resistant *Staphylococcus aureus* (MRSA) and *P aeruginosa* need to be covered empirically. Typically, pipericillin-tazobactam can be administered more rapidly than vancomycin, so it may be prudent to give pipericillin-tazobactam first.

Considerations specific to route of administration

Intravenous antimicrobials might be preferred to oral options when the need to achieve an effective therapeutic index rapidly is judged to be particularly pressing. Though somewhat controversial, a common strategy is to administer a single dose of intravenous antibiotics followed by an oral agent that provides similar coverage but requires more time to reach effective therapeutic levels. For example, a patient can be given a dose of intravenous ampicillin-sulbactam followed by oral amoxicillin-clavulanate. Although research to support this approach is limited, it arguably combines the desired effects of early arrival at an effective therapeutic level with the practical preference for outpatient management in appropriately selected patients.[10]

Mode of action: bactericidal versus bacteriostatic

Bactericidal drugs kill bacteria, whereas bacteriostatic drugs inhibit cell growth. Drugs that are bactericidal do not need to reach near the concentration that bacteriostatic drugs are required to reach to kill the organism. Bactericidal drugs often kill at 4 times the mean inhibitory concentration (MIC), whereas bacteriostatic drugs may not kill until they reach a concentration of 16 times the MIC. Therefore, when considering infections in locations with poor blood flow, such as the prostate, or when treating a patient with significant microvascular disease (eg, a person with poorly controlled diabetes), bactericidal drugs might be more beneficial in reaching effective concentrations in the host's infected tissues without reaching toxic levels in other organ systems.

Despite the 4-fold difference in efficacy, bacteriostatic drugs play an important role in treating infections. Bacteriostatic agents contain the growth of an organism and allow the host's immune system to fight the infection. Specific features of the patient must be considered when predicting whether the host will be able to mount a sufficient response to fight the infection that remains. Bactericidal agents are preferred for patients who are immunocompromised or neutropenic, and those who have endovascular infections (endocarditis, meningitis, or cerebral abscess) or osteomyelitis.[9] Bacteriostatic antibiotics can be particularly beneficial in disease processes caused by organisms that divide rapidly or produce toxins that are targeted by the antibiotic: for example, toxic shock syndrome is a systemic manifestation of group A streptococci (GAS) infection secondary to the toxin produced by the GAS. Clindamycin, though bacteriostatic, is the drug of choice in this situation, because its mechanism of action decreases toxin production and thereby lessens systemic symptoms (**Table 1**).

Table 1
Pharmacokinetic properties of major antibiotic classes

Antibiotic	Mechanism of Action	Targeted Microbes	Special Considerations
Penicillins (β-lactam)	BACTERICIDAL: Inhibit cell-wall synthesis, exposing unstable membranes, leading to cell lysis	Gram-positive, some gram-negative coverage	
β-Lactamase inhibitor (clavulanate, sulbactam, tazobactam)	Augment utility of β-lactam-ring–based antibiotics by inhibiting enzymatic breakdown	Extends spectrum of many penicillins to target resistant organisms and more gram-negative coverage	
Cephalosporins (β-lactam)	BACTERICIDAL: Inhibit cell-wall synthesis, exposing unstable membranes, leading to cell lysis, but less susceptible to β-lactamase		Some of the less commonly used inhibit vitamin K production and cause disulfiram-like reaction (eg, cefotetan)
	First generation (cephalexin, cefazolin)	Gram-positive cocci, gram-negative bacilli (Proteus, Escherichia coli, Klebsiella)	
	Second generation (cefaclor, cefuroxime, cefotetan, cefoxitin)	Gram-positive cocci, gram-negative cocci (Neisseria gonorrhoeae), gram-negative bacilli (Enterobacter, E coli, Haemophilus influenzae, Klebsiella, Proteus)	
	Third generation (cefdinir, cefixime, cefotaxime, cefpodoxime, ceftriaxone, ceftazidime)	Broader gram-negative coverage (Pseudomonas covered by ceftazidime)	Ceftriaxone is excreted in bile
	Fourth generation (cefepime)	Staphylococci, streptococci, and gram-negative bacilli (including Pseudomonas)	
	Fifth generation (ceftaroline)	Gram-positive cocci, gram-negative bacilli, MRSA (only SSTI)	

(continued on next page)

Table 1
(continued)

Antibiotic	Mechanism of Action	Targeted Microbes	Special Considerations
Carbapenems (meropenem, imipenem, ertapenem, doripenem)	BACTERICIDAL: Inhibit cell-wall synthesis, exposing unstable membranes, leading to cell lysis, but less susceptible to β-lactamase	Penicillinase gram-positive and gram-negative organisms, anaerobes, and *Pseudomonas*	
Monobactams (aztreonam)	BACTERICIDAL: Inhibit cell-wall synthesis, exposing unstable membranes, leading to cell lysis but less susceptible to β-lactamase	Gram-negative only, including pseudomonas	Should be reserved for identified resistance; limit empiric use.
Vancomycin	BACTERICIDAL: Inhibit cell-wall synthesis, exposing unstable membranes, leading to cell lysis but less susceptible to β-lactamase	Gram-positive, including MRSA and enterococci	Oral use reserved for *Clostridium difficile* infection only Very broad coverage when combined with aminoglycoside Administer 1 g/h to prevent red man syndrome
Tetracyclines (doxycycline, minocycline)	BACTERIOSTATIC: Inhibit protein synthesis by reversibly binding ribosomes blocking tRNA	Gram-positive and some gram-negative; atypical or intracellular organisms (such as *Chlamydia*, *Mycoplasma*, and tick-borne disease)	Substantial bacterial resistance TERATOGENIC: causes discoloration and hypoplasia of bones and teeth, fetal hepatotoxicity
Aminoglycosides (amikacin, gentamicin, tobramycin, streptomycin)	BACTERICIDAL (based on concentration and dosing intervals): Inhibit protein synthesis by binding to ribosome subunit, preventing full ribosome assembly	Gram-negative (includes *Pseudomonas*)	Activity augmented when preceded by a penicillin

Macrolides (erythromycin, clarithromycin, azithromycin, telithromycin)	BACTERIOSTATIC: Inhibit protein synthesis by irreversibly binding ribosomes, preventing translocation	Atypical or intracellular organisms (such as *Chlamydia, Legionella, Mycoplasma*)	
Clindamycin	BACTERIOSTATIC: Inhibit protein synthesis by binding ribosomes, preventing translocation	Gram-positive (including MRSA), anaerobic bacteria	Most frequent culprit of *C difficile* infection Used for toxin-producing infections such as toxic shock syndrome
Linezolid	BACTERIOSTATIC: Inhibit protein synthesis by preventing full ribosome complex formation (bactericidal against certain organisms)	Gram-positive (MRSA, VRE, *Listeria*)	
Fluoroquinolones (levofloxacin, moxifloxacin, ciprofloxacin)	BACTERICIDAL (dose dependent): Inhibit DNA gyrase and topoisomerase, preventing DNA replication causing cell death, and blocks cell division by not allowing new DNA to segregate	Gram-negative (some *Pseudomonas*), gram-positive (no MRSA) and atypical organisms	TERATOGENIC: affects connective tissue development
Sulfonamides (trimethoprim-sulfamethoxazole)	BACTERIOSTATIC: Inhibit synthesis of bacterial folic acid preventing formation of essential cofactors	Gram-positive (MRSA), limited gram-negative	Severe hypersensitivities including SJS Can elicit hemolytic anemia in patients with G6PD
Metronidazole	BACTERICIDAL: forms unstable molecules within DNA	Anaerobic bacteria and protozoa	Biliary excretion allows it to be effective against *C difficile*

Abbreviations: G6PD, glucose-6-phosphate dehydrogenase; MRSA, methicillin-resistant *Staphylococcus aureus*; SJS, Stevens-Johnson syndrome; VRE, vancomycin-resistant enterococci.

GROWING ANTIBIOTIC RESISTANCE IN THE UNITED STATES

Data from the Centers for Disease Control and Prevention (CDC) demonstrate that resistance persists as a growing public health concern. Unless significant action is taken in altering the way antibiotics are stewarded by physicians, organisms that are resistant to the newest and strongest antibiotics will continue to emerge. In November 2012, the National Institutes of Health (NIH) and the Pew Health Group published a study highlighting the absolute necessity of improving prescribing habits and educating patients.[11,12] Many Americans understand the importance of antibiotic resistance and know that the full course of prescribed antibiotics should be taken, even if they do not always comply with such recommendations. Patients believe that organisms are becoming resistant to antibiotics in the community, but they have low suspicion that the organisms will affect them or a family member.[11] As physicians, our role in patient education and taking responsibility to not overprescribe antibiotics is of the utmost importance. Prescribing rates for antibiotics have fallen 17% nationwide since 1999, although some states have had more progress than others.[13] Emergency physicians frequently feel pressured by patients to prescribe antibiotics.

The number of antibiotics and other antimicrobials being developed has fallen drastically over the past several decades. From 1983 to 1987, pharmaceutical companies introduced 16 new antimicrobial agents to the market. Since then there has been a steady decline in production; between 2003 and 2007, only 5 new antibiotics were introduced, and since 2007 only 1 new agent has been developed.[14] The Pew Health Group identified several challenges to antibiotic innovation. Scientifically, new classes of antibiotic with novel mechanisms of action are difficult to discover. Economically, antibiotics produce lower revenues than other pharmaceuticals. In addition, achieving approval for a new antibiotic from the US Food and Drug Administration (FDA) has become more challenging, because investigators find it difficult to amass a sufficient number of study subjects and regulatory measures are tighter, requiring that the new agent must show improved efficacy and decreased adverse reactions or toxicity.[13]

The financial burden associated with resistant organisms is increasing. The CDC estimates that each year, resistant infections account for about $20 billion management costs and contribute to an estimated 8 million additional hospital days.[14,15] An increasing number of organisms have been identified as having resistant strains in North America and abroad. The most prevalent drug-resistant pathogens cited by the CDC are *Acinetobacter*, group B streptococci, *Klebsiella pneumoniae*, MRSA, *Neisseria meningitidis*, *Shigella*, *S pneumoniae*, vancomycin-resistant enterococci, *Candida*, and the human immunodeficiency virus (HIV) and the organisms that cause anthrax, gonorrhea, tuberculosis, typhoid fever, influenza, and malaria.[16] Therefore, in times of increasing resistance, the most efficacious antibiotic should be deployed, which will create the least amount of inducible resistance within the host and deliver the most precise targeting to the susceptible organism and the affected organ system.

TARGETED ANTIMICROBIAL THERAPY BY SYSTEM
Central Nervous System

Meningitis and encephalitis
Meningitis and encephalitis secondary to bacterial infection confer significant risk of morbidity and mortality. Early diagnosis and treatment remain essential to averting death and disabling neurologic sequelae. Typical presentations warrant empiric treatment, including appropriately timed diagnostic studies and early antibiotics. Atypical presentations pose diagnostic challenges, emphasizing the importance of maintaining

a high index of suspicion for these conditions, and carefully considering the timing and sequencing of therapeutic efforts.

Although incidental cases of bacterial meningitis and encephalitis are relatively rare, they are considered true neurologic emergencies. When meningitis or encephalitis is suspected, empiric administration of the appropriate antibiotic should be seriously considered as early as possible. Proulx and colleagues[17] demonstrated that patients who receive antibiotics in the ED are significantly less likely to die than patients who do not receive antibiotics before arrival at the inpatient service (mortality rates of 7.9% and 29%, respectively). Other studies have shown a less robust effect of early antibiotic administration.[2] Typical manifestations of meningitis/encephalitis are fever, headache, nuchal rigidity, and altered mental status.[18] The clinical syndrome of fever and headache should prompt consideration of meningoencephalitis, although these symptoms are nonspecific.

Evaluation and diagnosis
Appropriate evaluation includes certain diagnostic tests that may cause significant delays in definitive therapy. In particular, the appropriateness and timing of computed tomography (CT) of the head, lumbar puncture, and blood cultures need to be considered in relation to the expected clinical benefits compared with earlier administration of antibiotics and, possibly, steroids. The Infectious Diseases Society of America (IDSA) guidelines for bacterial meningitis emphasize that blood cultures should be obtained and lumbar puncture performed promptly (before administration of parenteral antibiotics and steroids when it has been determined that a head CT scan is not needed).[19]

Analysis of cerebrospinal fluid
Analysis of CSF allows the differentiation of bacterial from viral meningitis. A positive Gram stain points convincingly toward a bacterial source, whereas a negative Gram stain cannot exclude an occult bacterial infection. CSF cell counts and chemistries are expected to demonstrate typical patterns corresponding to either a viral or bacterial source. Nevertheless, results sometimes will be equivocal. CSF cultures can also be useful, but require 24 to 48 hours to provide useful information.[20,21]

Other candidate markers in the CSF, including lactate and procalcitonin levels, are under active investigation as correlates of bacterial meningitis, but evidence to recommend their routine use is lacking.[19] Imperfect prediction of bacterial meningitis based on CSF analysis emphasizes the point that empiric therapy for bacterial infection could be prudent regardless of test results in selected cases.

Treatment
Cases requiring prompt treatment of bacterial meningitis have (1) typical presentations, (2) a typical or atypical presentation along with objective test results that raise concern, or (3) atypical features, including equivocal test results, in patients with additional unreassuring findings (eg, systemic inflammation, hypotension, or altered mental status). The common approach to antibiotic administration targeting meningeal infection is presented in **Table 2**.

RESPIRATORY INFECTIONS
Upper Respiratory Infections

Sinusitis
Fever is a common presenting symptom associated with acute maxillary sinusitis. Fever can be present whether the infection is caused by a virus (commonly rhinovirus) or a bacterium (commonly *S pneumoniae* and *H influenzae*). Therefore, the presence of

Table 2
Algorithm for the empiric treatment of meningitis

Risk Factors	Common Pathogens	Antimicrobial Therapy
<1 mo	*Streptococcus agalactiae, Escherichia coli, Listeria monocytogenes, Klebsiella*, herpes simplex virus, varicella zoster virus	Ampicillin[a] + cefotaxime; or ampicillin + aminoglycoside + acyclovir (as needed for viral suspicion)
1–23 mo	*Streptococcus pneumoniae, Neisseria meningitides, S agalactiae, Escherichia coli, Haemophilus influenzae*, herpes simplex virus, varicella zoster virus	Vancomycin + third-generation cephalosporin + acyclovir (as needed for viral suspicion)
2–50 y	*S pneumoniae, N meningitides*, herpes simplex virus, varicella zoster virus	Vancomycin + third-generation cephalosporin + acyclovir (as needed for viral suspicion)
>50 y	*S pneumoniae, N meningitides, L monocytogenes*, aerobic gram-negative bacilli, herpes simplex virus, varicella zoster virus	Vancomycin + third-generation cephalosporin + ampicillin + acyclovir (as needed for viral suspicion)
Trauma: basilar skull fracture	*S pneumoniae, H influenzae*, group A β-hemolytic streptococci	Vancomycin + third-generation cephalosporin
Trauma: penetrating trauma	*Staphylococcus aureus*, coagulase-negative staphylococcus (ie, *Staphylococcus epidermidis*), aerobic gram-negative bacilli (including *Pseudomonas aeruginosa*)	Vancomycin + cefepime[b] or ceftazidime[b] or meropenem[b]
Following neurosurgery	*S aureus*, coagulase-negative staphylococci (ie, *S epidermidis*), aerobic gram-negative bacilli (including *P aeruginosa*)	Vancomycin + cefepime[b] or ceftazidime[b] or meropenem[b]
CSF shunt	*S aureus*, coagulase-negative staphylococci (ie, *S epidermidis*), aerobic gram-negative bacilli (including *P aeruginosa*), *Propionibacterium acnes*	Vancomycin + cefepime[b] or ceftazidime[b] or meropenem[b]

[a] Ampicillin is added to specifically target *L monocytogenes*.
[b] Cefepime, ceftazidime, or meropenem is added to specifically target *P aeruginosa*.
Adapted from Tunkel AR, Hartman BJ, Kaplan SL, et al. Practice guidelines for the management of bacterial meningitis. Clin Infect Dis 2004;39:1267–84; with permission.

fever cannot be used to guide treatment. Most cases of acute rhinitis and sinusitis have a viral source and run a benign course. These facts, coupled with growing concern about bacterial resistance, have led the CDC to advise judicious use of antibiotics. Supportive care with decongestants should be sufficient to treat viral sinusitis.[22]

Longer duration of symptoms suggests a bacterial source. A course of antibiotics might be advisable when symptoms last longer than 10 days, the patient is febrile with severe symptoms of pain and purulent discharge, or the patient has experienced resolution of the symptoms of an upper respiratory infection only for headache, facial pain, or purulent nasal discharge to return. These infections are commonly caused by *S pneumoniae* or *H influenzae*, for which β-lactam with β-lactamase inhibitor is indicated.

Increasing resistance over the previous decade emphasizes the importance of selecting antibiotics that are effective against β-lactamase–producing organisms. In patients who are allergic to penicillin, doxycycline (preferred) or a fluoroquinolone is recommended. Resistance to macrolides is now so widespread that they cannot be recommended as first-line therapy. Empiric coverage for MRSA is not recommended.[23]

Pharyngitis

Adult pharyngitis is most frequently a viral infection, but adults, like children, remain susceptible to group A β-hemolytic streptococci. Gonococcal infection is a less common but nevertheless important cause of bacterial pharyngitis. Approximately 5% to 15% of cases of adult pharyngitis are secondary to group A streptococci and, of that group, 1 in 3000 is at risk for acute rheumatic fever.[24] The Centor criteria can usefully guide the diagnosis and treatment of acute pharyngitis:

1. History of fever
2. Absence of cough
3. Tonsillar exudates
4. Tender anterior cervical lymphadenopathy

When all 4 criteria are positive, patients should be treated empirically for GAS. Patients with 2 or more criteria should be tested with a rapid streptococcal antigen test. If this result is positive, the patient should be treated with penicillin (if the patient is allergic to penicillin, a macrolide may be used).[24]

Acute bronchitis

Acute bronchitis is an acute respiratory illness characterized by cough, with or without sputum production, lasting up to 3 weeks.[25] As with other upper respiratory infections, 90% of cases are viral in origin. The most common culprits are influenza, parainfluenza, respiratory syncytial virus, and adenovirus. When bacteria are implicated, the most common organisms are *Bordetella pertussis*, *Mycoplasma pneumoniae*, and *Chlamydia pneumoniae*.[26]

Routine empiric treatment with antimicrobials is not recommended for acute bronchitis. However, when patients present within 48 hours after symptom onset and a polymerase chain reaction of a nasal swab confirms influenza A or B, a neuraminidase inhibitor (ie, oseltamivir or zanamivir) may decrease the severity and duration of symptoms, and is therefore useful in selected populations.

The CDC recommends initiation of antiviral treatment as soon as possible for patients in whom influenza is suspected or confirmed, and who are hospitalized, have severe, complicated underlying progressive illness, or are at risk for influenza complications. The following groups are considered at high risk for complications: those at the extremes of age (<2 years or >65 years); those with significant chronic pulmonary disease, neurologic disease, diabetes, or an immunocompromised state; women who are pregnant or in the postpartum period (within 2 weeks after delivery); those who are younger than 19 years and on long-term aspirin therapy; American Indians/Alaska Natives; the morbidly obese (body mass index $\geq$40 kg/m^2); and residents of chronic care facilities.[27] The CDC no longer recommends treatment of influenza A with amantadine, because 100% of strains tested since 2008 were found to be resistant.

When a patient with apparent bronchitis experiences episodic worsening of the illness and has a persistent, high-pitched cough, the diagnosis of *B pertussis* should be entertained. For patients who have those characteristics and who either did not receive the pertussis vaccine or received it more than 10 years previously, empiric treatment with macrolides can be considered. Trimethoprim-sulfamethoxazole may be administered to patients who are allergic to macrolides.

LOWER RESPIRATORY INFECTIONS
Community-Acquired Pneumonia

Pneumonia is the eighth leading cause of death in the United States.[28] Given its epidemiologic significance, research and policy priorities have focused on early recognition and treatment. In 2002, the Joint Commission on Accreditation of Healthcare Organizations and the Center for Medicare and Medicaid Services identified early antibiotic administration in pneumonia as a core performance measure.[29] The relevant literature suggests real but limited benefit from early antibiotic administration in community-acquired pneumonia (CAP); benefits from earlier treatment in patients with nosocomial infections (health care–associated pneumonia and ventilator-associated pneumonia) are significant and apparent.[2] Patients with CAP often present with typical features, including fever, cough, and an infiltrate on chest film. If the illness is particularly severe or if the patient is immunocompromised, the presentation can be dominated by nonspecific features such as altered mental status, and atypical findings such hypothermia or the absence of fever.

CAP can be bacterial or viral in origin. The most commonly implicated bacteria are *S pneumoniae*, *Mycoplasma pneumoniae*, *C pneumoniae*, *H influenzae*, *Legionella pneumophila*, anaerobes from aspiration, and gram-negative bacilli. Viral causes include influenza virus, parainfluenza virus, respiratory syncytial virus, human metapneumovirus, hantavirus, coronavirus, varicella, and rubeola.[30]

The essential approach to suspected pneumonia requires estimation of its severity, including determination of whether inpatient or outpatient treatment is needed. The literature provides several prediction rules that may be helpful. The Pneumonia Severity Index (PSI), or PORT score, is one such commonly used tool.[31] The PSI includes 20 markers, and could therefore prove cumbersome for application in many clinical settings.

Another commonly used prediction rule is the CURB-65 method, promoted by the British Thoracic Society. This tool is less complex than the PSI, so its application is more feasible in clinical settings.[32] Each key element is given 1 point, as described:

C: Confusion, defined as disorientation to place, time, or person or another finding that causes concern during examination of mental status
U: Uremia, with blood urea nitrogen level higher than 7 mmol/L (20 mg/dL)
R: Respiratory rate 30 breaths/min or more
B: low Blood pressure (systolic <90 mm Hg or diastolic <60 mm Hg)
65: age 65 years or older.

The simplified recommendation is that patients with a total score of 0 or 1 can be treated on an outpatient basis, those with a score of 2 warrant admission to inpatient wards, and those with a score of 3 or more should be considered for care in the intensive care unit. No scoring system is sufficient to replace clinical judgment, but sufficient judgment might allow either of these tools to be useful in appropriately selected situations. In addition, the likely pathogens should be identified so that the appropriate spectrum of activity for antibiotic coverage can be determined. Toward this end, the American Thoracic Society (ATS) and the IDSA jointly published guidelines in 2007 (**Box 1**).[33]

Box 1
Treatment of community-acquired pneumonia

1. Outpatient treatment
   a. Previously healthy with no prior antimicrobials within 3 months
      i. Macrolide (unless in a region with high *Streptococcus pneumoniae* resistance)
      ii. Doxycycline
   b. Presence of chronic conditions and comorbidities or prior treatment with antimicrobial:
      i. Respiratory fluoroquinolone (moxifloxacin, gemifloxacin, or levofloxacin)
      ii. β-Lactam plus a macrolide
2. Inpatients, non-ICU treatment
   a. Respiratory fluoroquinolone
   b. β-Lactam plus a macrolide
3. Inpatients, ICU treatment
   a. β-Lactam (third-generation cephalosporin or ampicillin-sulbactam) plus fluoroquinolone or macrolide
      i. Penicillin allergic: fluoroquinolone plus aztreonam
   b. Pseudomonal risk (recent hospitalization or structural lung disease)
      i. Antipneumococcal/antipseudomonal β-lactam (pipericillin-tazobactam, cefepime, imipenem, or meropenem) plus fluoroquinolone (ciprofloxacin or levofloxacin)
      ii. Or the above β-lactam plus aminoglycoside plus azithromycin or fluoroquinolone
      iii. Penicillin allergic: aztreonam rather than above β-lactams
   c. Community-acquired MRSA risk, add vancomycin or linezolid to the above regimens

Abbreviation: ICU, intensive care unit.
Adapted from Centers for Disease Control and Prevention. Sexually transmitted diseases treatment guidelines, 2010: pelvic inflammatory disease. 2011. Available at: www.cdc.gov/std/treatment/2010/pid.htm. Accessed March 26, 2013.

Hospital-Acquired Pneumonia

The ATS and the IDSA divide hospital-acquired pneumonia into 2 categories: health care–associated pneumonia (HCAP) and ventilator-associated pneumonia (VAP). HCAP is a nosocomial infection acquired in an acute care hospital or a chronic care facility. VAP can occur in the acutely critically ill and in patients with chronic respiratory failure requiring mechanical ventilation. The most common multidrug-resistant gram-negative bacterial pathogen that causes hospital-acquired pneumonia is *P aeruginosa*. Other pathogens that should be considered are *K pneumoniae*, *Enterobacter*, *Serratia*, *Acinetobacter*, *Stenotrophomonas*, *Burkholderia cepacia*, MRSA, *S pneumoniae*, *H influenzae*, *Legionella*, *Candida*, *Aspergillus*, influenza, parainfluenza, adenovirus, measles, and respiratory syncytial virus.[34]

Treatment decisions are based on the patient's risk profile for drug-resistant organisms. Patients at highest risk are those who have been in chronic care facilities, who frequent dialysis centers, who were hospitalized for 2 or more days in the previous 90 days, who live in communities with a high prevalence of resistance, who have a family member with a known resistant organism, or who are immunosuppressed (**Table 3**).[34]

Table 3
Initial combination empiric therapy for hospital-acquired pneumonia in high-risk patients (options for treating each pathogen)

MDR/*Pseudomonas* #1[a]	Cephalosporin (cefepime or ceftazidime) OR	Carbapenem (imipenem or meropenem) OR	β-Lactam (piperacillin-tazobactam)
MDR/*Pseudomonas* #2[a]	Fluoroquinolone (ciprofloxacin or levofloxacin) OR	Aminoglycoside (amikacin, gentamicin, or tobramycin)	
MRSA	Linezolid OR	Vancomycin	
Legionella	Fluoroquinolone (ciprofloxacin or levofloxacin) OR	Azithromycin	

If a pathogen is suspected, each should be treated with one antimicrobial from each row.
[a] Given the increasing resistance patterns, multidrug-resistant (MDR) organisms/*Pseudomonas* should be covered with combination therapy and 2 antimicrobials (one from each row), in addition to coverage for MRSA and *Legionella*, if applicable.
Data from American Thoracic Society; Infectious Diseases Society of America. Guidelines for the management of adults with hospital-acquired, ventilator-associated, and healthcare-associated pneumonia. Am J Respir Crit Care Med 2005;171:388–416.

As discussed earlier, when treating drug-resistant organisms it is imperative to understand local resistance patterns, to be aware of institutional recommendations based on in-house epidemiologic studies and antibiograms, and, most importantly, to consider resistant patterns documented in a specific patient's medical history.

Tuberculosis

Because of the public health implications surrounding tuberculosis (TB), clinicians should maintain a high index of suspicion toward their patients' risk for this disease. The CDC has delineated the following high-risk populations: the immunocompromised, the incarcerated, international travelers, and immigrants from countries with a high prevalence of TB.[35] High clinical suspicion for active TB in a patient being assessed in the ED warrants initiation of appropriate precautions and treatment. Because the prevalence of organisms resistant to isoniazid is so high, the World Health Organization recommends administration of 4 antimicrobials to patients suspected of having active TB for the first 2 months of treatment: ethambutol, isoniazid, rifampin, and pyrazinamide.[36]

CARDIAC

Establishing the diagnosis of infective endocarditis is particularly challenging early in the course of illness. The Duke criteria should be useful in guiding the decision to begin empiric therapy in the ED (**Table 4**). This approach recommends initiation of treatment in the ED for cases that meet 2 major criteria, 1 major and 3 minor criteria, or 5 minor criteria.

Empiric therapy is not typically instituted unless the patient has become acutely ill and is exhibiting signs of sepsis. Before treatment is initiated, a serious effort to identify the infectious source should be undertaken. An appropriate blood culture is essential in this effort, using at least 3 samples from 3 sites, if possible. The most common offending organism is *S aureus*.

For patients with native valves, initial treatment with ampicillin-sulbactam combined with gentamicin is recommended in most cases. For patients who are allergic to

Table 4	
Modified Duke criteria	
Major Criteria	**Minor Criteria**
Blood culture positive: viridans streptococci, *Streptococcus bovis*, HACEK group, *Staphylococcus aureus*, enterococci OR persistently positive blood cultures OR a single positive blood culture for *Coxiella burnetii* or anti–phase 1 IgG antibody titer >1:800	Predisposing heart condition or intravenous drug use
Echocardiogram positive for infective endocarditis (TEE is the most sensitive)	Fever >38°C
	Vascular phenomena; major arterial emboli, septic pulmonary infarcts, mycotic aneurysms, intracranial hemorrhage, conjunctival hemorrhage, Janeway lesions
	Immunologic phenomena: glomerulonephritis, Osler nodes, Roth spots, rheumatoid factor
	Blood culture positive that does not meet major criteria

Abbreviations: HACEK, *Haemophilus, Actinobacillus, Cardiobacterium hominis, Eikenella corrodens, Kingella kingae*; IgG, immunoglobulin G; TEE, transesophageal echocardiography.
Adapted from Baddour LM, Wilson WR, Bayer AS, et al. Infective endocarditis: diagnosis, antimicrobial therapy, and management of complications. Circulation 2005;111:e394–433; with permission.

penicillins, treatment with vancomycin combined with gentamicin and ciprofloxacin can be considered. When endocarditis develops in an intravenous drug abuser, the infective organism is usually *S aureus*; vancomycin is commonly recommended in this patient population. The clinician should remain alert to the possibility of polymicrobial infections in these patients.[37]

Patients with prosthetic valves should receive broader coverage administered aggressively. Coverage of *Bartonella* species, in particular, should be ensured. Common recommendations are ceftriaxone with gentamicin with or without doxycycline. When patients are not actively symptomatic and their clinical condition remains stable, admission for further workup to establish the diagnosis definitively is recommended if endocarditis is suspected.[37]

ABDOMINAL INFECTIONS

Intraluminal intestinal flora is the most common cause of intra-abdominal infection. The Surgical Infection Society and the IDSA jointly issued recommendations pertaining to patients with abdominal infections. When abdominal infection is suspected and signs of systemic inflammation or hypoperfusion are present, administration of antibiotics should begin empirically in parallel with efforts to definitively identify the source.[38] When an intra-abdominal source of infection is suspected, surgical consultation is necessary to plan the treatment course.

DIVERTICULITIS, APPENDICITIS, AND BOWEL ISCHEMIA

The most common microbial causes of abdominal infections are enteric gram-negative aerobic and facultative bacilli, and enteric gram-positive streptococci.

Antimicrobial treatment should include coverage for those organisms and, when the distal small bowel, appendix, or colon is involved, obligate anaerobic bacilli should also be covered. Current guidelines suggest that routine blood cultures tend to not be helpful. Blood cultures are more likely to be helpful when patients are exhibiting signs of sepsis or are immunocompromised, and when resistant organisms are suspected.[38] Standard recommendations for empiric coverage in adult patients with mild or moderate disease call for administration of cefoxitin, ertapenem, moxifloxacin, tigecycline, or ticarcillin–clavulanic acid. When the illness is judged to be severe or when the patient's vulnerability is judged to be high (in someone at an advanced age or in an immunocompromised host), broader coverage is typically advisable.[38]

Decisions regarding the treatment of nosocomial infections should be guided by culture data and local resistance patterns. Broad-spectrum antibiotics are typically needed. Treatment decisions must be adapted when uncommon sources are suspected; fungal infection (commonly *Candida albicans*) might require the addition of fluconazole, and resistant *Staphylococcus* species might require vancomycin or linezolid.[38]

Diverticulitis is a relatively common abdominal infection that can be treated medically, and on an outpatient basis in selected cases. General recommendations suggest that uncomplicated cases (ie, patients with diverticulitis for the first time, those without bowel perforation or abscess formation, patients who can hydrate orally, and those who can achieve sufficient pain control) can be discharged with instructions to obtain outpatient treatment and follow-up. Oral treatment regimens should include moxifloxacin, ciprofloxacin plus metronidazole, levofloxacin plus metronidazole, or amoxicillin–clavulanic acid.[38]

BILIARY INFECTIONS

The organisms that typically cause acute cholecystitis and acute cholangitis are slightly different from those associated with other intra-abdominal infections. Antimicrobial therapy does not need to cover anaerobes unless a biliary-enteric anastomosis is present. An enterococcal infection should be considered if the patient has received an organ transplant or is otherwise immunocompromised. Therefore, targeted organisms usually include enteric gram-negative aerobic and facultative bacilli, and enteric gram-positive streptococci (**Table 5**).

Special Case: Diarrhea

Diarrhea is a common complaint among ED patients. Most cases pose little risk to life or health, but diarrheal illness causes significant discomfort and distress. When diarrhea is profuse and persistent, the patient faces the risk of dehydration and hypovolemia. Most patients require only supportive care. Some require rehydration (either orally or intravenously). Antimicrobial therapy should be reserved for patients with fever or hemorrhagic features.[39]

When antimicrobial therapy is contemplated, the decision to obtain targeted stool studies should be made in tandem. Determining which stool studies are needed is linked to clinical suspicion. If an inflammatory cause is possible, a stool sample should be examined for fecal polymorphonuclear leukocytes. If the patient is hemorrhagic and a shiga-toxin–producing *Escherichia coli* (*E coli* O157) is suspected, a test specific for that organism can be requested.[39] In patients with community-acquired or traveler's diarrhea, infection secondary to *Salmonella*, *Shigella*, *Campylobacter*, *E coli* O157:H7, or *Clostridium difficile* should be considered.

Table 5
Antimicrobial considerations in intra-abdominal infections

Infection	Regimen
Community-acquired acute cholecystitis of mild to moderate severity	First-, second-, or third-generation cephalosporin (cefazolin, cefuroxime, or ceftriaxone)
Community-acquired acute cholecystitis with toxic appearance, shock, advanced age, or immunocompromised condition	Carbapenems, piperacillin-tazobactam, levofloxacin, cefepime, COMBINED WITH metronidazole
Acute cholangitis following bilioenteric anastomosis of any severity	Carbapenems, piperacillin-tazobactam, levofloxacin, cefepime, COMBINED WITH metronidazole
Health care–associated biliary infection of any severity	Carbapenems, piperacillin-tazobactam, levofloxacin, cefepime, COMBINED WITH metronidazole AND vancomycin

Data from Solomkin JS, Mazuski JE, Bradley JS, et al. Diagnosis and management of complicated intra-abdominal infection in adults and children: guidelines by the Surgical Infection Society and the Infection Diseases Society of America. Clin Infect Dis 2010;50:133–64.

Diarrhea secondary to *Salmonella* and *Shigella* should be treated with fluoroquinolones in adults and trimethoprim-sulfamethoxazole in children. *Campylobacter* has increasing antimicrobial resistance, and should be treated with a macrolide. *E coli* O157 should be suspected in patients who are afebrile but have hemorrhagic diarrhea. Given the significant risk of hemolytic uremic syndrome from shiga-toxin release, diarrhea suspected to be secondary to *E coli* O157 should not be treated with antimicrobial therapy. Supportive care alone is recommended. *C difficile* should be considered in immunosuppressed patients with acute diarrhea and in those who have been recently treated with antimicrobials for another infection. Initial therapy should include oral metronidazole.[39]

When diarrhea begins after a recent hospitalization, infection with *C difficile* should be considered.[39] When diarrhea persists for more than 7 days, parasitic infections or other inflammatory processes should be considered.

PELVIC INFECTIONS
Genitourinary Infections

Uncomplicated urinary tract infections
In 2010 the IDSA, in conjunction with the American Congress of Obstetricians and Gynecologists, the American Urological Society, the Association of Medical Microbiology and Infectious Disease—Canada, and the Society for Academic Emergency Medicine, updated guidelines for the treatment of uncomplicated cystitis and pyelonephritis in otherwise healthy premenopausal women.[40] In otherwise young healthy patients, uncomplicated cystitis is not usually associated with fever. However, if a patient with urinary tract symptoms has a fever or complains of back pain, pyelonephritis or complicated urinary tract infection (UTI) should be considered.

When treating cystitis, community and hospital antibiograms should be reviewed. The vast majority of UTIs in the community are caused by *E coli*; the remainder is caused by other gram-negative pathogens, including *Proteus mirabilis* and *K pneumoniae*, or gram-positive *Staphylococcus saprophyticus*. Resistance patterns in communities change frequently. Following the best practices and recommendations in one's community ensures the best targeting of treatment. If a local antibiogram is not available, the IDSA guidelines can be followed (**Box 2**). These guidelines state that, in some communities, resistance is so common that community-specific resistance data really are necessary for the treatment of UTIs.

Complicated urinary tract infections

Pyelonephritis Pyelonephritis should be considered in patients with symptoms of cystitis paired with systemic symptoms of fever, malaise, and flank or back pain. Treatment should be targeted to the specific pathogen; therefore, cultures are generally advisable. As for the treatment of uncomplicated cystitis, empiric antibiotics should be chosen based on local resistance patterns.

When treating empirically, several options are available. In areas where the local resistance is less than 10%, fluoroquinolones are commonly recommended for outpatient treatment.[8] The current guidelines recommend oral ciprofloxacin, 500 mg 2 times a day for 7 days.[40] If the resistance exceeds 10% or if the patient has an intolerance or hypersensitivity to quinolones, trimethoprim-sulfamethoxazole can be used for outpatient therapy. When admission is necessary, intravenous antibiotics are recommended, typically a third-generation quinolone.

Catheter-associated urinary tract infection Catheterized patients are at risk of infection secondary to different microbes compared with typical UTIs. In general, the patient remains at risk for the typical organisms but are also at increased risk of *staphylococcus* and *streptococcal* infections given the instrumentation of the urethral tract. Unfortunately, some of the typical symptoms that concern providers for UTI may not be appreciated in patients with catheters. For example, urgency, frequency and dysuria will not be present. Therefore, one must have a high index of suspicion in a patient with a catheter and proceed systematically to reach the diagnosis.

In patients with suspected catheter associated infections, if unable to simply remove the foley and attempt a trial of void to obtain a sample, the catheter should be removed and replaced. The cultures should then be sent from the new catheter.[41] The ideal is to treat a positive urine culture. However, as frequently mentioned in this

---

Box 2
Treatment algorithm for uncomplicated UTI in otherwise healthy young females

1. Initial treatment options[a]

   a. Nitrofurantoin/monohydrate, 100 mg twice daily for 5 days

   b. Trimethoprim-sulfamethoxazole, 160/800 mg (double-strength tablet) twice daily for 3 days

2. If the patient cannot tolerate the initial treatment options or if the initial treatment failed, consider the following[b]:

   a. Fluoroquinolone

   b. β-Lactam

   c. First-generation cephalosporins

[a] Do not use in patients who might have early pyelonephritis.
[b] These options are less desirable because of the resistance they can induce and because of population effects.
Data from Gupta K, Hooton TM, Naber KG, et al. International clinical practice guidelines for the treatment of acute uncomplicated cystitis and pyelonephritis in women: a 2010 update by the Infectious Diseases Society of America and the European Society for Microbiology and Infectious Diseases. Clin Infect Dis 2011;52(5):e103–20.

review, cultures are less than ideal in the emergency department. The urine leukocyte count, presence of nitrites, and urine appearance and odor may help direct clinical suspicion.

Treatment should be targeted at the possible infecting organisms. Because chronically ill populations often have chronic indwelling catheters, the prior culture data from the patient's chart should be reviewed if available. The prevalence of the resistant organisms and fungal infections is much greater in this population, and if that prior data is available in the ED it should be used to help direct treatment.[41] Otherwise, as discussed above, treatment should focus on the organisms that are at risk for infecting the patient and be relatively broad in coverage to cover gram positive, gram negative and anearobic organisms.

Prostatitis Acute bacterial prostatitis frequently presents with concomitant UTI: hematuria, dysuria, frequency, suprabic or rectal pain, etc, however, it is extremely important to try differentiate between a simple UTI and an associated prostatitis. In general, otherwise healthy men have minimal risk for a UTI. Although acute bacterial prostatitis is uncommon, the overall prevalence of prostatitis is high and estimated at approximately 9.7% of males.[42,43] If acute bacterial prostatitis is suspected, it is imperative that emergency physicians start appropriate treatment as the incidence of recurrence with progression to chronic bacterial prostatitis is extremely high and estimated at 20–50%.[43] Initial treatment should seek to optimize clearance of the offending organism in hopes of decreasing the potential for recurrence. Duration of treatment is often four weeks, so if discharged home, the patient should have prompt primary care follow up.

As mentioned above, the prostate is an organ with relatively limited blood flow. Therefore, penetration of antibiotics can be difficult and an agent that is bactericidal should be used. The most common microbes are *E coli* (87.5%), *Pseudomonas*, *Proteus*, *Klebsiella*, and polymicrobial infections.[44] Therefore, antibiosis should target these gram negative organisms. The most highly recommended agent is levofloxacin.[42,44] It has significant gram negative coverage, is bactericidal, and is renally excreted while also withstanding the low pH of the prostate and can therefore reach desired levels in prostatic tissue (see **Table 1**). Other agents that may be considered in the setting of hypersentivity to flouroquinolones include aminoglycosides with or without a penicillin like ampicillin, or a third-generation cephalosporin with or without an aminoglycoside.[45] Patients who have been instrumented or are immunocompromised may be at risk of different organisms and should be covered more broadly to ensure sufficient coverage of gram-positive organism like *S Aureus*, including addressing the possibility of resistant organisms.

Gynecologic Infections

The presence of fever in the setting of a gynecologic infection is relatively rare; however, infection of the gynecologic tract is relatively common. Given the increasing resistance of *Neisseria gonorrhoeae*, attention to antibiotic coverage updates is important. The CDC has liberalized its recommendations regarding the treatment of pelvic inflammatory disease (PID) in an effort to improve control.

The presentation of PID can range from pelvic pain with minimal tenderness to fever, a toxic appearance, and shock. Although fever is the focus of this discussion, it is imperative to stress that pelvic pain in a young sexually active female without a clear cause should raise suspicion for PID. PID includes all infections of the upper gynecologic tract: endometritis, salpingitis, and tubo-ovarian abscess.

Treatment of PID (mild to severe) should be directed at *N gonorrhoeae*, *Chlamydia trachomatis*, and anaerobes such as *Bacteroides fragilis*. Regimens are dependent on the severity of the illness. Treatment of sexual partners is advised (**Table 6**).[46] Pregnant patients with suspected PID should be hospitalized and receive parenteral antibiotics.

SKIN AND SOFT-TISSUE INFECTIONS

The management of skin and soft-tissue infections can pose diagnostic challenges. In particular, acute infection superimposed on chronic changes associated with wounds or venous stasis might not always be easily detected.[47] Severe cases manifest with systemic signs, including fever, and should be easier to detect. Once systemic manifestations occur, intravenous antibiotics are needed; surgical treatment might also be necessary. IDSA guidelines emphasize the importance of key signs consistent with severe cases, including pain disproportionate to examination findings, violaceous bullae, cutaneous hemorrhage, skin sloughing, anesthesia, rapid progression, and gas in the tissue.[47]

Cellulitis

Cellulitis is most commonly caused by gram-positive organisms. Streptococci (most often group A β-hemolytic streptococci) and staphylococci are the most prevalent causes of soft-tissue infections in otherwise healthy individuals. The approach to distinguishing staphylococcal from streptococcal cellulitis is based on clinical findings. *S aureus* is often associated with furuncles, carbuncles, and abscesses. When cellulitis is not associated with a clear portal of entry and diffuse erythema is found, *Streptococcus* species are more likely. Blood cultures are not routinely useful.[47]

Simple cellulitis should be treated empirically with a penicillinase-resistant penicillin or a first-generation cephalosporin. Penicillin-allergic patients should be treated with clindamycin or vancomycin when inpatient treatment is required. The prevalence of community-acquired MRSA is increasing across the United States. In settings where prevalence is high, the threshold to cover should be low. Clindamycin, trimethoprim-sulfamethoxazole, and tetracyclines are effective for community-acquired MRSA. In

Table 6 Treatment of pelvic inflammatory disease (PID)	
Severity	**Regimen**
Mild PID	Ceftriaxone, 250 mg IM single dose, PLUS doxycycline, 100 mg PO BID for 14 d, PLUS metronidazole,[a] 500 mg PO BID for 14 d Alternative: ceftriaxone, 250 mg IM single dose, PLUS azithromycin, 1 g PO once a week for 2 wk, PLUS metronidazole,[a] 500 mg PO BID for 14 d
Moderate to severe PID, or with tuboovarian abscess	Cefotetan, 2 g IV every 12 h, OR cefoxitin, 2 g IV every 6 h, PLUS doxycycline, 100 mg IV every 12 h Alternative: clindamycin, 900 mg IV every 8 h, PLUS gentamicin (varied dosing recommendations)

Abbreviations: BID, twice daily; IM, intramuscular; IV, intravenous; PO, by mouth.
    [a] Metronidazole is recommended for concomitant treatment of bacterial vaginosis (a single 2-g dose of metronidazole can also be considered).
    Adapted from Centers for Disease Control and Prevention. Sexually transmitted diseases treatment guidelines, 2010: pelvic inflammatory disease. 2011. Available at: www.cdc.gov/std/treatment/2010/pid.htm. Accessed March 26, 2013.

inpatient settings, vancomycin remains the antimicrobial of choice although other options do show promise, including linezolid, daptomycin, and tigecycline.[48,49]

Necrotizing Infections

Emergency physicians should maintain a high index of suspicion for necrotizing infections. Features that should engender concern include pain out of proportion to appearance, skin necrosis, crepitus or gas detected on imaging, bullae, skin sloughing, marked edema or firmness of subcutaneous tissue extending beyond erythema, cutaneous anesthesia, rapid progression, and evidence of sepsis.[47] Necrotizing infections can develop in any patient, but those with vascular insufficiency are at heightened risk (eg, diabetics and patients with venous stasis, lymphedema, or peripheral vascular disease). Antibiotic therapy is required. Emergency surgical source control is the cornerstone of therapy.

These infections can be caused by a single organism (eg, *Streptococcus pyogenes*, *Vibrio vulnificans*, *Aeromonas hydrophila*, or MRSA), but polymicrobial infections are more common. Patients with penetrating trauma and a concomitant reduction in blood flow are at increased risk for gas gangrene, a particularly worrisome polymicrobial infection often caused by *Clostridium* species.[47]

Broad-spectrum antibiotics, covering gram-positive organisms, gram-negative organisms, aerobes, and anaerobes, are required. The current treatment recommendation for mixed infections indicates penicillin with β-lactamase inhibition combined with clindamycin and ciprofloxacin.

Fournier gangrene should be considered in patients with perineal cellulitis/necrotizing fasciitis, with perianal or complex UTI, or with a history of trauma that may have allowed the entry of bacteria into the genital fascial planes.[47] Aggressive intravenous administration of antibiotics, specifically covering *Pseudomonas*, is required. Debridement is the definitive treatment.

SUMMARY

The choice and timing of antimicrobial therapy are challenging for the acute care physician. The resistance that antimicrobials have developed to certain pathogens has changed the emergency physician's approach to patients and the process by which priorities are determined. The role of emergency physicians as stewards of health care resources is growing. In all cases, an organized approach to evaluation, diagnosis, and treatment is helpful. Using antimicrobials rationally means ensuring that the right treatments are available to the right people at the right time and in the right place.

REFERENCES

1. Centers for Disease Control, National Center for Health Statistics. National Hospital Ambulatory Medical Care Survey: 2009 emergency department summary tables. Available at: www.cdc.gov/nchs/data/ahcd/nhamcs_emergency/2009_ed_web_tables.pdf. Accessed March 25, 2013.
2. Pines JM. Timing of antibiotics for acute severe infections. Emerg Med Clin North Am 2008;26:245–57.
3. The Joint Commission for the Accreditation of Hospitals and Organization. Specifications manual for national hospital inpatient quality measures. Available at: www.jointcommission.org/specifications_manual_for_national_hospital_inpatient_quality_measures.aspx. Accessed March 25, 2013.

4. Kumar A, Haery C, Paladuga B, et al. The duration of hypotension before the initiation of antibiotic treatment is a critical determinant of survival in a murine model of *Escherichia coli* septic shock: association with serum lactate and inflammatory cytokine levels. J Infect Dis 2006;193:51–8.

5. Rivers E, Nguyen B, Havstad S, et al. Early goal-directed therapy in the treatment of severe sepsis and septic shock. N Engl J Med 2001;345:1368–77.

6. Faieski D, Mikkelsen M, Band R, et al. Impact of time to antibiotics on survival in patients with severe sepsis or septic shock in whom early goal-directed therapy was initiated in the emergency department. Crit Care Med 2010; 38(4):1045–53.

7. Dillinger P, Levy M, Rhodes A, et al. Surviving Sepsis Campaign: international guidelines for management of severe sepsis and septic shock: 2012. Crit Care Med 2013;41(2):580–637.

8. Deresinski S. Principles of antibiotic therapy in severe infections: optimizing the therapeutic approach by use of laboratory and clinical data. Clin Infect Dis 2007;45(Suppl 3):S177–83.

9. Sharma S, Kumar A. Antimicrobial management of sepsis and septic shock. Clin Chest Med 2008;29:677–87.

10. Hoang KD, Pollack CV. Antibiotic use in the emergency department, IV: single-dose therapy and parenteral-loading dose therapy. J Emerg Med 1996;14(5): 619–28.

11. Hart Research Associates and Public Opinion Strategies. Americans' knowledge of and attitudes toward antibiotic resistance: a report of findings from a national survey and two focus groups. Available at: www.pewhealth.org/uploadedFiles/PHG/Content_Level_Pages/In_the_News/abx-poll-summary.pdf. Accessed March 25, 2013.

12. Painter K. Southeast paying health price for high antibiotic use. USA Today; 2012. Available at: http://www.usatoday.com/story/news/nation/2012/11/12/antibiotic-resistance-infections-southeast-pew-survey/1699953/. Accessed August 19, 2013.

13. Pew Health Group. The superbug threat: as drug-resistant bacteria spread, the pipeline for new antibiotics is drying up. Available at: http://www.pewhealth.org/reports-analysis/issue-briefs/the-superbug-threat-85899374353. Accessed April 5, 2013.

14. Centers for Disease Control. World Health Day: media fact sheet: antimicrobial resistance: no action today, no cure tomorrow. Available at: www.cdc.gov/media/releases/2011/f0407_antimicrobialresistance.pdf. Accessed March 25, 2013.

15. Pew Health Group. The superbug threat: the emergence of antibiotic-resistant bacteria and its impact on human health. Available at: http://www.pewhealth.org/uploadedFiles/PHG/Supporting_Items/FactSheet_Threat.pdf. Accessed April 5, 2013.

16. Centers for Disease Control and Prevention. Antibiotic/antimicrobial resistance: diseases/pathogens associated with antimicrobial resistance. July 19, 2010. Available at: www.cdc.gov/drugresistance/DiseasesConnectedAR.html. Accessed March 26, 2013.

17. Proulx N, Frechette D, Toye B, et al. Delays in the administration of antibiotics are associated with mortality from adult acute bacterial meningitis. QJM 2005;98(4): 291–8.

18. Van de Beek D, de Gans J, Spanjaard L, et al. Clinical features and prognostic factors in adults with bacterial meningitis. N Engl J Med 2004;351(8):1849–59.

19. Tunkel AR, Hartman BJ, Kaplan SL, et al. Practice guidelines for the management of bacterial meningitis. Clin Infect Dis 2004;39:1267–84.
20. Bonadio WA. The cerebrospinal fluid: physiologic aspects and alterations associated with bacterial meningitis. Pediatr Infect Dis J 1992;11(6):423–31.
21. Short WR, Tunkel AR. Timing of administration of antimicrobial therapy in bacterial meningitis. Curr Infect Dis Rep 2001;3(4):360–4.
22. Hickner JM, Bartlett JG, Besser RE, et al. Principles of appropriate antibiotic use for acute rhinosinusitis in adults: background. Ann Emerg Med 2001;37(6):703–10.
23. Chow AW, Benninger MS, Brook I, et al. IDSA clinical practice guideline for acute bacterial rhinosinusitis in children and adults. Clin Infect Dis 2012;54:e72–112.
24. Cooper RJ, Hoffman JR, Bartlett JG, et al. Principles of appropriate antibiotic use for acute pharyngitis in adults: background. Ann Emerg Med 2001;37(6):711–9.
25. Braman SS. Chronic cough due to acute bronchitis: ACCP evidence-based clinical practice guidelines. Chest 2006;129(1S):95S–103S.
26. Gozales R, Bartlett JG, Besser RE, et al. Principles of appropriate antibiotic use for treatment of uncomplicated acute bronchitis: background. Ann Emerg Med 2001;37(6):720–7.
27. Centers for Disease Control and Prevention. influenza antiviral medications: summary for clinicians: current for the 2012-2013 influenza season. Available at: www.cdc.gov/flu/pdf/professionals/antivirals/antiviral-summary-clinicians.pdf. Accessed March 25, 2013.
28. Heron M. Deaths: leading causes for 2009. Natl Vital Stat Rep 2012;61(7):1–95.
29. The Joint Commission for the Accreditation of Hospitals and Organization. Comprehensive Review of Development and Testing for National Implementation of Hospital Core Measures, November 3, 2010.
30. Plouffe JF, Martin DR. Pneumonia in the emergency department. Emerg Med Clin North Am 2008;26(2):389–411.
31. Fine MJ, Auble TE, Yealy DM, et al. A prediction rule to identify low-risk patients with community-acquired pneumonia. N Engl J Med 1997;336:243–50.
32. Ebell MH. Outpatient vs inpatient treatment of community acquired pneumonia. Fam Pract Manag 2006;13(4):41–4.
33. Mandell LA, Wunderink RG, Anzueto A, et al. Infectious Diseases Society of America/American Thoracic Society consensus guidelines on the management of community-acquired pneumonia in adults. Clin Infect Dis 2007;44(S2):S27–72.
34. American Thoracic Society, Infectious Diseases Society of America. Guidelines for the management of adults with hospital-acquired, ventilator-associated, and healthcare-associated pneumonia. Am J Respir Crit Care Med 2005;171:388–416.
35. Centers for Disease Control and Prevention. Tuberculosis: TB in specific populations. Available at: www.cdc.gov/tb/topic/populations/default.htm. Accessed March 25, 2013.
36. American Thoracic Society, CDC, Infectious Diseases Society of America. Treatment of tuberculosis. MMWR Recomm Rep 2003;52(RR11):1–77.
37. Baddour LM, Wilson WR, Bayer AS, et al. Infective endocarditis: diagnosis, antimicrobial therapy, and management of complications. Circulation 2005;111:e394–433.
38. Solomkin JS, Mazuski JE, Bradley JS, et al. Diagnosis and management of complicated intra-abdominal infection in adults and children: guidelines by the Surgical Infection Society and the Infection Diseases Society of America. Clin Infect Dis 2010;50:133–64.

39. Guerrant RL, Van Gilder T, Steiner TS, et al. Practice guidelines for the management of infectious diarrhea. Clin Infect Dis 2001;32:331–50.
40. Gupta K, Hooton TM, Naber KG, et al. International clinical practice guidelines for the treatment of acute uncomplicated cystitis and pyelonephritis in women: a 2010 update by the Infectious Diseases Society of America and the European Society for Microbiology and Infectious Diseases. Clin Infect Dis 2011;52(5): e103–20.
41. Hooton TM, Bradley SF, Cardenas DD, et al. Diagnosis, prevention, and treatment of catheter-associated urinary tract infection in adults: 2009 International Clinical Practice Guidelines from the Infectious Diseases Society of America. Clin Infect Dis 2010;50:625–63.
42. Lummus WE, Thompson I. Genitourinary emergencies: prostatitis. Emerg Med Clin North Am 2001;19(3):691–707.
43. Nickel JC. Special report on prostatitis: state of the art. Rev Urol 2001;3(2):94–8.
44. Ramakrishnan K, Salinas RC. Prostatitis: acute and chronic. Prim Care 2010;37: 547–63.
45. Grabe M, Bishop MC, Bjerklund-Johansen TE, et al. Guidelines on urological infections. European Association Urology 2009;1–109. Available at: www.uroweb. org/fileadmin/tx_eauguidelines/2009/Full/Urological_Infections.pdf. Accessed March 27, 2013.
46. Centers for Disease Control and Prevention. Sexually transmitted diseases treatment guidelines, 2010: pelvic inflammatory disease. Last updated January 28, 2011. Available at: www.cdc.gov/std/treatment/2010/pid.htm. Accessed March 26, 2013.
47. Stevens DL, Bisno AL, Chambers HF, et al. Practice guidelines for the diagnosis and management of skin and soft-tissue infections. Clin Infect Dis 2005;41: 1373–406.
48. Stryjewski ME, Chambers HF. Skin and soft tissue infections causes by community-acquired methicillin-resistant *Staphylococcus aureus*. Clin Infect Dis 2008;46(S5):S368–77.
49. Ellis MW, Lewis JS. Treatment approaches for community-acquired methicillin-resistant *Staphylococcus aureus* infections. Curr Opin Infect Dis 2005;18: 496–501.

Endocrine Causes of Dangerous Fever

Andrea G. Tenner, MD, MPH[a],*, Karin M. Halvorson, MD[b]

KEYWORDS

- Fever • Hyperthermia • Endocrine • Hyperthyroidism • Thyroiditis • Thyroid storm
- Adrenal insufficiency • Pheochromocytoma

KEY POINTS

- Fever in endocrinopathies is often multifactorial and is poorly understood.
- Thyroid storm is a true emergency that often presents with fever, and primarily is a clinical diagnosis.
- If a febrile patient has hypotension that is unresponsive to fluids and vasopressors, adrenal insufficiency should be considered and steroids should be given empirically.
- Pheochromocytoma can cause a wide variety of clinical syndromes including pheochromocytoma multisystem crisis, which is defined by fever, multisystem organ failure, and vascular lability, and is associated with a high mortality rate.

Because most patients presenting to emergency departments (EDs) with fever have an underlying infection, noninfectious causes of elevated body temperatures are often overlooked. However, life-threatening endocrinopathies also can cause hyperthermia. The purpose of this article is to provide an overview of serious endocrine derangements that can present with a febrile syndrome.

Fever, in the traditional sense, occurs when the "set point" of the hypothalamic thermoregulatory center is raised, causing the regulatory functions of the hypothalamus to maintain a higher core temperature. Endocrinopathies generally do not change the hypothalamic set point. Rather, they tend to cause hyperthermia, an elevated body temperature that overwhelms the body's regulatory mechanisms. The distinction between Fever and hyperthermia is usually not clinically relevant in the ED. It is difficult to differentiate fever from hyperthermia during a typical ED assessment, but the distinction could explain some of the clinical manifestations and assist in the formulation of

The authors have no funding sources or conflicts of interest to disclose.
[a] Department of Emergency Medicine, University of Maryland, 110 South Paca Street, 6th Floor, Suite 200, Baltimore, MD 21201, USA; [b] Department of Pulmonary & Critical Care, Brown University, 593 Eddy Street, Providence, RI 02903, USA
* Corresponding author.
E-mail address: atenner@umem.org

treatment plans. Because the hypothalamic set point is not elevated in hyperthermia, patients exhibit signs associated with the body's attempt to decrease temperature, such as sweating, flushing, and tachypnea.[1] In general, hyperthermia does not respond to antipyretics but fever often will.[1] Conversely, some endocrinopathies cause secretion of cytokines, which can elevate the hypothalamic set point and cause true fever. In patients with endocrine dysfunction that induces the release of pyrogens (ie, cytokines, interleukin), the resulting fever can be indistinguishable from the fever that accompanies acute infection; however, the hyperthermia/fever syndrome is often multifactorial and therefore the fever still might not respond to antipyretics.[2] Because the distinction between an elevated set point (fever) and elevated temperature from other causes (hyperthermia) is unlikely to be made in the acute care setting, and most hyperthermia is called "fever" in the ED as well as in the literature, the terms are used interchangeably in this article.

Thyrotoxicosis (specifically thyroid storm), adrenal insufficiency, and pheochromocytoma constitute the primary endocrine causes of dangerous fever. Other less acute endocrine causes of febrile syndromes exist, but this article focuses on those that must be identified and treated acutely to avoid serious morbidity and mortality. The action of thyroid hormone on adenosine triphosphatase (ATPase) in the sodium/potassium pump of plasma membranes in the normal state contributes the majority of basal heat production. When abnormal amounts of thyroid hormone are present, the hypermetabolic state (caused partly by an increase in pump activity) that ensues can cause hyperthermia. Often the body's mechanisms to diffuse excess heat (primarily sweating and peripheral vasodilation) suffice to maintain a near-normal body temperature; however, these mechanisms can be overwhelmed.[3]

The pathophysiology of elevated body temperature resulting from adrenal insufficiency and pheochromocytoma is not as well understood. The mechanism by which adrenal insufficiency causes hyperthermia is not well known.[3] Patients with adrenal insufficiency have increased susceptibility to infection and can have fevers caused by infectious processes. However, these patients can also have fevers unrelated to infection, which resolve only with appropriate steroid treatment.[3–5] Pheochromocytoma is generally believed to cause hyperthermia because an excess of catecholamines increases metabolism and heat production, combined with generalized vasoconstriction that prohibits the heat from being dissipated into the environment.[3]

Patients with all 3 of these conditions (thyrotoxicosis, adrenal insufficiency, and pheochromocytoma) can present acutely to the ED in extremis with a nonspecific febrile illness. The astute clinician must be aware of these noninfectious causes of febrile illness and their presentations as all 3 of them, if left untreated, can be rapidly fatal. The causes, clinical presentations, diagnosis, and management of the febrile patient with thyroid storm, adrenal insufficiency, and pheochromocytoma are described herein.

THYROID CAUSES OF FEVER
Etiology and Pathophysiology

Thyrotoxicosis is caused by dysregulation of the feedback loops between the hypothalamus, pituitary gland, thyroid gland, and peripheral circulating thyroid hormone. In homeostatic states, thyrotropin-releasing hormone (TRH) from the hypothalamus regulates the release of thyroid-stimulating hormone (TSH) from the anterior pituitary gland. TSH regulates the synthesis and release of thyroid hormone from the thyroid gland. Thyroid hormone then is able to act on various organ systems. Free triiodothyronine (T_3) and free L-thyroxine (T_4) also participate in a negative feedback loop on the anterior pituitary to ensure a steady state of secretion of thyroid hormone (**Fig. 1**).[6]

The actions of thyroid hormones are varied. T_3 is the most biologically active of the thyroid hormones, and T_4 is secreted from the thyroid in the largest amounts. Peripherally, T_4 is converted to T_3 via 5'-iodinase. T_3 is involved in growth, maturation of the central nervous system, regulation of the basal metabolic rate (BMR), metabolism, and modification of cardiac output. One of the main actions of T_3 is to increase the activity of ATPase. Through this upregulation, thyroid hormones increase oxygen consumption, BMR, and heat production (**Fig. 2**).[6]

The most common endocrine diseases are those associated with thyroid dysfunction. The hyperthyroid state causes derangements in temperature regulation and eventual hyperpyrexia (**Box 1**).

Although hyperthermia can occur with hyperthyroid states (states of excessive thyroid gland function), dangerous febrile syndromes occur primarily with thyrotoxicosis (a state of thyroid-hormone excess that may or may not be related to increased gland function). Thyrotoxicosis is caused mainly by primary hyperthyroidism (increased production/secretion of thyroid hormone from the gland independent of TSH [most commonly Graves disease]) and secondary hyperthyroidism (increased stimulation of the thyroid by TSH or other substances produced by the pituitary). It can also be induced by thyroiditis, exogenous intake of thyroid hormone, and other causes of acute inflammation of the thyroid gland.[7]

Graves disease is the most common cause of primary hyperthyroidism and is the culprit in 60% to 80% of cases of thyrotoxicosis. Biologically active autoantibodies mimic TSH in this disease. These autoantibodies stimulate the thyroid gland to release thyroid hormone.[7] Thyroid nodules are another form of primary hyperthyroidism that can cause thyrotoxicosis. In patients with long-standing nodules within the thyroid, autonomous nodules that can secrete excess thyroid hormone also emerge. Toxic nodular goiter is a hyperfunctioning autonomous follicular adenoma that, again, secretes excess hormone.[8,9]

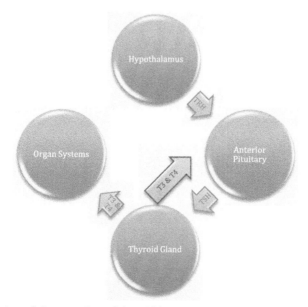

Fig. 1. Regulation of the secretion of thyroid hormone.

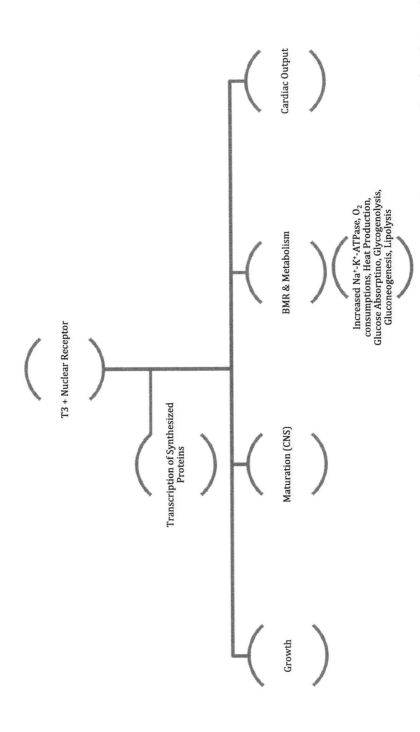

Fig. 2. Action of thyroid hormone. ATPase, adenosine triphosphatase; BMR, basal metabolic rate; CNS, central nervous system. (*Data from* Costanzo L. Physiology. 4th edition. Oxford (United Kingdom): Elsevier Ltd; 2010.)

Box 1
Causes of thyrotoxicosis

Primary Hyperthyroidism

- Graves disease
- Toxic multinodular goiter
- Toxic adenoma
- Thyroiditis
- Thyroid cancer

Secondary Hyperthyroidism

- Pituitary adenoma
- Thyroid hormone resistance syndrome

Thyrotoxicosis Without Thyroid Dysfunction

- Factitious thyroid ingestion
- Amiodarone
- Lithium
- Radiation

Data from Bahn RS, Burch HB, Cooper DS, et al. Hyperthyroidism and other causes of thyrotoxicosis: management guidelines of the American Thyroid Association and American Association of Clinical Endocrinologists. Endocr Pract 2011;17:456–520; and Ingbar SH. Classification of the causes of thyrotoxicosis. In: Ingbar SH, Braverman LE, editors. The thyroid. Philadelphia: Lippincott; 1986. p. 809.

TSH-secreting pituitary adenomas (secondary hyperthyroidism) are rare causes of thyrotoxicosis. In the absence of Graves disease, the predominant causes of thyrotoxicosis are thyroiditis and exogenous thyroid hormone, or excess iodine intake. Hyperthyroidism (excessive thyroid function, as described earlier) is absent in these cases. The clinical symptoms are caused by direct action of the thyroid hormone (see later discussion), with no increased function in the gland. In thyroiditis, the thyroid gland is being damaged and stored hormone is released prematurely. Active production of thyroid hormone does not increase, but the end organs see higher levels of thyroid hormone when hormone that would normally be stored is released. Similarly, with exogenous ingestion of thyroid hormone, the gland is producing the same or smaller amounts of hormones, but the rest of the body sees higher levels of thyroid hormone.[7] With ingestion of iodine, maximal hormone production is achieved with normal gland function, leading to excess thyroid hormone.[7,10]

Many of these cases are not acute emergencies but should be on the differential for the ED physician. However, life-threatening thyroid storm can arise from any of these causes of thyroid dysfunction, so the recognition, diagnosis, and treatment of storm must be in the ED physician's repertoire.

Clinical Features

The clinical features of thyrotoxicosis, regardless of its cause, are similar (**Box 2**). Patients usually have warm, moist skin, and complain of sweating and heat intolerance (generally related to their increased metabolic rate and heat production in the absence of a change in the hypothalamic set point). Other signs of thyroid disease

---

Box 2
Clinical features of thyrotoxicosis

- Fever
- Heat intolerance
- Sweating
- Tremor
- Palpitations
- Nervousness
- Fatigue
- Weight loss
- Hyperdefecation
- Tachycardia
- Wide pulse pressure with increased systolic blood pressure
- Ophthalmopathy
- Lid retraction
- Hyperreflexia
- Increased cardiac output

Data from Bahn RS, Burch HB, Cooper DS, et al. Hyperthyroidism and other causes of thyrotoxicosis: management guidelines of the American Thyroid Association and American Association of Clinical Endocrinologists. Endocr Pract 2011;17:456–520; and Ingbar SH. Classification of the causes of thyrotoxicosis. In: Ingbar SH, Braverman LE, editors. The thyroid. Philadelphia: Lippincott; 1986. p. 809.

---

include unexplained weight loss (despite increased appetite, resulting from increased metabolic rate) or weight gain (this occurs in 5% of patients because of increased food consumption). Lid retraction that leads to a "staring" appearance can occur in any form of thyrotoxicosis, but Graves disease causes a specific type of ophthalmopathy that enlarges the extraocular muscles, possibly leading to proptosis (exophthalmos). Exophthalmos can be detected by observing a rim of sclera between the lower border of the iris and the eyelid when the patient is looking directly forward.[7]

The most dreaded manifestation of thyrotoxicosis is thyroid storm, a medical emergency that requires timely identification and specific intervention. Many factors can precipitate thyroid storm, including infection, surgery, stroke, myocardial infarction, pulmonary embolism, and even palpation of the thyroid. Patients with thyroid storm may experience pyrexia (often with temperatures >40°C [104°F]) and delirium that may lead to coma. Patients can have such high metabolic rates that they develop high-output cardiac failure. Thyroid storm, however, is not a separate entity in and of itself, but rather occurs at the far end of the spectrum of thyrotoxicosis.[11] This scenario can present some difficulty in identifying patients who are suffering an immediately life-threatening storm versus those who have severe thyrotoxicosis and need to be treated urgently. Four main features characterize thyroid storm: fever; sinus tachycardia or supraventricular arrhythmias, with or without heart failure; central nervous system dysfunction such as agitation, psychosis, or seizures; and gastrointestinal dysfunction such as diarrhea, vomiting, or jaundice.[11,12]

Diagnosis

Thyroid storm is often diagnosed based on clinical features alone, because it often takes considerable time for the confirmatory laboratory test results to return. The Burch-Wartofsky score[12] was developed to evaluate patients for thyroid storm (**Table 1**). A cumulative score of greater than 45 is highly suggestive of thyroid storm,

Table 1 Burch-Wartofsky score	
Parameters	**Scoring System**
Thermoregulatory Dysfunction Oral temperature (°F)	
99–99.9	5
100–100.9	10
101–101.9	15
102–102.9	20
103–103.9	25
≥104	30
Cardiovascular Dysfunction	
Tachycardia	
99–109	5
110–119	10
120–129	15
130–139	20
≥140	25
Congestive Heart Failure	
Absent	0
Mild (pedal edema)	5
Moderate (bibasilar rales)	10
Severe (pulmonary edema)	15
Atrial fibrillation	
Absent	0
Present	10
Central Nervous System Dysfunction	
Absent	0
Mild (agitation)	10
Moderate (delirium, psychosis, extreme lethargy)	20
Severe (seizures, coma)	30
Gastrointestinal/Hepatic Dysfunction	
Absent	0
Moderate (diarrhea, nausea/vomiting, abdominal pain)	10
Severe (unexplained jaundice)	20
Precipitating Event	
Absent	0
Present	10

Data from Refs.[10–12]

a score of 25 to 44 suggests "impending storm," and a score of less than 25 is unlikely to be thyroid storm.[8,11–20]

In general, thyrotoxicosis can be diagnosed via low levels of TSH and high levels of T_3 and T_4. The diagnosis of thyroid storm, as a spectrum of thyrotoxicosis, is supported by these laboratory values, but the diagnosis of storm itself, as already stated, is based on clinical findings. Laboratory test results are usually not available in time for the ED diagnosis, but the results should be forwarded to the clinicians who are taking care of these patients after they have been treated for the acute crisis and have been admitted to the hospital (**Fig. 3**).[8,11,21]

Treatment

The mortality rate for thyroid storm is high, ranging from 20% to 30%. Thus, patients presenting with thyroid storm must be managed aggressively in the ED and the intensive care unit (ICU). Treatment of thyroid storm is aimed at reversing complications of elevated levels of thyroid hormone, treating the precipitating underlying condition, and lowering circulating levels of T_3 and T_4, thus blocking the peripheral effects of these hormones. Initiation of β-adrenergic blockade helps to decrease the cardiac symptoms of thyrotoxicosis. Propranolol has the theoretical added benefit of blocking peripheral T_4-to-T_3 conversion, making it the drug of choice for β-blockade. Supportive care is important as well, and treatment of the fever, associated fluid losses, and underlying cause are essential. Cooling blankets might be necessary, and administration of acetaminophen can be attempted (although it has variable efficacy, depending on

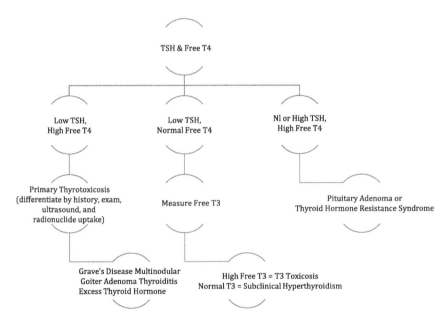

Fig. 3. Diagnostic evaluation of thyrotoxicosis. Nl, normal; T3, triiodothyronine; T4, L-thyroxine; TSH, thyroid-stimulating hormone. (*Data from* Bahn RS, Burch HB, Cooper DS, et al. Hyperthyroidism and other causes of thyrotoxicosis: management guidelines of the American Thyroid Association and American Association of Clinical Endocrinologists. Endocr Pract 2011;17:456–520; and Ingbar SG, Freinkel N. Simultaneous estimation of rates of thyroxine degradation and thyroid hormone synthesis. J Clin Invest 1955;34:808–19.)

the patient's mechanism of hyperthermia). Salicylates should be avoided, as they can cause an increase in levels of free thyroid hormone. Intravenous fluids with dextrose should be given to replenish glycogen stores. Infection is thought to be the most common underlying cause of thyroid storm; therefore, infectious causes must be sought aggressively and ruled out, and the clinician should maintain a low threshold for starting antibiotics if indicated.[10,11]

Levels of circulating thyroid hormone can be decreased by propylthiouracil (PTU) or methimazole, which both inhibit hormone synthesis. PTU is theorized to have the additional effect of inhibiting peripheral conversion of T_4 to T_3, and thus is generally regarded as the treatment of choice for acute medical care. Glucocorticoids have been used as adjunctive medications because they decrease peripheral conversion of T_4 to T_3 and treat possible relative adrenal insufficiency (see later discussion).[10] Iodine therapy augments the effects of PTU and methimazole by blocking the release of hormone from the thyroid gland; however, iodine given before PTU or methimazole can actually induce production of thyroid hormone. Both PTU and methimazole take approximately 1 hour to begin to block synthesis; therefore, iodine therapy should not be given any earlier than 60 minutes after the dose of synthetic blockade has been given (**Box 3**).[10]

Box 3
Treatment of thyrotoxicosis

Decrease thyroid hormone synthesis

- PTU, 600 to 1000 mg PO loading dose, then 200 to 250 mg PO every 4 hours[8,22]
- Alternative: methimazole, 40 mg PO loading dose, then 25 mg PO every 4 hours[22]

Corticosteroids

- Hydrocortisone, 300 mg load, then 100 mg IV every 8 hours[8]
- Alternative: dexamethasone, 2 mg IV every 6 hours[22]

β-Blockade[22]

- Propranolol, 1 to 2 mg IV every 10 to 15 minutes PRN (up to 480 mg/d)
- Alternatives include esmolol drip (500 μg/kg bolus, then 50–200 μg/kg/min)

Prevent release of hormone (wait at least 1 hour after antithyroid drugs)[22]

- Iodine: iapanoic acid, 1 g IV every 8 hours for 24 hours, then 500 mg IV BID, or potassium iodide, 5 drops PO every 6 hours, or Lugol solution, 8 to 10 drops PO every 6 hours
- Alternative: lithium carbonate, 300 mg PO every 6 hours (1200 mg/d PO)

Supportive care[8,10,11,22]

- IV fluids with dextrose
- Supplemental O_2 (or airway protection if mental status is severely deranged)
- Close telemetry monitoring

Consider antipyretic therapies[10,11,22]

- Cooling blanket
- Acetaminophen, 650 mg PO every 4 hours

Abbreviations: BID, twice daily; IV, intravenous; PO, by mouth; PRN, as needed; PTU, propylthiouracil.

ADRENAL CAUSES OF FEVER
Etiology and Pathophysiology

Normal cortisol production relies on a tightly regulated feedback loop. Stress and normal circadian rhythms stimulate the hypothalamus to release corticotropin-releasing hormone (CRH) which, in turn, stimulates the production of adrenocorticotropic hormone (ACTH or corticotropin) in the anterior pituitary. ACTH then travels to the adrenal gland to stimulate cortisol production. Cortisol feeds back on the anterior pituitary and hypothalamus, regulating CRH and ACTH.[23] Cortisol has several direct physiologic effects. First, it increases levels of blood glucose and improves glucose delivery to cells during stress. Second, it is essential for the normal response of cardiovascular tissues to catecholamines and angiotensin II. Finally, cortisol decreases responsiveness to nitric oxide, limiting vasodilation. In addition, cortisol has important anti-inflammatory properties, exerting at least some effect on virtually all cells that participate in the inflammatory process through inhibition of cytokines, chemokines, complement, and other inflammatory mediators, and stimulation of anti-inflammatory factors.[24]

Mineralocorticoids are produced via the renin-angiotensin-aldosterone system (RAAS), which is regulated primarily by renal production of renin. Renin release results in the cleavage of angiotensin I, which is then converted to angiotensin II. Angiotensin II activates the angiotensin II receptor type 1 (AT1 receptor), causing aldosterone to be produced. Aldosterone increases sodium retention by the kidneys (and therefore increases potassium excretion), resulting in expansion of blood volume. This feedback loop is controlled primarily by effects of aldosterone and AT1 receptor on renal perfusion pressure.

Adrenal insufficiency can be divided into primary and secondary insufficiency. Primary adrenal insufficiency (Addison disease), or the inability of adrenal glands to produce cortisol, is the most common cause of decreased cortisol production.[23,25] ACTH and angiotensin II are produced normally; however, the adrenal gland is unable to respond. Thus, aldosterone levels are low (causing renal sodium losses and retention of potassium) and, more importantly, circulating levels of cortisol are inadequate to respond to stress.[23] The decreased cortisol levels can cause life-threatening hypotension and hypoglycemia as well as impaired immune function.[23] The major cause of primary adrenal insufficiency in the developed world is autoimmune adrenalitis, but it can also be caused by tuberculosis, the human immunodeficiency virus, and fungal infections (more commonly seen in low-income and middle-income countries).[23,25]

Suppressed ACTH production manifests as secondary adrenal insufficiency and, because of exogenous steroid use and withdrawal, has become the most common form of adrenal insufficiency. The remaining cases are caused by tumors of the pituitary or hypothalamus, or tumor treatment by surgery or radiation.[23] Because, by definition, secondary adrenal insufficiency derives from lesions above the adrenal gland, this entity can be differentiated from primary adrenal insufficiency by intact mineralocorticoid production.[23]

Clinical Manifestations

Signs of life-threatening adrenal crisis are listed in **Box 4**. Many of these signs and symptoms are very similar to those of other shock states, making them difficult to differentiate. Signs of preexisting primary adrenal insufficiency are chronic skin hyperpigmentation (due to ACTH excess)[25] or, conversely, paleness in secondary adrenal insufficiency (due to lack of ACTH secretion).[23] However, patients with cushingoid features can still have adrenal crisis in response to abrupt withdrawal

---

Box 4
Clinical manifestations, diagnosis, and treatment of adrenal crisis

Clinical features

- Orthostatic hypotension
- Confusion/agitation
- Fever
- Abdominal pain
- Myalgia/joint pain
- Nausea/vomiting/diarrhea
- Circulatory collapse poorly responsive to intravenous fluids or vasopressors
- Hyponatremia
- Hypoglycemia
- Hyperkalemia
- Eosinophilia, lymphocytosis, anemia
- Hyperpigmentation/pallor

Diagnosis

- Hypotension poorly responsive to fluids and vasopressors
- Adjuncts
  - Cosyntropin stimulation test
  - Depressed random cortisol level

Acute treatment

- Hydrocortisone, 100 mg every 8 hours (alternative: hydrocortisone, 50 mg every 6 hours)
- Treat any underlying infection or the precipitating cause of the adrenal crisis if known

Data from Refs.[23–25]

(or insufficient stress dose) of replacement steroids. Patients with chronic adrenal insufficiency can have symptoms of disruption of other axes as well (eg, hypothyroidism, hypogonadism). The classic signs of hyponatremia and hyperkalemia occur only in association with primary adrenal insufficiency (due to the loss of mineralocorticoid production as well as glucocorticoid). Thus they are helpful if present, but their absence does not exclude adrenal insufficiency. Patients with secondary adrenal insufficiency tend to present with fatigue, myalgia or joint pain, fever, low blood pressure, mild hyponatremia (without hyperkalemia, owing to loss of feedback inhibition of release of antidiuretic hormone, causing a mild syndrome of inappropriate antidiuretic hormone secretion [SIADH]), and hypoglycemia. Those with primary adrenal insufficiency tend to present with the same symptoms of glucocorticoid deficiency as in secondary adrenal insufficiency, but with more abdominal pain, nausea/vomiting, hyperpigmentation, and hyperkalemia, and more prominent dizziness and postural hypotension.[23]

Diagnosis

Diagnosis of acute adrenal insufficiency can be challenging and is much disputed. The 2 most commonly used methods are measurement of a random cortisol level[24] and the cosyntropin stimulation test.[23–25] Both tests are based on a predicted increase in cortisol levels with stress.

The traditional test of choice to evaluate the body's ability to produce ACTH is the cosyntropin stimulation test (**Box 5**). Inadequate secretion of ACTH, or an inadequate response to it, is indicated in critically ill patients with a baseline cortisol level of less than 10 µg/dL and in those who fail to achieve an increase of at least 9 µg/dL sampled 30 to 60 minutes after cosyntropin administration.[26,27] For the random cortisol level, some investigators suggest that a level lower than 25 µg/dL in a critically ill patient indicates adrenal insufficiency. Patients with normal cortisol release should be able to mount a response to at least this level.[24]

Both of these tests have drawbacks, and experts still debate which one to use.[23–25] The random cortisol level could be affected by the normal diurnal rhythm, and some patients could have adequate baseline levels but fail to mount a response to stress. Also, the test measures total cortisol; tests that measure free cortisol (which is biologically active, dependent on protein binding, and difficult to predict in acute illness) are not widely available.[27] Proponents of random cortisol measurements argue that the diurnal variation is lost in critical illness, and that any patient with an intact stress response mechanism should at least mount a response of 25 µg/dL to the stress of illness alone.[24] The cosyntropin stimulation test also has some drawbacks in that it takes at least 30 to 60 minutes to perform and requires several blood draws. In addition, some experts believe that if the initial cortisol level in a seriously ill patient is less than 25 µg/dL no further studies are needed, and that patients who have severe physiologic stress and an elevated cortisol level could be responding adequately but are at the upper limit of what the adrenals are able to produce. Therefore, a change of in the cortisol level less than 9 µg/dL does not necessarily mean that the response is inadequate.[24]

Realistically, administration of fluids and vasopressors should be initiated for critically ill hypotensive patients. If the hypotension remains unresponsive to this treatment, adrenal insufficiency should be suspected and treated with moderate-dose hydrocortisone therapy. There is evidence of improved outcomes in patients with septic shock with the use of moderate-dose steroids in both nonresponders and responders to cosyntropin stimulation. However, recommendations still include determining the pretreatment cortisol level and obtaining cosyntropin stimulation

---

Box 5
Cosyntropin stimulation test

Procedure

1. Measure baseline cortisol level.

2. Immediately after blood draw, administer 250 µg of synthetic corticotropin (cosyntropin) intravenously.

3. Measure cortisol level 30 minutes after cosyntropin administration.

4. Measure cortisol level 60 minutes after cosyntropin administration if the cortisol level is lower than 20 µg/dL or the cortisol level has not changed more than 9 µg/dL.

Results

- If the cortisol level is lower than 20 µg/dL 30 to 60 minutes after cosyntropin administration or the change in cortisol levels is less than 9 µg/dL, the likelihood of adrenal insufficiency is high.

Data from Marik PE, Zaloga GP. Adrenal Insufficiency in the critically ill: a new look at an old problem. Chest 2002;122:1784–96.

testing, if possible, to help the inpatient team with subsequent management of the patient. If the patient is in extremis and the result is lower than 25 μg/dL, or the cosyntropin stimulation test shows an increase of less than 9 μg/dL, the diagnosis of adrenal insufficiency is supported.

Treatment

The treatment of acute adrenal crisis is summarized in **Box 4**. Hydrocortisone is the treatment of choice.[23–25] The recommended dose of 200 to 300 μg/d (100 μg every 8 hours [most commonly] or 50 μg every 6 hours) is based on an approximation of the maximal daily cortisone secretion under stress.[27,28] For patients with chronic renal insufficiency, the baseline dose of chronic steroids is often based on clinical judgment.[28,29] This point is important to remember because even patients on replacement can be underdosed (even if they take additional steroids during periods of stress). If they present in crisis, it is always better to err on the side of giving higher-dose steroids.

It is not necessary to replace mineralocorticoids acutely in adrenal crisis because hydrocortisone doses of greater than 50 mg provide sufficient mineralocorticoid activity. Of the glucocorticoids, only hydrocortisone and cortisone have effective mineralocorticoid activity, and they must be used at high doses for this benefit to be seen. However, patients on baseline replacement doses need mineralocorticoid supplementation. Methylprednisolone has only minimal mineralocorticoid activity, and dexamethasone has none. However, if cortisol levels or a cosyntropin stimulation test cannot be performed initially, dexamethasone can be given temporarily because a single dose does not cross-react with future cortisol assays. Dexamethasone does not have any mineralocorticoid activity and should be switched to hydrocortisone as soon as possible, or if continued should be given with fludrocortisone.[24,28]

Hahner and colleagues[29] demonstrated that infection is the most common trigger for adrenal crisis. Thus, although adrenal insufficiency and crisis alone can cause fever, it is important to remember that these patients are immunosuppressed and more susceptible to infection. Sources of infection should therefore be evaluated, and a combination of steroids and antibiotics is often necessary to treat the patient appropriately.[23]

PHEOCHROMOCYTOMA AS A CAUSE OF FEVER
Etiology and Pathophysiology

A pheochromocytoma is a catecholamine-producing tumor of the sympathetic or parasympathetic nervous system. Typically the term pheochromocytoma is used to refer to clinically active tumors that arise from sympathetic tissue, and this interpretation is used in this article.

Most pheochromocytomas (80%–85%) secrete norepinephrine, whereas the remainder secrete epinephrine or are clinically silent dopamine-secreting tumors.[30,31] The mechanism of fever production is not well described but is thought to be related to several factors, including: the induced hypermetabolic state and decreased ability to dissipate heat because of impaired vasodilation; tumor necrosis; release of hormones or other biologically active substances from the tumor; a complication of an inciting stressor; or the biological actions of the tumor itself (eg, induced rhabdomyolysis, myocardial infarction, cerebrovascular accident).[32] A case report describing a patient with an interleukin-6–producing pheochromocytoma suggests that at least some pheochromocytomas can stimulate fever directly via production of proinflammatory factors.[2] Epinephrine-secreting tumors have a strong association with fever.[3,31]

Clinical Manifestations

Pheochromocytomas are difficult to diagnose, and are known as "great masquer-aders" because of the variety of symptoms with which they present. Palpitations, headaches, and profuse sweating constitute the classic triad and raise concerns for pheochromocytoma, especially if the patient also presents with hypertension.[33]

The clinical manifestations and treatment of pheochromocytomas are outlined in **Box 6**. The predominant sign is hypertension, which may be episodic or sustained. The triad of headache, diaphoresis, and tachycardia has sensitivity of 90% and spec-ificity of 93.8%.[31] Catecholamine crisis can also lead to heart failure, pulmonary edema, arrhythmia, and intracranial hemorrhage. Hypertensive crisis can be

---

Box 6
Clinical features, diagnosis, and treatment of pheochromocytoma

Clinical Features

- Hypertension (episodic or sustained)
- Headache
- Anxiety
- Diaphoresis
- Palpitations and tachycardia
- Pallor (often followed by flushing)
- Nausea/vomiting
- Dyspnea
- Fever
- Hyperglycemia

Diagnosis

- Plasma free metanephrines
  - Alternative: 24-hour urine testing for vanillylmandelic acid, metanephrines, and catecholamines
- Computed tomography with low-osmolar contrast, or magnetic resonance imaging with gadolinium

Treatment

- Surgery is the definitive treatment; all other treatments are administered to control symptoms in preparation for surgery
- Acute blood pressure reduction
  - Phentolamine, 2.5- to 5-mg intravenous boluses (given at a rate of 1 mg/min) followed by a drip titrated to blood pressure
  - Alternatives
    - Sodium nitroprusside, nicardipine, nitroglycerine dosed as for other hypertensive emergencies
- Control of tachycardia (only after α-blockade is achieved to avoid uncontrolled hypertension)
  - β-Blocker (propranolol, metoprolol, esmolol drip) intravenously

Data from Refs.[30–35]

stimulated by a variety of stressors and generally lasts less than an hour.[30,33] However, the crises tend to increase in frequency, duration, and severity over time.[30]

Tumors that secrete norepinephrine cause elevations in the systolic and diastolic blood pressure. By contrast, those that secrete epinephrine cause elevation of only systolic blood pressure.[31,34] Although epinephrine-secreting tumors are rarer, patients with such tumors exhibit more of the "classic" pheochromocytoma signs: palpitations, headache, anxiety, hyperthermia, and hyperglycemia.[34] Patients with epinephrine-secreting tumors can also experience hypotension and shock after α-blockade, because of the β-adrenergic effects of the epinephrine.[30] Patients with norepinephrine-secreting pheochromocytomas tend to experience sustained hypertension (due to continuous catecholamine excess) but can have episodes of paroxysmal hypertension.[34] Patients with both types of tumors (norepinephrine-secreting and epinephrine-secreting) can also experience orthostatic hypotension as a result of blunting of sympathetic reflexes and constriction of vascular volume by high levels of circulating catecholamines.[30,34]

Pheochromocytoma multisystem crisis (PMC) is defined by multiple organ system failure, temperature higher than 40°C, encephalopathy, and vascular lability (hypertension and/or hypotension). Patients with PMC tend to have large tumors with high levels of epinephrine secretion, do not do well on medical therapy alone, and need emergent surgical intervention because of their high mortality rate.[32,34,36,37]

Pheochromocytoma has also been linked to shock. This presentation represents one of the most difficult diagnostic challenges of pheochromocytoma in the ED. Pheochromocytoma should be suspected when there is no other explanation for circulatory collapse, especially when the patient presents with abdominal pain, pulmonary edema, intense mydriasis, weakness, diaphoresis, cyanosis, hyperglycemia, and leukocytosis.[24]

Diagnosis

Diagnosis of pheochromocytoma is confirmed by catecholamine and metanephrine testing. Twenty-four-hour assessment of vanillylmandelic acid, total or fractionated metanephrines, and catecholamines are the most widely available tests.[33] However, measurement of free plasma metanephrines has become the test of choice, because it is more convenient and is the most sensitive (and much easier to obtain in the acute setting). If the metanephrine level is elevated, diagnostic imaging should be performed, especially in patients with PMC, as surgery is the definitive treatment.[31–33,36,37] Computed tomography (CT) with contrast and magnetic resonance imaging (MRI) with gadolinium have been shown to be similar in sensitivity; thus, in an ED setting CT with contrast would likely be the most efficient test.[31,33] There have been reports of worsening symptoms with intravenous contrast administration when higher osmolar formulations were used, but low-osmolar contrast has been well tolerated and should be used when performing CT in patients with suspected pheochromocytoma.[34] MRI, however, has been shown to be slightly better at locating extra-adrenal pheochromocytomas.[33,35]

The tumors themselves can be asymptomatic for many years. It is thought that they need to reach a certain size before they produce enough catecholamines to cause symptoms. Thus, the diagnosis of pheochromocytoma should be considered in patients with adrenal "incidentalomas" who present with hypertension that is difficult to control or other symptoms that cause concern.[33]

Treatment

Surgery is the definitive treatment for pheochromocytoma (and, in the case of PMC, must be performed emergently, as it is the only effective treatment).[33,36] Given the catecholamine surge caused by surgery, patients must be stabilized and prepared appropriately. The primary goal is a blood pressure consistently below 160/90 mm Hg and a heart rate lower than 100 beats/min.[30,33,34]

The first principle of treatment is that α-blockade must be initiated before β-blockade to avoid hypertensive crisis.[35] If the patient is not in crisis, α-adrenergic blockade with phenoxybenzamine is the treatment of choice. Start phenoxybenzamine at low doses (5–10 mg 3 times daily with goal dose of 20–30 mg 3 times daily) to minimize orthostatic hypotension. For hypertensive crisis, intravenous phentolamine (given in 2.5- to 5-mg boluses at 1 mg/min followed by a drip [the half-life is 3–5 minutes]) has traditionally been given to manage paroxysms, but other drugs such as sodium nitroprusside, nitroglycerine, or nicardipine can also be used.[34] β-Blockers can be started after α-blockade (most commonly propranolol, 10 mg 3 times daily or 4 times daily in the stable patient, or intravenously in unstable or preoperative patients); the dose can be increased as needed for tachycardia.[33] Orthostatic hypotension should be treated with volume replacement. Steroids have been linked to severe adverse reactions (thought to be caused by induction of production and secretion of catecholamines), and should not be given to patients with pheochromocytoma.[34]

SUMMARY

Although endocrinopathies are less common causes of hyperthermia than infectious disease, they are important factors to consider when evaluating febrile, critically ill patients. The most dangerous endocrine causes of fever are thyroid storm, adrenal crisis, and PMC. All 3 of these are clinical diagnoses in the ED; confirmatory laboratory tests should be obtained to aid in management of the patient once the acute crisis is over. These diagnoses are uncommon, but lack of recognition by the ED physician and delay in treatment could prove rapidly fatal for the patient.

ACKNOWLEDGMENTS

The authors would like to thank Laura Tenner, MD, for her assistance in editing this article.

REFERENCES

1. Dinarello CA, Porat R. Fever and hyperthermia. In: Fauci AS, Kasper DL, Jameson JL, et al, editors. Harrison's principles of internal medicine. 18th edition. New York: McGraw-Hill; 2012. Chapter 16. Available at: www.accesspharmacy.com/content.aspx?aID=9095580. Accessed March 7, 2013.
2. Taranoglu O, Yarman S, Altun E, et al. Interleukin-6-producing pheochromocytoma presenting with fever of unknown origin. Endocr Abstr 2007;14:496.
3. Gilboa Y, Horer B, Isaac B. Fever in endocrinologic disorders. In: Isaac B, Kernbaum S, Burke MJ, editors. Unexplained fever: a guide to the diagnosis and management of febrile states in medicine, surgery, pediatrics and subspecialties. Boca Raton (FL): CRC Press; 1991. p. 225–32.
4. Hahner S, Allolio B. Management of adrenal insufficiency in different clinical settings. Expert Opin Pharmacother 2005;6:2407–17.
5. Hatton MP, Durand ML, Burns SM, et al. Exaggerated postsurgical inflammation in a patient with insufficiently treated Addison disease. Ophthal Plast Reconstr Surg 2009;25:67–9.

6. Costanzo L. Physiology. 4th edition. Oxford (United Kingdom): Elsevier Limited; 2010.
7. Jameson JL, Weetman AP. Disorders of the thyroid gland. In: Fauci AS, Kasper DL, Jameson JL, et al, editors. Harrison's principles of internal medicine. 18th edition. New York: McGraw-Hill; 2012. Chapter 341. Available at: www.accesspharmacy.com/content.aspx?aID=9140510. Accessed March 7, 2013.
8. Bahn RS, Burch HB, Cooper DS, et al. Hyperthyroidism and other causes of thyrotoxicosis: management guidelines of the American Thyroid Association and American Association of Clinical Endocrinologists. Endocr Pract 2011;17: e1–65.
9. Ingbar SH. Classification of the causes of thyrotoxicosis. In: Ingbar SH, Braverman LE, editors. The thyroid. Philadelphia: Lippincott; 1986. p. 809.
10. Nayak B, Burman K. Thyrotoxicosis and thyroid storm. Endocrinol Metab Clin North Am 2006;35:663–86.
11. Migneco A, Ojetti V, Testa A, et al. Management of thyrotoxic crisis. Eur Rev Med Pharmacol Sci 2005;9:69–74.
12. Burch HB, Wartofsky L. Life-threatening thyrotoxicosis: thyroid storm. Endocrinol Metab Clin North Am 1993;22:263–77.
13. Arem R, Karlsson F, Deppe S. Intravenous levothyroxine therapy does not affect survival in severely ill intensive care unit patients. Thyroidol Clin Exp 1995;7:79.
14. Nicoloff JT. Thyroid storm and myxedema coma. Med Clin North Am 1985;69: 1005–17.
15. Tietgens ST, Leinung MC. Thyroid storm. Med Clin North Am 1995;79:169.
16. Kudrjavcev T. Neurologic complications of thyroid dysfunction. Adv Neurol 1978; 19:619–36.
17. Parfitt AM, Dent CE. Hyperthyroidism and hypercalcemia. Q J Med 1970;39: 171–87.
18. Sellin JH, Vassilopoulou-Sellin R, Lester R. The gastrointestinal tract and liver. In: Ingbar SH, Braverman LE, editors. The thyroid. Philadelphia: Lippincott; 1986. p. 871.
19. Wartofsky L. Thyrotoxic storm. In: Ingbar SH, Braverman LE, editors. The thyroid. Philadelphia: Lippincott; 1986. p. 974.
20. Parker JL, Lawson PH. Death from thyrotoxicosis. Lancet 1974;2:894.
21. Ingbar SG, Freinkel N. Simultaneous estimation of rates of thyroxine degradation and thyroid hormone synthesis. J Clin Invest 1955;34:808–19.
22. Tintinalli J, Stapczynski J, Ma OJ, et al, editors. Tintinalli's emergency medicine: a comprehensive study guide. 7th edition. New York: McGraw-Hill; 2010.
23. Arlt W. Disorders of the adrenal cortex. In: Fauci AS, Kasper DL, Jameson JL, et al, editors. Harrison's principles of internal medicine. 18th edition. New York: McGraw-Hill; 2012. Chapter 342. Available at: www.accesspharmacy.com/content.aspx?aID=9140931. Accessed December 31, 2012.
24. Marik PE, Zaloga GP. Adrenal insufficiency in the critically ill: a new look at an old problem. Chest 2002;122:1784–96.
25. Nieman LK, Chanco Turner ML. Addison's disease. Clin Dermatol 2006;24: 276–80.
26. Moraes RB, Czepielewski MA, Friedman G, et al. Diagnosis of adrenal failure in critically ill patients. Arq Bras Endocrinol Metabol 2011;55:295–302.
27. Marik PE, Pastores SM, Annane D, et al. Recommendations for the diagnosis and management of adrenal insufficiency in critically ill adult patients: consensus statements from an international task force by the American College of Critical Care Medicine. Crit Care Med 2007;36:1937–49.

28. Schimmer BP, Funder JW. ACTH, adrenal steroids, and pharmacology of the adrenal cortex. In: Chabner BA, Burnton LL, Knollmann BC, editors. Goodman & Gillmans's the pharmacological basis of therapeutics. 12th edition. New York: McGraw-Hill; 2011. Chapter 42. Available at: www.accesspharmacy.com/content.aspx?aID=16674048. Accessed March 8, 2013.

29. Hahner S, Loeffler M, Bleicken B, et al. Epidemiology of adrenal crisis in chronic adrenal insufficiency: the need for new prevention strategies. Eur J Endocrinol 2012;162:597–602.

30. Walther MM, Keiser HR, Linehan WM. Pheochromocytoma: evaluation, diagnosis, and treatment. World J Urol 1999;17:35–9.

31. Zapanti E, Illias I. Pheochromocytoma: physiopathologic implications and diagnostic evaluation. Ann N Y Acad Sci 2006;1088:346–60.

32. Gordon DL, Atamian SD, Brooks MH, et al. Fever in pheochromocytoma. Arch Intern Med 1992;152:1269–72.

33. Neumann HP. Pheochromocytoma. In: Fauci AS, Kasper DL, Jameson JL, et al, editors. Harrison's principles of internal medicine. 18th edition. New York: McGraw-Hill; 2012. Chapter 343. Available at: www.accesspharmacy.com/content.aspx?aID=9141133. Accessed March 8, 2013.

34. Prejbisz A, Lenders JW, Eisenhofer G, et al. Cardiovascular manifestations of phaeochromocytoma. J Hypertens 2011;29:2049–60.

35. Shah U, Giubellino A, Pacak K. Pheochromocytoma: implications in tumorigenesis and the actual management. Minerva Endocrinol 2012;37:141–56.

36. Newell KA, Prinz RA, Pickleman J, et al. Pheochromocytoma multisystem crisis: a surgical emergency. Arch Surg 1988;123:956–9.

37. Davlouros PA, Velissaris D, Tsiola A, et al. Case reports: fever with multiple organ failure: not always sepsis. Anaesth Intensive Care 2010;38:1090–3.

Fever and Neurologic Conditions

Aisha T. Liferidge, MD, MPH*, Janaé E.P. Dark, MD, MPH

KEYWORDS

- Fever • Neurologic conditions • Neurologic abnormalities

KEY POINTS

- Neurologic conditions can be categorized into 2 broad categories: (1) those that cause a change in mental status and (2) those that create a focal finding on physical examination.
- The cause of a neurologic abnormality associated with fever can be a primary neurologic condition or a condition that does not originate in the central nervous system.
- Optimal management of neurologic conditions associated with fever requires high clinical suspicion and a broad differential diagnosis, which facilitates rapid recognition and effective treatment.
- A thorough history and physical examination are key determinants in accurately diagnosing neurologic conditions associated with fever, often requiring acquisition of collateral information from persons other than the patient.

Fever in a patient with neurologic abnormalities can be the manifestation of a wide range of illnesses. The physician responsible for the care of a febrile patient with neurologic manifestations must have a thoughtful and clear approach to a constellation of symptoms. Although it may be tempting to attribute the patient's complaints to an intracranial source, the clinician must avoid premature closure and consider a broad differential diagnosis. Careful attention must be paid to the patient's history and physical examination in guiding the direction of the diagnostic workup. In addition, serial examinations might be necessary to elicit important clues to the cause of the patient's presentation.

HISTORY

Two separate processes are occurring in patients with fever and neurologic changes. Therefore, the history should be approached in a manner that addresses each symptom individually, despite their apparent association. By giving equal attention to both groups of symptoms, the health care provider can gather subtle clues that will elucidate the primary disorder. Depending on the nature of the neurologic involvement, the

Department of Emergency Medicine, George Washington University School of Medicine, 2120 L Street Northwest, Suite 450, Washington, DC 20037, USA
* Corresponding author.
E-mail address: aliferidge@mfa.gwu.edu

Emerg Med Clin N Am 31 (2013) 987–1017
http://dx.doi.org/10.1016/j.emc.2013.07.005
0733-8627/13/$ – see front matter © 2013 Elsevier Inc. All rights reserved.

patient might not be able to provide sufficient information, so collateral sources might be necessary.

Appropriate characterization of the fever is of utmost importance. Specifically, the details surrounding its onset and course should be clarified. A 3-week history of waxing and waning fevers leads the care provider in a different direction than does a persistent fever of 2 days' duration. The maximum temperature, if known, should be noted as well as the patient's response, if any, to antipyretic therapy. The timing and amount of the last dose of an antipyretic should be determined.

Neurologic conditions can be classified into 2 broad categories: those that alter mental status and those that cause focal deficits. Changes in mental status can be further classified as either altered level of consciousness (lethargy) or altered sensorium (disorientation). As stated earlier, changes in mental status can obfuscate the history and physical, so friends or family members with knowledge of the patient's baseline mental status should be queried. Questions should be directed at determining the onset (sudden vs gradual) and course (intermittent vs persistent) of the symptoms. A specific inquiry should be made regarding the timing of the neurologic changes in relation to the onset of fever.

In the patient with focal deficits and fever, clear identification of the time of onset is critical. Information regarding the initial neurologic manifestation should also be well defined. For example, if a patient initially manifested a facial droop that was seen by family members but now has unilateral hemiparesis, the change in symptoms is certainly clinically relevant. The patient and witnesses should be asked specifically about improving or worsening symptoms since the onset of illness.

The emergency physician should also investigate potentially significant patient characteristics or comorbidities. A history of malignancy, immunosuppression, arrhythmia, cerebrovascular accident, intravenous drug abuse, anticoagulation, or recent infection should be elicited. Other pertinent facts, such as the use of new medications, sick contacts, and recent camping, hiking, or international travel (and corresponding vaccinations or chemoprophylaxis) should be ascertained. Associated signs and symptoms such as rash, skin changes, headache, nausea, vomiting, back pain, and urinary or upper respiratory symptoms should also be documented.

PHYSICAL EXAMINATION

In the hyperthermic patient with neurologic involvement, vital signs can provide insight into hemodynamic instability as well as evidence of the involvement of other organ systems. The vital signs should be recorded before or immediately following bedside evaluation of the patient, and repeat measurements should be taken after any intervention.

The mental status can be evaluated quickly on initial examination. Lethargy or decreased activity will be obvious; disorientation may be more difficult to determine. Use of the Glasgow Coma Scale can provide significant insight into the patient's mental state. The rest of the neurologic examination might yield suboptimal results if the patient's mental status does not allow him or her to fully participate in the examination. Close attention should be paid to motor and sensory function. The patient's ability to spontaneously and grossly move all extremities should be noted, even if a detailed motor and sensory examination is not feasible. Cranial nerve deficits can be demonstrated with a thorough examination, and the absence of a gag reflex might indicate the need for intubation. Evidence of meningismus should be sought.

The remaining organ systems should also be evaluated. The HEENT (head, ears, eyes, nose, and throat) examination should include an evaluation of pupillary size and reactivity. The mastoid processes should be palpated and both ears should be inspected. All sinuses should be assessed for tenderness to palpation. The neck should be examined for meningismus. Auscultation of heart sounds should assess for the absence or presence of a murmur as well as tachycardia. Hypoventilation might represent the need for intubation, and rhonchi might indicate aspiration secondary to decreased mental status. Evaluation of the gastrointestinal system may warrant a rectal examination to assess adequate tone. Concomitant assessment for saddle anesthesia should be done at this time. The musculoskeletal examination should include palpation of the entire spine to determine focal midline tenderness or detect signs of infection. Lastly, the skin should be inspected carefully for the presence of a rash or mottling.

DELIRIUM

Delirium is a disorder primarily involving alterations in the level of consciousness. It is characterized by an acute onset of global cognitive dysfunction and manifests as impaired attention, cognition, and orientation.[1,2] It has a waxing and waning course and is often accompanied by autonomic system involvement. Most importantly, delirium indicates an underlying process and should be viewed as a symptom rather than the primary condition. Although commonly observed in patients, delirium should be considered a neurologic emergency.[3]

The overall incidence of delirium in emergency department (ED) patients is unknown, but several studies have found that 7% to 20% of elderly patients who come to EDs are delirious.[2–6] As the elderly are vulnerable to delirium, much focus has been placed on detecting it among older patients. Unfortunately, the diagnosis is often missed: emergency physicians diagnose delirium appropriately only 16% to 25% of the time.[4,7,8] These missed diagnoses are not without consequence, as the literature demonstrates that patients with delirium have a longer length of stay in hospital,[9] a higher mortality rate,[10] and higher health care costs.[11] Thus, it would be ideal for emergency physicians to be able to make this diagnosis in a timely fashion in an effort to improve outcomes.

Pathophysiology

The pathophysiology of delirium is complex. Patients can have intrinsic predisposing characteristics or might be subject to biochemical insults that precipitate development of the illness.[12,13] In febrile patients, delirium has numerous causes. Urinary tract infection, pneumonia, and other infections; medication side effects (with or without concomitant infection); hyperthermia; thyroid dysfunction; substance abuse; and primary central nervous system (CNS) infection should all be thoughtfully considered.[13] A more comprehensive list of the causes of delirium is presented in **Table 1**.[2,12–14]

Clinical Presentation

Delirious patients have a variety of presentations. While fully awake, the patient might show signs of inattention or be unable to perform simple tasks. Memory and perception might be altered, and hallucinations can occur. Hallucinations associated with delirium are usually visual, but can be auditory as well.[2] Psychomotor agitation can be present in 1 of 3 forms: hypoactive, hyperactive, or mixed.[15] Hypoactive delirium manifests as quiet somnolence or sedation; the hyperactive subtype is exemplified by agitation and increased motor activity. The mixed form is an alteration of hypoactive and hyperactive behavior, and the clinician might witness both during the same ED visit.

Table 1 **Predisposing factors and causes of delirium**	
Predisposing Factors	**Organic Causes (I WATCH DEATH)**
Age >65 y	Infectious Urinary tract infection Pneumonia Meningitis/encephalitis Sepsis Syphilis
Male gender	Withdrawal Alcohol Barbiturates Benzodiazepines Illicit substances
Comorbid conditions	Acute metabolic
Chronic kidney disease	Electrolyte abnormality (Na, Ca, Mg)
End-stage liver disease	Acidosis
Dementia	Hypoglycemia
Hearing or visual impairment	Hepatic failure (hepatic encephalopathy)
Terminal illness	Renal failure (uremia) Hyper/hypothyroidism
Multiple comorbidities	Trauma Head injury Burns
Functional dependence or immobility	Central nervous system disease Intracranial hemorrhage Subarachnoid hemorrhage Subdural/epidural hematoma Stroke Seizure Mass lesion Vasculitis
Dehydration	Hypoxia Acute hypoxia (pulmonary embolus, congestive heart failure) Chronic lung disease Hypotension (myocardial infarction)
Malnutrition	Deficiencies Thiamine (Wernicke encephalopathy) B_{12} Niacin
Polypharmacy	Environmental Hypo-/hyperthermia Excessive noise or other stimuli Interrupted sleep Physical restraints
	(continued on next page)

Table 1 (continued)	
Predisposing Factors	**Organic Causes (I WATCH DEATH)**
History of alcohol or substance abuse	Acute vascular
	Hypertensive encephalopathy
	Sagittal vein thrombosis
	Toxins/drugs
	Alcohols
	Anticholinergics
	Antihistamines
	Antipsychotics
	Antidepressants
	Antiparkinsonian agents
	Histamine H_2 blockers
	Sedative-hypnotics
	Narcotic analgesics
	Solvents
	Pesticides
	Carbon monoxide
	Illicit substances
	Heavy metals
	Lead
	Mercury

Data from Refs.[2,12–14]

Diagnosis

Delirium is diagnosed based on the clinical presentation. Laboratory test results and imaging might point to the underlying cause, but no one diagnostic tool will confirm delirium. Key factors are found in the history and physical examination. As mentioned earlier, delirium is poorly diagnosed in the ED, so clinicians must have a high suspicion for it. A concerted effort must be made to evaluate patients' mental status. Routine screening for delirium is recommended. The Mini-Mental Status Examination (MMSE) has been used conventionally to screen patients for delirium; however, this tool is impractical for use in the ED because it takes approximately 7 to 10 minutes to complete, requires the patient to be able to read and write, and poorly detects mild alterations in mental status.[16] Consequently, newer tools for the evaluation of mental status have been devised and validated for use in the ED. The Quick Confusion Scale,[17,18] the Six-Item Screener,[16,18,19] and the Confusion Assessment Method for the Intensive Care Unit[8] have all been proved to be appropriate substitutes for the MMSE in the emergency setting The components of these tests are presented in **Fig. 1**.[8,17,19]

Treatment

The definitive therapy for delirium is treatment of the underlying cause. Despite prompt recognition and treatment of the primary pathologic process, delirium can persist for months. Supportive measures such as the creation of a calm and soothing environment, avoidance of restraints, minimization of indwelling lines (such as Foley catheters), and consistent reorientation should be provided when possible.[14,20] Pharmacologic therapy should be initiated as needed. Haloperidol is considered first-line treatment, as it is the most studied antipsychotic for the management of delirium.[2,20]

A

Instructions to the patient: I would like to ask you some questions that may ask you to use your memory. I am going to name three objects. Please wait until I say all three words, then repeat them. Remember these words for me: GRASS – PAPER – SHOE. (May repeat names 3 times if necessary, repetition not scored).

1) What year is this?
2) What month is this?
3) What is the day of the week?
After one-minute. What are the three objects that I asked you to remember?
4) [Grass]
5) [Paper]
6) [Shoe]

Each correct response is awarded one-point. Two or more errors is considered high-risk for cognitive impairment.

B

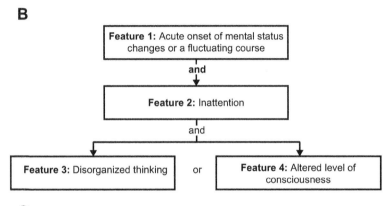

C

The QCS (and its scoring) can be summarised in seven questions:
- What year is it now? (2 points)
- What month is it? (2 points)
- Repeat this phrase after me and remember it: "John Brown, 42 Market Street, New York."
- About what time is it? (2 points)
- Count backwards from 20 to 1. (2 points)
- Say the months in reverse. (2 points)
- Repeat the memory phrase. (5 points)

Fig. 1. Mental status evaluation tools for the emergency department. These tools have been shown to be suitable alternatives to the Mini-Mental Status Examination. (*A*) Delirium is suspected when 2 or more errors are made on the Six-Screener Examination. (*B*) The Confusion Assessment Method for the Intensive Care Unit (CAM-ICU) diagnoses delirium when Features 1 and 2 are present in addition to either Feature 3 or 4. (*C*) The Quick Confusion Scale designates clinically significant cognitive impairment with a score of 11 or less. ([*A*] *From* Carpenter CR, DesPain B, Keeling TN, et al. The Six-Item Screener and AD8 for the detection of cognitive impairment in geriatric emergency department patients. Ann Emerg Med 2011;57:653–61; with permission; [*B*] *From* Han JH, Zimmerman EE, Cutler N, et al. Delirium in older emergency department patients: recognition, risk factors, and psychomotor subtypes. Acad Emerg Med 2009;16:193–200; with permission; [*C*] *From* Huff JS, Farace E, Brady WJ, et al. The quick confusion scale in the ED: comparison with the mini-mental state examination. Am J Emerg Med 2001;19(6):461–4; with permission.)

Appropriate dosing starts with 5 to 10 mg orally, intravenously, or intramuscularly, with reduced dosages in the elderly. Benzodiazepines may be used in conjunction with haloperidol to achieve rapid sedation.[21] Atypical antipsychotics can be used to combat agitation.[2,13,21]

THROMBOTIC THROMBOCYTOPENIC PURPURA

Thrombotic thrombocytopenic purpura (TTP) is a rare, life-threatening disorder of hemostasis. Because of its multisystem organ involvement, it often has a rapidly progressive course, and outcomes have been poor in the past. In the pretreatment era, the mortality rate was 90%. Improved awareness and treatment modalities have reduced the mortality rate to approximately 20%.[22] Despite these advances in the management of TTP, difficulties in making the diagnosis and initiating early treatment continue to challenge clinicians who encounter patients with this disease.

TTP primarily affects women, African Americans, and young adults.[22] It has been shown in retrospective analysis to have an increased occurrence in the summer, suggesting an environmental or infectious association with the season.[23] It is known to be associated with numerous drugs and medical conditions such as pancreatitis, infection with the human immunodeficiency virus, and pregnancy.[24–27]

Pathophysiology

The metalloproteinase ADAMTS-13 (**a d**isintegrin **a**nd **m**etalloproteinase with **t**hrombo**s**pondin type 1 motif, member 13) lies at the center of the pathophysiology of TTP.[28] This protein is responsible for cleaving von Willebrand factor (vWF). Patients with TTP have either a diminished level of ADAMTS-13 or autoantibodies to it. Without adequate concentrations of the fully functional compound, multiple vWF monomers form vWF multimers, resulting in the accumulation of multimers in the microcirculation and subsequent microthrombus formation. Concomitant platelet aggregation results in exhaustion of the body's platelets, leading to thrombocytopenia. The shearing of red blood cells (RBCs) produces microangiopathic hemolytic anemia (MAHA). Eventually these intravascular abnormalities coalesce, resulting in end-organ damage.

Clinical Presentation

TTP is characterized by the classic pentad of fever, anemia, thrombocytopenia, and renal and neurologic involvement.[28,29] It should be noted, however, that only 5% of patients present with all symptoms of the pentad.[30] Data from the Oklahoma TTP-HUS (hemolytic uremic syndrome) Registry reveal that 66% of patients presented with some neurologic abnormality, and symptoms ranged from minor complaints such as confusion or headache to more serious conditions such as focal deficits, seizure, stroke, and coma.[30] In addition, multiple reports have described atypical presentations of TTP, including acute coronary syndrome and primary vision changes.[31]

Diagnosis

Part of the difficulty in diagnosing TTP is its overlap with other serious illnesses. Malignant hypertension, sepsis, hemolytic uremic syndrome, disseminated intravascular coagulation, HELLP (**h**emolysis, **e**levated **l**iver enzymes, **l**ow **p**latelets) syndrome, and systemic lupus erythematosus all resemble TTP.[22,32]

Because of the high mortality rate associated with a missed diagnosis, efforts have been made to relax the diagnostic criteria for TTP, leading to the recommendation that the presence of unexplained thrombocytopenia and MAHA should prompt the clinician to consider TTP. Ultimately, the diagnosis is made based on the patient's history and the findings on physical examination, in conjunction with laboratory findings. In addition to the aforementioned thrombocytopenia and anemia, the peripheral blood smear will contain schistocytes, which denote MAHA. Levels of serum lactate dehydrogenase will be markedly elevated while coagulation panel tests will be normal. ADAMTS-13 levels will not be readily available in the emergency care setting, and thus should not be expected to guide care.[22]

Treatment

The primary focus of the treatment of TTP is plasma exchange, and once the diagnosis is made it should be initiated immediately.[33] This treatment modality removes autoantibodies to ADAMTS-13 and replenishes the metalloproteinase level. If plasmapheresis cannot be started in a timely manner, the clinician may begin plasma infusion as a temporizing measure.[22,30] Patients with severely low levels of ADAMTS-13 should be managed with steroids: either prednisone, methylprednisolone, or dexamethasone.[22,33] As the emergency physician will not know the ADAMTS-13 level, steroid administration is recommended.[30] Despite the natural inclination to transfuse platelets for profound thrombocytopenia, platelet transfusion is not recommended for patients with TTP because it can worsen outcomes.[33] However, in the event of intracranial hemorrhage or other life-threatening bleeding, platelet transfusion is considered appropriate.[32] Emergent consultation with a hematologist is warranted for the treatment of TTP.

HYPERTHERMIA IN TRAUMATIC BRAIN INJURY

Posttraumatic hyperthermia (PTH), also known as neurogenic fever, is a noninfectious elevation in body temperature, which often negatively influences outcome after traumatic brain injury (TBI). TBI is a major cause of death and disability worldwide, particularly among children and young adults. It results in functional and chronic deficits in 70,000 to 90,000 survivors every year, who require continued treatment and care.[34] TBI-related morbidity and poor outcome are associated with hyperthermia in the acute postinjury phase. PTH persists for weeks to months in 4% to 37% of patients with moderate to severe TBI.[35]

Pathophysiology

Thermoregulation of the human body is maintained by a complex interaction of autonomic, endocrine, and behavioral processes.[36] The preoptic region of the hypothalamus of the brain is the primary thermoregulator, and serves as the thermostat that manages mechanisms for heat dissipation. Stimulation studies suggest that temperature regulation is controlled by a hierarchy of neural structures, consisting of a coordinating center in the ventromedial preoptic region of the anterior hypothalamus and effector areas for specific thermoregulatory responses throughout the brainstem and spinal cord (**Fig. 2**).[37]

The neurons of the preoptic region are sensitive, and respond to subtle changes in the hypothalamus or core temperature. These neurons receive somatosensory input from skin, spinal thermoreceptors, and endogenous substances such as pyrogens, which they use to compare and integrate central and peripheral thermal information. Endogenous substances such as pyrogens and antipyretics additionally affect the activity of preoptic thermosensitive neurons, resulting in thermoregulation. It is thought that these substances trigger the release of mediators such as prostaglandin, which produce fever by inhibiting preoptic neurons, which suppress heat-loss responses and elevate the hypothalamic set-point temperature.[37]

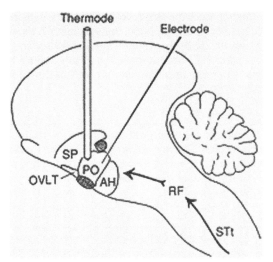

Fig. 2. Sagittal view of mammalian hypothalamus structures, including the organum vasculosum lamina terminalis (OVLT), the septum (SP), the preoptic region (PO) with an implanted thermode used to warm and cool for experimental purposes, the anterior hypothalamus (AH), the reticular formation (RF), and the lateral spinothalamic tract (STt). (*From* Boulant JA. Role of the preoptic-anterior hypothalamus in thermoregulation and fever. Clin Infect Dis 2000;31(Suppl 5):S157–61; with permission.)

Disruption of the preoptic region by injury may result in heat intolerance or thermostatic dysfunction. The hypothalamus and brainstem contain pathways for autonomic and behavioral thermoregulation; if they are injured, hypothermia, poikilothermia, or hyperthermia can result.[36] Animal and human studies have suggested that TBI might result in hypothermia or hyperthermia. One study of severely brain-injured rats found that 69% developed profound hypothermia followed by a slow and gradual return to baseline temperature, and that 27% experienced 2 or more days of PTH associated with loss of circadian rhythm. Another study found that activation of certain hypothalamic receptors in rabbits decreases heat production and increases heat loss, resulting in hypothermia, and that inhibiting such receptors conversely results in hyperthermia.[38]

The inflammatory response to brain injury consists of astrocytosis and the infiltration of neutrophils, microglia, and macrophages. The infiltration of inflammatory mediators is accompanied by an upregulation of proinflammatory cytokines, which activates thermosensitive neurons in the ventromedial preoptic nucleus and paraventricular nucleus of the anterior hypothalamus, resulting in fever and increased body temperature.

Hyperthermia results in increased metabolic expenditure, glutamate release, and neutrophil activity, which can further compromise the function of an injured brain while increasing the vulnerability of the brain-injured patient to secondary pathogenic events.[35] For every 1°C increase in body temperature there is a 13% increase in metabolic rate, which exacerbates stress on the body and its energy stores.[39] Furthermore, body temperatures higher than 43°C can cause neuronal injury to the brain, and prolonged periods of moderate hyperthermia to 40°C can alter brain structure and function.[39]

Clinical Presentation

PTH is characterized by relative bradycardia, lack of diurnal variation in temperature, a notable absence or paucity of perspiration, and relative resistance to antipyretic medications.[39] These features primarily differentiate PTH from fever among TBI patients.

Fever is a regulated increase in the preoptic temperature set point in response to circulating pyrogenic cytokines. Unlike fever, in hyperthermia there is no resetting of a temperature set point; instead, thermoregulatory mechanisms are overwhelmed by excessive heat production, heat storage, or dysfunctional heat dissipation.[36] Neurogenic fever can also be associated with a prolonged decrease in awareness, coma, or diabetes insipidus.[39]

Diagnosis

PTH is largely a diagnosis of exclusion, often requiring extensive preliminary diagnostic testing to rule out other sources of fever.[39] Given the typically lengthy diagnostic period, PTH is rarely diagnosed in the ED. The prolonged time to diagnosis often results a delay in rehabilitation because patients are categorized as medically unstable during the fever workup.[39]

Treatment

The initial treatment of PTH consists of external cooling methods until an accurate diagnosis can be made and appropriate drug therapy started. Based on anecdotes and case reports, several drugs have been used successfully to treat neurogenic fever, including bromocriptine, amantadine, dantrolene, and propranolol. Given that these medications are associated with potentially significant side effects such as hypotension and gastrointestinal bleeding, they should be used judiciously and only after a firm diagnosis of neurogenic fever has been made.[39]

Efforts are needed to better elucidate the cellular mechanisms of PTH to aid in the compilation of a diagnostic algorithm, improve its treatment, and minimize its negative effects.

BACTERIAL MENINGITIS

Meningitis is an inflammatory disease of the leptomeninges. In bacterial meningitis, the arachnoid mater of the meninges and the cerebrospinal fluid (CSF) in both the subarachnoid space and cerebral ventricles are infected with a bacterial agent.

Each year, approximately 1.2 million cases of bacterial meningitis occur worldwide; about 135,000 of them are fatal, making meningitis 1 of the 10 most common infectious causes of death. Despite the availability of effective antibiotics for clearing bacteria from the CSF, bacterial meningitis continues to cause significant morbidity and mortality. Large case series found a case-fatality rate for adults with bacterial meningitis as high as 25%, with 21% to 18% of survivors sustaining transient or permanent neurologic morbidity.[40]

Pathophysiology

Streptococcus pneumoniae is the most common bacterial source of community-acquired meningitis among adults (71%). The high frequency of pneumococcal meningitis is thought to reflect the relatively high rate of general pneumococcal infection in the community. Other causes are[40]:

- *Neisseria meningitidis* (12%)
- Group B streptococci (7%)
- *Haemophilus influenzae* (6%)
- *Listeria monocytogenes* (4%)

In adults 60 years or older, *L monocytogenes* is the second most common culprit, responsible for up to 20% of cases.[40] The causes of nosocomial bacterial meningitis include staphylococci and aerobic gram-negative bacilli. These infections usually occur in patients who have internal or external ventricular drains after neurosurgical procedures, and in those who have sustained head trauma.

Clinical Presentation

Patients with bacterial meningitis often appear very ill and typically seek medical attention soon after the onset of symptoms. One study found that the median duration of symptoms before admission was only 24 hours.[41] Classically patients with bacterial meningitis present with the triad of fever, nuchal rigidity, and change in mental status; however, a significant percentage of patients do not present with all 3 classic features.

Abnormality of mental status tends to be present initially in about 78% of cases.[42] High fever (>38°C) is common, with a reported sensitivity of 85%.[43] A small percentage of patients present with hypothermia. Almost no one with bacterial meningitis presents with a normal temperature.[44]

Nuchal rigidity, which is present initially in 88% of cases, can be demonstrated in the clinical setting by actively or passively flexing the patient's neck. If the patient cannot touch the chin to the chest, nuchal rigidity is likely. Use of lateral neck motion to assess nuchal rigidity is less reliable than flexion. Tests that elicit the Brudzinski sign or Kernig sign can be used to demonstrate meningeal irritation. A positive Brudzinski sign refers to spontaneous hip flexion during passive flexion of the neck. A lack of or limited extension of the knee when the hip is flexed to 90° indicates a positive Kernig sign. These examinations were developed more than a century ago and were tested in patients with severe, late-stage meningitis. Therefore, they might have limited reliability among broader patient groups. An additional maneuver known as jolt accentuation can be used to examine a patient in whom bacterial meningitis is highly suspected. This test consists of rotating the patient's head horizontally 2 to 3 times per second, which might significantly exacerbate the headache of a patient who truly has bacterial meningitis.

Critical and comprehensive appraisal of the literature has found that essentially all patients with bacterial meningitis have at least 1 feature of the classic triad (99%–100% sensitivity).[40] Therefore the absence of fever, nuchal rigidity, and altered mental status essentially excludes the diagnosis of bacterial meningitis. Older patients, particularly those with underlying diabetic and cardiopulmonary conditions, may present in an atypical fashion, with more insidious symptoms such as lethargy, no fever, and variable signs of meningeal inflammation. Severe, diffuse headache is also commonly associated with bacterial meningitis.

In addition to classic and common findings, other neurologic and nonneurologic manifestations might occur with bacterial meningitis. Examples of such complications include:

- Seizure
- Focal neurologic deficits such as cranial nerve palsies
- Papilledema
- Hearing loss
- Skin manifestations such as petechiae and palpable purpura
- Arthritis
- Features of source infection such as otitis or sinusitis

Patients with *Listeria* meningitis are more likely to have seizures and focal neurologic deficits early in the course of infection. Some may even present with rhombencephalitis, manifested as a syndrome of ataxia, cranial nerve palsies, or nystagmus. Skin changes are more likely to present with *N meningitidis* than with other types of bacterial meningitis. Petechiae, palpable purpura, and maculopapular rashes are examples of skin manifestations.

Diagnosis

The diagnostic management of bacterial meningitis consists of laboratory evaluation of the blood and CSF. Although serum blood tests rarely yield any significant abnormality that would affect management, the white blood cell (WBC) count might be elevated with a left shift toward immature forms, or leukopenia might be evident, indicating more severe infection. The platelet count might be decreased. Leukopenia and thrombocytopenia are associated with poor outcomes in patients with bacterial meningitis. Blood cultures are often positive in these patients, and can be particularly helpful if CSF was not obtained before the administration of antibiotics. Therefore, 2 sets of blood cultures should always be obtained from patients suspected of having bacterial meningitis. Obtaining 2 sets rather than 1 improves sensitivity and affords more accurate interpretation of ambiguous results associated with contamination.

Lumbar puncture should be performed to obtain CSF so as to diagnose bacterial meningitis definitively. Relative contraindications to lumbar puncture include evidence of elevated intracranial pressure, thrombocytopenia, bleeding diathesis, or spinal epidural abscess. Brain imaging is often obtained as a screening test for increased intracranial pressure before performing the lumbar puncture, but should not delay the collection of CSF or administration of antimicrobial therapy. Most patients with suspected meningitis do not need brain imaging before lumbar puncture, because such scans rarely reveal any significant abnormality.[45] The types of patients for whom lumbar puncture is warranted before computed tomography (CT) are listed in **Box 1**.[46]

If the lumbar puncture is delayed or deferred, blood cultures should be obtained and antibiotics administered empirically, followed by puncture as soon as possible. Dexamethasone should be administered just before or at the same time as the antibiotics. If the patient has received antimicrobial therapy, steroids should be withheld, because their administration is unlikely to improve outcome.[47] Administration of antimicrobials tends to have little effect on chemistry and cytology findings, but it might reduce the yield of the Gram stain and culture. In most cases, a pathogen can still be cultured from CSF for several hours after antibiotics are administered.[48,49] Patients with

---

Box 1
Bacterial meningitis: conditions for which a brain CT scan is warranted before lumbar puncture

- History or suspicion of central nervous system disease such as a mass lesion, stroke, or focal infection
- Seizure (ie, prolonged, within 30 minutes of presentation, tonic)
- Papilledema
- Abnormal or deteriorating level of consciousness, particularly if the Glasgow Coma Scale score is less than 11
- Focal neurologic deficit or abnormality (eg, pupillary changes, posturing, recent seizure)
- Irregular respirations
- Hypertension with bradycardia

From Joffe AR. Lumbar puncture and brain herniation in acute bacterial meningitis: a review. J Intensive Care Med 2007;22(4):194–207; with permission.

meningococcal infection, however, tend to have a lower yield of positive CSF analysis when the fluid is obtained after antibiotic administration.[48]

CSF Analysis

Opening pressure tends to be high in patients with bacterial meningitis. One study found that the mean opening pressure in cases of bacterial meningitis was 350 mm H_2O (normal up to 250 mm H_2O). Bacterial meningitis can be differentiated from viral meningitis by performing a Gram stain and culture on the CSF in addition to reviewing the results of cell-count studies. Normal CSF values are compared with typical values from patients with bacterial meningitis in **Table 2**.

Concentrations of CSF lactate are useful in differentiating bacterial from viral meningitis. Some studies have concluded that the diagnostic accuracy of CSF lactate is superior to that of CSF WBC count, glucose, and protein concentrations[50,51]; however, the sensitivity of CSF lactate concentration in differentiating bacterial from viral meningitis is lower in patients who have received antibiotics before lumbar puncture. In addition, CNS diseases other than bacterial meningitis might elevate the CSF lactate concentrations.[50,51]

Pleocytosis, or an elevated WBC count in the CSF, can have causes other than true infection. Traumatic lumbar puncture, intracranial hemorrhage, and seizure can all result in pleocytosis. When related to an excess of RBCs in the CSF, the following formula can be used to determine the true WBC count in the CSF:

$$\text{True WBC in CSF} = \text{Actual WBC in CSF} - \text{WBC in blood} \times \text{RBC in CSF/RBC in blood}$$

Generalized seizures can also induce a transiently elevated WBC count in the CSF. In these cases, the WBC count should not exceed 80/μL, the fluid should be clear and colorless, the opening pressure and glucose concentration should be within normal limits, and a Gram stain should be negative.[41] Even with careful analysis of the CSF in the search for evidence of bacterial meningitis, the diagnosis remains challenging because of the wide range of values (some being only mildly abnormal) and the effects of antibiotic administration; in addition, some patients are generally neutropenic.

A Gram stain should be obtained from the CSF of all patients suspected of having bacterial meningitis. The sensitivity of the stain ranges from 60% to 90%, and its specificity approaches 100%.[41] Use of the Gram stain is additionally advantageous because it might suggest a bacterial source before culture results become available. Ten percent to 15% of patients who have bacterial meningitis but negative CSF cultures (perhaps because they received antibiotic therapy before lumbar puncture) have a positive Gram stain. In the absence of a positive Gram stain, in the setting of

Table 2		
Comparison of normal CSF values and values from patients with bacterial meningitis		
	Normal	**Bacterial Meningitis**
Protein	<50 mg/dL	100–500 mg/dL
CSF to serum glucose ratio	>0.6	<0.4[a]
White blood cell count	<5/μL	1000–5000/μL[b]
Lactate concentration	<3.5 mEq/L	See text

[a] Glucose <40 mg/dL.
[b] Range, <100 to >10,000; neutrophils usually >80%.

an elevated CSF WBC count, no single CSF biochemical variable can reliably exclude bacterial meningitis.[52–54] Common results of Gram staining and their interpretations are presented in **Table 3**.

Meningitis Versus Encephalitis

The distinction between meningitis and encephalitis is based primarily on the clinical presentation. Meningitis is an infection of the meninges, and encephalitis is an infection of the brain parenchyma. Patients with meningitis typically present with malaise, lethargy, severe headache, and nuchal rigidity, but their cerebral brain function remains normal.[55] Patients with encephalitis, on the other hand, typically present with abnormal brain function such as altered mental status, motor or sensory deficits, abnormal behavior and personality changes, and speech or movement disorders. More severe neurologic manifestations such as hemiparesis, flaccid paralysis, and paresthesias can also be present in patients with encephalitis. Seizure is more likely to occur with encephalitis, but can also be associated with meningitis. Patients with both meningeal and parenchymal involvement can present with clinical characteristics that overlap the classic symptoms of meningitis and encephalitis. In these instances, the syndrome is referred to as meningoencephalitis.[55] The distinction between meningitis and encephalitis is important because the causative agents are different, requiring specific treatment.

Clues from the patient's history that suggest encephalitis are[56–58]:

- Unusual exposure history or a characteristic clinical presentation
- Epidemiologic information, such as seasonal occurrence or exposure to conditions transmitted via ticks, such as arboviruses (eastern equine, western equine, St Louis, Venezuelan equine encephalitis, and West Nile virus), Colorado tick fever (western United States), or nonviral causes such as Lyme disease or Rocky Mountain spotted fever
- History of exposure to animals or of being bitten could suggest rabies encephalitis

Results from the physical examination that suggest encephalitis are[59,60]:

- Parotitis strongly suggests mumps encephalitis in an unvaccinated patient with mental status changes
- Flaccid paralysis that evolves into encephalitis strongly suggests West Nile virus infection
- Tremors of the eyelids, tongue, lips, and extremities suggest St Louis encephalitis or West Nile encephalitis in the appropriate geographic location or in a patient with a relevant travel history
- Hydrophobia, aerophobia, pharyngeal spasms, and hyperactivity suggest encephalitic rabies

Table 3	
Bacterial meningitis: interpretation of common Gram stain results	
Finding	Indication
Gram-positive diplococci	Pneumococcal infection
Gram-negative diplococci	Meningococcal infection
Small pleomorphic gram-negative coccobacilli	*Haemophilus influenzae* infection
Gram-positive rods and coccobacilli	*Listeria* infection

- Grouped vesicles in a dermatomal pattern could suggest varicella zoster virus (VZV), which can occasionally cause encephalitis (absence of rash does not eliminate VZV)

The characteristics of viral CNS infections/encephalitis are:

- Increased WBC count (usually <250/mm^3) with predominance of lymphocytes; early infection could be associated with a predominance of neutrophils
- Elevated protein concentration (usually <150 mg/dL)
- Glucose concentration is usually normal (>50% of blood value); moderately reduced values are seen occasionally with herpes simplex virus (HSV), mumps, and some enteroviruses
- Red cells are usually absent (in a nontraumatic tap); their presence suggests HSV-1 infection or other necrotizing encephalitides

Treatment

Bacterial meningitis is a potentially life-threatening condition. Delay in the administration of antibacterial medication is associated with a worse prognosis. When bacterial meningitis is suspected, therapy should be started as soon as possible, and not delayed by awaiting the results of CSF analysis. An antibiotic should be chosen based on the specific type of causative bacterial agent. While awaiting CSF culture results (which can require up to 48 hours), empiric therapy that treats the most common causes of bacterial meningitis should be administered. The mainstay of treatment is a cephalosporin, such as ceftriaxone or cefotaxime, as well as additional gram-positive coverage with vancomycin, given increasing cephalosporin resistance. Chloramphenicol plus ampicillin has also been found to be effective.[40] In patients who are 50 years or older, as well as the immunocompromised, ampicillin should be added to cover *L monocytogenes*. The key to effective treatment of bacterial meningitis is timely and adequate penetration of the blood-brain barrier and meninges. Not all antibiotics have sufficient CSF penetration.

Adjuvant treatment with corticosteroids such as dexamethasone or an equivalent has been shown to be beneficial, particularly in cases of pneumococcal meningitis. Some studies have shown, for example, that the incidence of hearing loss, short-term neurologic sequelae, and even death is decreased when a corticosteroid is given. It is recommended that the corticosteroid be given just before the first dose of antibiotic, and continued for 4 days.[40] The presumed mechanism is suppression of inflammation.

Prognosis

Untreated bacterial meningitis is almost always fatal when antibiotics are not administered, whereas viral meningitis tends to resolve spontaneously with supportive management. Prognosis is determined by the patient's age, the presence of comorbidities, and the length of time for the pathogen to be cleared from the CSF. A poorer prognosis is associated with more severe illness, decreased level of consciousness, abnormally low number of WBCs in the CSF, and delayed antibiotic administration. Meningitis caused by *H influenzae* and meningococci carries a better prognosis than cases caused by group B streptococci, coliforms, and *S pneumoniae*.[61,62]

SPINAL EPIDURAL ABSCESS

Spinal epidural abscess (SEA) is a rare disorder of the CNS. Although it accounts for fewer than 2 per 10,000 hospital admissions, the incidence of SEA has been climbing over the past 2 decades.[63,64] Multiple theories have been postulated to explain the increase in SEA, including growth in the number of patients undergoing neurosurgical procedures and surges in intravenous drug use (IVDU).[65]

Pathophysiology

The spinal epidural space becomes infected in the same manner as intracranial suppurative processes. Inoculation arises from hematogenous spread, local extension, or direct implantation. Hematogenous seeding is the most common method of translocation, accounting for nearly 50% of SEA cases.[66] The skin and soft tissue are frequently the primary sites of infection. In approximately 30% of cases, local extension occurs and can arise from an abscess of the psoas muscle, an infected vertebral body, or an inflamed disk.[65,67] The remaining cases are secondary to direct implantation. Regardless of the mechanism of infection, the focal infection typically encompasses 3 to 5 segments of the spinal cord.[68] Patients with diabetes, alcoholism, IVDU, immunosuppression, chronic renal failure, or a history of undergoing a neurosurgical procedure, as well as the elderly have an increased risk for SEA.[64,69]

Clinical Presentation

Patients with SEA most commonly complain of back pain, which accompanies up to 90% of cases.[70] The classic triad of fever, back pain, and neurologic deficit is present in less than 20% of patients, but fever has been documented in up to 70% of cases.[68] Spinal tenderness to palpation and focal neurologic deficit have been observed in approximately 30% of patients.[66,70]

Diagnosis

The diagnosis of SEA is confirmed by neuroimaging. Gadolinium-enhanced magnetic resonance imaging (MRI) offers the greatest sensitivity and specificity, and is therefore the preferred choice for imaging.[68,70] If MRI is contraindicated, CT myelography can be performed instead. Laboratory testing is expected to reveal leukocytosis and an elevated erythrocyte sedimentation rate, although neither test is specific for SEA.[69]

Treatment

SEA requires immediate neurosurgical consultation. Surgical decompression must be completed promptly to prevent impending neurologic decline. Antibiotics should be started empirically based on the likely culprits. *Staphylococcus aureus* is the causative agent in the majority (60%–90%) of cases.[67] Initial antibiotic coverage should be broad spectrum, so vancomycin, metronidazole, and a third- or fourth-generation cephalosporin are first-line therapy for the treatment of SEA.[65]

INTRACRANIAL SUPPURATIVE DISEASE

Intracranial suppurative disease can occur in the form of abscess or empyema. An abscess is a discrete collection of purulence surrounded by a capsule. Intracranial abscesses are found primarily in the brain parenchyma or within the epidural space (**Fig. 3**).[71,72] An empyema is a less-localized collection of purulent material, most commonly found between the dura mater and arachnoid mater (ie, the subdural space).[71] Although intracranial suppurative disorders are rare, they are life threatening and are often initially missed. Therefore, a high index of suspicion is necessary to make the appropriate diagnosis.

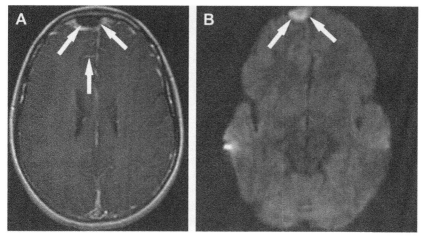

Fig. 3. (*A, B*) Intracranial epidural abscess. A 15-year-old girl who was taking oral antibiotics for acute sinusitis experienced a rapid decline in her clinical status over the course of 12 hours. Magnetic resonance imaging studies revealed an epidural abscess (*arrows*). (*From* Hoxworth JM, Glastonbury CM. Orbital and intracranial complications of acute sinusitis. Neuroimaging Clin N Am 2010;20:511–26; with permission.)

Pathophysiology

Intracranial suppurative disease occurs by 1 of 3 mechanisms: hematogenous spread, local extension, or direct implantation.[73] Hematogenous spread usually gives rise to multiple brain abscesses and can originate from remote sites such as intra-abdominal, pulmonary, or cardiac sources.[74] The lesions are typically found in territories supplied by the middle cerebral artery. Infectious spread from nearby structures can arise from complications of sinusitis, dental infection, or otitis media.[75–85] Direct implantation can be caused by indwelling neurosurgical hardware, such as a halo device, or penetrating trauma.[86]

Clinical Presentation

The presentation of intracranial suppurative disease is variable and depends on the number, location, and size of the lesions. Headache is the most common symptom, and fever is usually present but might be absent.[71,87] The nature of the neurologic examination depends on the anatomic location of the lesions.

Epidural abscesses tend to have an indolent course because of the confined nature of infection.[76] The epidural space is tightly contained between the calvarium and the dura mater; an insidious onset of headache and fever points to this disease. Alternatively, a subdural empyema can present with a rapidly progressive course because purulent material flows freely into the subdural space. Without the natural barrier present in the epidural space, the purulent collection will give rise to focal deficits as well as meningeal signs and increased intracranial pressure.[76] A solitary brain abscess can have a slowly progressive course similar to that of an epidural abscess, but it can also be accompanied by signs of elevated intracranial pressure, focal deficits, and seizures. Multiple processes can occur simultaneously: patients could have an empyema with concomitant abscess. Patients with an intracranial suppurative process might have normal results on neurologic examination, so the clinician should not dismiss the possibility of infection based merely on a lack of physical findings.

Diagnosis

The diagnosis of intracranial suppurative disease is confirmed by neuroimaging. Contrast-enhanced CT of the brain allows visualization of ring-enhancing masses and fluid collections. However, MRI is more sensitive and can be used when clinically appropriate.[88] In the emergent setting, the more practical initial imaging tool is contrast-enhanced CT, because of its shorter time to completion and greater availability.

Treatment

Intracranial suppuration is a neurosurgical emergency. Antibiotic therapy is directed toward likely causative agents, and should be started immediately. In the setting of trauma or an indwelling neurologic device, *S aureus* is most common. Patients with risk factors for an odontogenic or otorhinolaryngeal source of infection require treatment with coverage against anaerobes such as *Bacteroides*, *Fusobacterium*, *Actinomyces*, and anaerobic streptococci. Seeding from remote sites warrants treatment against *Streptococcus anginosus* (formerly *Streptococcus milleri*), *Streptococcus viridans*, enteric gram-negative bacilli, and anaerobes such as *Bacteroides*, *Peptostreptococcus*, *Actinomyces*, and *Fusobacterium* (**Table 4**).[64,74,89,90] A neurosurgeon should be consulted immediately to evaluate the strategy for drainage. Antiepileptics should not be administered unless the patient is actively seizing or has provided a history of seizure, or unless the consulting neurosurgeon or neurologist advises prophylaxis.

BOTULISM

Botulism is a rare, but potentially lethal, toxin-mediated condition that affects the neuromuscular junction. About 145 cases are reported annually in the United States, the majority of which (65%) are infantile botulism. Botulism is caused by the toxin produced by the anaerobic, spore-forming bacterium *Clostridium botulinum*.[91,92]

Pathophysiology

The toxin binds irreversibly to the presynaptic membrane of nerves, resulting in the inhibition of acetylcholine release at the peripheral nerve synapse. The cholinergic synapses of the cranial nerves, autonomic nerves, and neuromuscular junctions are affected predominantly, resulting in cranial nerve palsies, parasympathetic blockade, and descending flaccid paralysis, respectively. Once affected by the toxin, the nerve is permanently damaged; recovery requires time for axonal regeneration and formation of new synapses.[93]

Clinical Presentation

Botulism causes descending, symmetric, flaccid paralysis, which can progress to respiratory failure. Cranial nerves tend to be affected first, resulting in diplopia, dysarthria, dysphagia, and vertigo.[91] The upper extremities and proximal muscles are affected more than the lower extremities and more distal muscles.[92] Although 14% of patients subjectively report paresthesias, botulism causes no sensory loss or pain. Patients often present with anticholinergic symptoms such as constipation, urinary retention, dry skin and mucous membranes, fever, and postural dizziness.[94]

Types of Botulism

Some infants with botulism have ingested honey, corn syrup, soil, or vacuum-cleaner dust, but often the source is never discovered. The spores that they ingest are able to germinate and produce toxin in the high-pH environment of the intestinal tract in

Table 4
Antimicrobial therapy for intracranial suppurative infections

Clinical Setting	Pathogen	Antibiotic Regimen
Local Extension		
Odontogenic infection (often polymicrobial)	Anaerobes (*Fusobacterium, Actinomyces, Bacteroides, Prevotella* spp), streptococci	Cefotaxime, 2 g IV every 6 h, and metronidazole, 500 mg IV every 6 h
Otogenic infection	Streptococci, anaerobes (*Bacteroides, Prevotella* spp), aerobic gram-negative bacilli (*Proteus, Klebsiella, Pseudomonas, Haemophilus* spp)	Cefotaxime, 2 g IV every 6 h, and metronidazole, 500 mg IV every 6 h
Paranasal sinusitis (often polymicrobial)	Streptococci, anaerobes (*Bacteroides, Fusobacterium, Peptostreptococcus* spp), aerobic gram-negative bacilli (*Haemophilus, Klebsiella* spp), *Staphylococcus aureus*	Cefotaxime, 2 g IV every 6 h, and metronidazole, 500 mg IV every 6 h
Direct Implantation		
Recent neurosurgical procedure	*S aureus*	Vancomycin, 15 mg/kg IV every 12 h, cefepime, 2 g IV every 8 h, and metronidazole, 500 mg IV every 6 h
Penetrating trauma	*S aureus*	Vancomycin, 15 mg/kg IV every 12 h, ceftazidime, 2 g IV every 8 h, and metronidazole, 500 mg IV every 6 h
Hematogenous Spread		
Urinary tract infection	Enteric gram-negative bacilli (*Bacteroides* spp)	Cefotaxime, 2 g IV every 6 h, and metronidazole, 500 mg IV every 6 h
Endocarditis	*Streptococcus viridans, S aureus,* enterococcus	Vancomycin, 15 mg/kg IV every 12 h, cefotaxime, 2 g IV every 6 h, and metronidazole, 500 mg IV every 6 h
Pulmonary infection	Streptococci, anaerobes (*Fusobacterium, Prevotella, Bacteroides, Actinomyces* spp), *Nocardia*	Cefotaxime, 2 g IV every 6 h, and metronidazole, 500 mg IV every 6 h
Intra-abdominal infection	Enteric gram-negative bacilli (*Bacteroides* spp), anaerobes (*Peptostreptococcus, Veillonella, Actinomyces, Propionibacterium* spp), *Enterococcus*	Vancomycin, 15 mg/kg IV every 12 h, cefotaxime, 2 g IV every 6 h, and metronidazole, 500 mg IV every 6 h

Abbreviation: IV, intravenously.
Data from Refs.[64,73,74,87,89,90]

infants. Spores are not active in the intestines of adults because of the lower pH and the presence of gut flora.[95] Infantile botulism typically causes constipation, poor feeding, lethargy, a weak cry, hypotonia, and respiratory failure (in 50% of cases) (**Fig. 4**).[92]

A food-borne bacterium accounts for 15% of botulism cases. This type of botulism emerges within 6 to 48 hours after a preformed toxin (rather than the spores or live bacteria) is ingested. The toxin is heat labile and can survive at temperatures of up to 85°C, but is not destroyed by digestive enzymes. Food contaminated with the toxin can appear and taste normal, or might exhibit signs of spoilage.[95,96] Symptoms include nausea, vomiting, abdominal cramping, diarrhea, or constipation in 50% of cases. Neurologic symptoms can begin at the same time as the gastrointestinal symptoms; their onset can also be delayed for a few days.

Twenty percent of botulism cases arise from a wound. This type of botulism has an incubation period of 4 to 14 days, during which toxin is produced within the wound. IVDU is the most common cause of wound botulism. Wounds directly inoculated with *C botulinum* spores can also become infected (**Fig. 5**).[93,94]

Iatrogenic botulism occurs when patients are injected intentionally with botulinum toxin to treat movement disorders such as dystonia or for cosmetic purposes. This type of exposure can inadvertently cause generalized or focal weakness.

Given that the botulinum toxin is highly toxic and easy to produce, it makes an ideal weapon of bioterrorism. Aerosolized botulinum toxin can be absorbed systemically through the respiratory tract. An intravenous dose as small as 0.09 to 0.15 μg or inhalation of 0.7 to 0.9 μg can cause death in a 70-kg human. Affected people would be expected to go to an ED within 12 to 72 hours after exposure.[96–98]

Diagnosis

Botulism is primarily a clinical diagnosis. The clinician should have a high index of suspicion for it when assessing a patient with symmetric, descending, flaccid paralysis. In adults, the "4 Ds" of botulism are often present: dry mouth, diplopia, dysphagia, and dysarthria. Other key findings include nausea, vomiting, and dilated and fixed pupils.

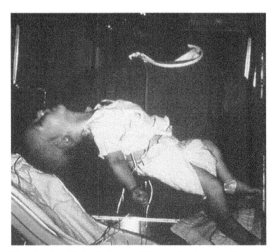

Fig. 4. A 6-week-old infant with botulism, with marked loss of muscle tone, particularly in the head and neck region. (*From* CDC Public Health Image Library. Available at http:// phil.cdc.gov/phil/home.asp.)

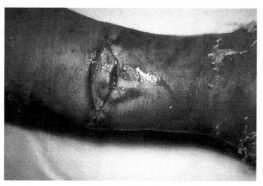

Fig. 5. Wound botulism in a 14-year-old boy who fractured his right ulna and radius. (*From* CDC Public Health Image Library. Available at http://phil.cdc.gov/phil/home.asp.)

Diagnostic laboratory testing includes checking the serum and stool for the presence of botulinum toxin. Other diseases might be excluded by checking the CSF for infection and protein elevation, by conducting Tensilon testing for myasthenia gravis (which may be minimally positive in botulism), and by performing neuroimaging to rule out focal brain and spine lesions or abnormalities.[91] Other diagnostic tests to consider include serial measurement of vital capacity to detect deteriorating ventilator status, and electromyography to determine muscle action potential by repetitively stimulating the nerve.[93,94,96] However, a normal electromyogram does not exclude the diagnosis.

Treatment

Management of botulism consists of several approaches. First, the airway must be stabilized. Early endotracheal intubation is encouraged if the patient's vital capacity is less than 12 mL/kg. In some cases, mechanical ventilation is performed while the toxin wears off (over the course of 2–8 weeks). Supportive management such as nasogastric suctioning to treat ileus or bladder catheterization to treat urinary retention might be helpful. Decontamination of the intestines with saline enemas or cathartics is also suggested, although this practice should be avoided if an ileus has developed. Magnesium-containing cathartics should be avoided, because hypermagnesemia exacerbates muscle weakness.[93,94,96]

Equine trivalent antibotulism toxin can be obtained from the Centers of Disease Control and Prevention (CDC) or the state health department. In patients with suspected botulism, one vial (10 mL) is diluted with 0.9% saline in a 1:10 ratio and administered slowly intravenously. Before receiving the antitoxin, patients should have skin testing done to determine if they are hypersensitive to it. The health care provider should also ascertain whether the patient has a history of asthma or hay fever or develops distress when in proximity to horses, because these individuals could develop serious anaphylactic reactions. The antitoxin should not be used in cases of infantile botulism, because it has not been found to be efficient and is associated with an increased risk of anaphylaxis. The antitoxin shortens the disease course and prevents progression of paralysis, but does not reverse it. Wounds that are infected with *C botulinum* should be debrided after the antitoxin is administered. Human botulism immunoglobulin can also be administered, as it decreases length of hospitalization and mechanical ventilation. Administration of anticholinesterases and antibiotics has not been found to be effective. In fact, tetracyclines and aminoglycosides have been shown to impair neuron calcium entry, which actually exacerbates the effects of botulinum toxin.

Disposition and Prognosis

All suspected and confirmed cases of botulism must be reported to the hospital epidemiologist or infection control practitioner, local and state health departments, or the CDC. These patients should be admitted to the intensive care unit. Respiratory failure and death caused by muscle weakness and aspiration pneumonia resulting from the loss of airway protective reflexes are potential major complications. The overall mortality rate associated with botulism is 8%, although patients' prognosis has improved significantly in recent years with advances in treatment.[92] Recovery requires the regeneration of neuromuscular connections. Muscle strength and endurance might not fully return to normal for up to 1 year.

INTRACRANIAL SHUNTS
Shunt Devices

CSF shunts are used to divert excess fluid associated with hydrocephalus away from the brain and to a different part of the body, where it is then absorbed. The proximal portion of the shunt catheter is typically placed in one of the cerebral ventricles, but it can also be placed in an intracranial cyst of the lumbar subarachnoid space. The distal portion of the catheter can be internalized, typically in the peritoneum (ie, a ventriculoperitoneal [VP] shunt) or vascular space (ie, a ventriculoatrial [VA] shunt), or externalized into a drain (**Fig. 6**). The externalized configuration is sometimes used temporarily in patients with acute hydrocephalus to monitor and decrease intracranial pressure. This type of device can also be placed for interim antibiotic treatment of infected internal devices.

Any of these devices can become infected and cause fever. Internalized shunt devices become infected at rates ranging from 5% to 15%. Rates of infection among externalized devices are lower, at 5% to 10%.[97] Risk factors for shunt infection are listed in **Box 2**.

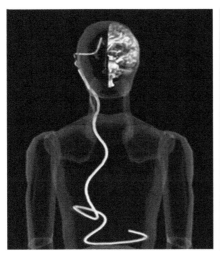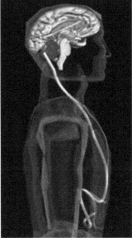

Fig. 6. Front and side views of ventriculoperitoneal shunt.

| **Box 2** |
| **Risk factors for shunt infection** |

- Recent placement of the device (ie, within the past month)
- Serial shunt revisions
- Revision of the device following treatment of shunt infection
- Intraventricular hemorrhage
- Subarachnoid hemorrhage
- Cranial fracture with CSF leak
- Craniotomy
- Ventriculostomy catheter irrigation
- Duration of catheterization (higher risk if device has been in place for >3 days)

Pathophysiology

Shunt infections frequently result from colonization of the proximal end of the device with flora from the overlying or adjacent skin. Early shunt infections are common, occurring at the time of surgery or postoperatively. The pathogen most commonly associated with shunt infections is *Staphylococcus*. Approximately half of all shunt infections are caused by coagulase-negative staphylococci, and *S aureus* is the culprit in about one-third of cases. Other associated pathogens might include diphtheroids such as *Propionibacterium acnes* and *Corynebacterium jeikeium*.[99]

The distal end of the shunt catheter can become contaminated directly or via hematogenous seeding. For example, distal-end VP shunt infections can result from bowel perforation or peritonitis. Infections of externalized devices tend to result from catheter irrigation or tracking of microorganisms along the exit site. These infections tend to occur months after shunt placement and can involve a variety of organisms, such as streptococci, gram-negative bacteria such as *Pseudomonas aeruginosa*, anaerobes, mycobacteria, and fungi.

Clinical Presentation

Although some patients with shunt infections present with fever, others have few or no symptoms at all. In some cases, symptoms develop only after the infection has led to shunt obstruction and subsequent malfunction. Shunt malfunction can produce clinical symptoms of increased intracranial pressure such as nausea, vomiting, headache, lethargy, and altered mental status. Meningeal symptoms might be absent, because there is no communication between the ventricles and meninges when a shunt is present. Common symptoms of distal catheter infection are listed in **Table 5**.

Diagnosis

If a shunt infection is suspected, a diagnostic evaluation (CSF analysis and blood culture) should be performed and imaging should be obtained. CSF should be obtained by direct aspiration of the shunt, when possible, rather than via ventricular aspiration or lumbar puncture. A cell count with differential, glucose and protein concentrations, Gram stain, and culture should be obtained from the CSF.

Interpretation of CSF parameters in the setting of a shunt infection can be challenging. No single laboratory parameter can reliably predict or exclude a shunt infection.[100] Infections related to CNS devices typically induce less inflammation than does

Table 5
Common symptoms of distal catheter infection

Device	Symptoms of Infection
Ventriculoperitoneal shunt	Peritonitis: fever, abdominal pain, anorexia; large loculated pockets of poorly absorbed CSF in the peritoneum
Ventriculoatrial shunt	Fever; bloodstream infection resulting from hematogenous spread of infected CSF or an infected thrombus at the catheter tip; endocarditis and associated sequelae such as septic pulmonary emboli; antibody-mediated sequelae such as glomerulonephritis and dermatologic manifestations
Distal external shunt	Soft-tissue infection: erythema, focal tenderness, purulent drainage, swelling, warmth

bacterial meningitis; therefore, cell-count abnormalities tend to be less pronounced, more subtle, and difficult to differentiate from postoperative inflammation. The WBC count differential might be useful in determining whether infection is present.[101,102] One report found that a WBC count differential with more than 10% neutrophils was 90% sensitive for predicting infection. The presence of eosinophils in CSF is rare and is more likely related to inflammation due to shunt malfunction rather than infection. CSF culture is critical for identifying a causative organism and directing antibiotic treatment. In cases where there is concern for false-positive cultures, antibiotic therapy should be started empirically and the CSF culture analysis repeated.

Blood cultures should be obtained when a shunt infection is suspected. The yield of such analysis is much higher in patients with VA shunts than in those with VP shunts. In one series it was reported that positive blood cultures were associated with shunt infections in 95% of VA cases versus 23% of VP cases.[103,104]

Imaging might also be helpful when shunt infection is suspected. Brain imaging might reveal signs of ventriculitis or CSF obstruction (**Fig. 7**). Radiographs of the shunt can reveal kinking and coiling of the catheter. Abdominal imaging via CT or ultrasonography may reveal loculations of CSF at the distal ends of VP shunts.

Treatment

Treatment of shunt infections should include removal of the device, external drainage, administration of parenteral antibiotic therapy, and shunt replacement

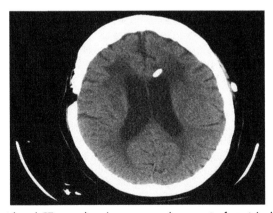

Fig. 7. Noncontrast head CT scan showing proper placement of ventriculoperitoneal shunt catheter within ventricle.

Table 6
Antibiotic therapy cocktails for shunt infections

Adults	Vancomycin plus gram-negative coverage (eg, ceftazidime, cefepime, meropenem)
Children	Vancomycin plus gram-negative coverage (eg, ceftazidime, cefepime, meropenem)
Methicillin-sensitive pathogens	Adjunctive nafcillin
Complicated cases of resistance	Adjunctive oral rifampin
Other adjunctive therapies	Oral rifampin, quinupristin-dalfopristin, gentamicin, tobramycin

once the CSF becomes sterile again. The length of time that the CSF should be sterile before replacement of the device varies, based on the type of contaminating organism. If removal of the device is not feasible, intraventricular antibiotic administration can be useful. The antibiotic therapy should be chosen based on the CSF Gram stain and culture reports. Pending these results, vancomycin plus antibiotic coverage for gram-negative pathogens can be started empirically. Suggested empiric therapy for various groups is presented in **Table 6**.[105] Once the culture results and associated antibiotic susceptibilities are available, therapy should be tailored accordingly.

No randomized trials on intraventricular antibiotic administration have been conducted. Because they are potentially toxic, intraventricular antibiotics should be reserved for circumstances wherein the conventional route of intravenous therapy has failed to sterilize the CSF. When it is not feasible to remove a shunt device, intraventricular antibiotics can be used additionally as a last alternative. The duration of antibiotic therapy is summarized in **Box 3**.

Patients with shunts are at increased risk for intracranial infections, which can lead to long-term cognitive defects and neurologic problems.[106] These patients may present with fever and other clinical manifestations such as nausea, vomiting, and meningismus. CSF analysis should be conducted to confirm the presence of shunt infection. Once confirmed, these patients should be admitted to the hospital to receive parenteral antibiotic therapy providing gram-positive and gram-negative coverage. If suspicion for shunt infection is moderate to high, empiric antibiotic coverage should be started while awaiting the results of CSF analysis.

Box 3
Duration of antibiotic therapy for patients with infected ventricular shunts

Coagulase-negative staphylococci plus abnormal CSF studies

- Administer for as long as the contaminated device is in place, plus 1 additional week following its removal

Staphylococcus aureus

- Administer for at least 10 days

Gram-negative bacilli

- Administer for 14 to 21 days

Contaminated device not removed

- Administer for at least 7 to 10 days after CSF becomes sterile

REFERENCES

1. Smith J, Seirafi J. Delirium and dementia. In: Marx JA, Hockberger RS, Walls RM, et al, editors. Rosen's emergency medicine: concepts and clinical practice. 7th edition. Philadelphia: Mosby Elsevier; 2009. p. 1367–78.
2. Huff JS. Altered mental status and coma. In: Tintinalli JE, Stapczynski JS, Cline DM, et al, editors. Tintinalli's emergency medicine: a comprehensive study guide. 7th edition. New York: McGraw-Hill; 2011. p. 1135–42.
3. D'Onofrio G, Jauch E, Jagoda A, et al. NIH roundtable on opportunities to advance research on neurologic and psychiatric emergencies. Ann Emerg Med 2010;56:551–64.
4. Barron EA, Holmes J. Delirium within the emergency care setting, occurrence and detection: a systematic review. Emerg Med J 2013;30:263–8.
5. Hustey FM, Meldon SW. The prevalence and documentation of impaired mental status in elderly emergency department patients. Ann Emerg Med 2002;39:248–53.
6. Élie M, Rousseau F, Cole M, et al. Prevalence and detection of delirium in elderly emergency department patients. CMAJ 2000;163:977–81.
7. Hustey FM, Meldon SW, Smith MD, et al. The effect of mental status screening on the care of elderly emergency department patients. Ann Emerg Med 2003;41:678–84.
8. Han JH, Zimmerman EE, Cutler N, et al. Delirium in older emergency department patients: recognition, risk factors, and psychomotor subtypes. Acad Emerg Med 2009;16:193–200.
9. Han JH, Eden S, Shintani A, et al. Delirium in older emergency department patients is an independent predictor of hospital length of stay. Acad Emerg Med 2011;18:451–7.
10. Han JH, Shintani A, Eden S, et al. Delirium in the emergency department: and independent predictor of death within 6 months. Ann Emerg Med 2010;56:244–52.
11. Milbrandt EB, Deppen S, Harrison PL, et al. Costs associated with delirium in mechanically ventilated patients. Crit Care Med 2004;32:955–62.
12. Gower LE, Gatewood MO, Kang CS. Emergency department management of delirium in the elderly. West J Emerg Med 2012;13:194–201.
13. Han JH, Wilson A, Ely EW. Delirium in the older emergency department patient: a quiet epidemic. Emerg Med Clin North Am 2010;28:611–31.
14. Miller MO. Evaluation and management of delirium in hospitalized older patients. Am Fam Physician 2008;78:1265–70.
15. Meagher DJ, Trzepacz PT. Motoric subtypes of delirium. Semin Clin Neuropsychiatry 2000;5:75–85.
16. Carpenter CR. Does this patient have dementia? Ann Emerg Med 2008;52:554–6.
17. Stair TO, Morrissey J, Jaradeh I, et al. Validation of the Quick Confusion Scale for mental status screening in the emergency department. Intern Emerg Med 2007;2:130–2.
18. Sanders AB. Mental status assessment in emergency medicine. Intern Emerg Med 2007;2:116–8.
19. Carpenter CR, DesPain B, Keeling TN, et al. The Six-Item Screener and AD8 for the detection of cognitive impairment in geriatric emergency department patients. Ann Emerg Med 2011;57:653–61.
20. Alici-Evcimen Y, Breitbart W. An update on the use of antipsychotics in the treatment of delirium. Palliat Support Care 2008;6:177–82.

21. Nassisi D, Okuda Y. ED management of delirium and agitation. Emerg Med Pract 2007;9:1–20.
22. George JN. Evaluation and management of patients with thrombotic thrombocytopenic purpura. J Intensive Care Med 2007;22:82–91.
23. Park YA, Poisson JL, McBee MT, et al. Seasonal association of thrombotic thrombocytopenic purpura. Transfusion 2012;52:1530–4.
24. Muñiz AE, Barbee RW. Thrombotic thrombocytopenic purpura (TTP) presenting as pancreatitis. J Emerg Med 2003;24:407–11.
25. Stead LG, Lock BG. Thrombocytopenia and altered mental status in an HIV positive woman. J Emerg Med 2002;22:367–9.
26. Scott SB. Emergency department management of hematologic and oncologic complications in the patient infected with HIV. Emerg Med Clin North Am 2010;28:325–33.
27. Stella CL, Dacus J, Guzman E, et al. The diagnostic dilemma of thrombotic thrombocytopenic purpura/hemolytic uremic syndrome in the obstetric triage and emergency department: lessons from 4 tertiary hospitals. Am J Obstet Gynecol 2009;200:381.e1–6.
28. Klap PC, Hemphill RR. Acquired hemolytic anemia. In: Tintinalli JE, Stapczynski JS, Cline DM, et al, editors. Tintinalli's emergency medicine: a comprehensive study guide. 7th edition. New York: McGraw-Hill; 2011. p. 1488–93.
29. Janz TG, Hamilton GC. Disorders of hemostasis. In: Marx JA, Hockberger RS, Walls RM, et al, editors. Rosen's emergency medicine: concepts and clinical practice. 6th edition. Philadelphia: Mosby Elsevier; 2006. p. 1892–906.
30. George JN. How I treat patients with thrombotic thrombocytopenic purpura: 2010. Blood 2010;116:4060–9.
31. Sarode R. Atypical presentations of thrombotic thrombocytopenic purpura: a review. J Clin Apher 2009;24:47–52.
32. Kessler CS, Khan BA, Lai-Miller K. Thrombotic thrombocytopenic purpura: a hematological emergency. J Emerg Med 2012;43:538–44.
33. Scully M, Hunt BJ, Benjamin S, et al, on behalf of British Committee for Standards in Haematology. Guidelines on the diagnosis and management of thrombotic thrombocytopenic purpura and other thrombotic microangiopathies. Br J Haematol 2012;158:323–35.
34. Centers for Disease Control and Prevention. Injury prevention and control: traumatic brain injury. Available at: www.cdc.gov/traumaticbraininjury. Accessed April 1, 2013.
35. Thompson HJ, Tkacs NC, Saatman KE, et al. Hyperthermia following traumatic brain injury: a critical evaluation. Neurobiol Dis 2003;12(3):163–73.
36. MacKenzie MA, Pieters GF, Hermus AR. The neurologic basis of fever [letter to the editor]. N Engl J Med 1944;331(19):1308.
37. Boulant JA. Role of the preoptic-anterior hypothalamus in thermoregulation and fever. Clin Infect Dis 2000;31(Suppl 5):S157–61.
38. Won SJ, Lin MT. 5-Hydroxytryptamine receptors in the hypothalamus mediate thermoregulatory responses in rabbits. Naunyn Schmiedebergs Arch Pharmacol 1988;338(3):256–61.
39. Thompson HJ, Pinto-Martin J, Bullock MR. Neurogenic fever after traumatic brain injury: an epidemiological study. J Neurol Neurosurg Psychiatry 2003;74:614–9.
40. Tunkel AR. Clinical features and diagnosis of acute bacterial meningitis in adults. UpToDate. Available at: www.uptodate.com/contents/clinical-features-and-diagnosis-of-acute-bacterial-meningitis-in-adults?source=search_result&;search=meningitis&selectedTitle=1~150. Accessed April 1, 2013.

41. Durand ML, Calderwood SB, Weber DJ, et al. Acute bacterial meningitis in adults: a review of 493 episodes. N Engl J Med 1993;328(1):21–8.

42. de Gans J, van de Beek D, European Dexamethasone in Adulthood Bacterial Meningitis Study Investigators. Dexamethasone in adults with bacterial meningitis. N Engl J Med 2002;347(20):1549–56.

43. Attia J, Hatala R, Cook DJ, et al. The rational clinical examination: does this adult patient have acute meningitis? JAMA 1999;282:175–81.

44. Domingo P, Mancebo J, Blanch L, et al. Fever in adult patients with acute bacterial meningitis. J Infect Dis 1988;158(2):496.

45. Hasbun R, Abrahams J, Jekel J, et al. Computed tomography of the head before lumbar puncture in adults with suspected meningitis. N Engl J Med 2001; 345(24):1727–33.

46. Joffe AR. Lumbar puncture and brain herniation in acute bacterial meningitis: a review. J Intensive Care Med 2007;22(4):194–207.

47. Tunkel AR, Hartman BJ, Kaplan SL, et al. Practice guidelines for the management of bacterial meningitis. Clin Infect Dis 2004;39(9):1267–84.

48. Kanegaye JT, Soliemanzadeh P, Bradley JS. Lumbar puncture in pediatric bacterial meningitis: defining the time interval for recovery of cerebrospinal fluid pathogens after parenteral antibiotic pretreatment. Pediatrics 2001;108(5): 1169–74.

49. Talan DA, Hoffman JR, Yoshikawa TT, et al. Role of empiric parenteral antibiotics prior to lumbar puncture in suspected bacterial meningitis: state of the art. Rev Infect Dis 1988;10(2):365–76.

50. Huy NT, Thao NT, Diep DT, et al. Cerebrospinal fluid lactate concentration to distinguish bacterial from aseptic meningitis: a systemic review and meta-analysis. Crit Care 2010;14(6):R240.

51. Sakushima K, Hayashino Y, Kawaguchi T, et al. Diagnostic accuracy of cerebrospinal fluid lactate for differentiating bacterial meningitis from aseptic meningitis: a meta-analysis. J Infect 2011;62(4):255–62.

52. Spanos A, Harrell FE Jr, Durack DT. Differential diagnosis of acute meningitis: an analysis of the predictive value of initial observations. JAMA 1989;262:2700–7.

53. Fitch MT, van de Beek D. Emergency diagnosis and treatment of adult meningitis. Lancet Infect Dis 2007;7:191–200.

54. Negrini B, Kelleher KJ, Wald ER. Cerebrospinal fluid findings in aseptic versus bacterial meningitis. Pediatrics 2000;105:316–9.

55. Johnson RP, Gluckman SJ. Viral encephalitis in adults. Available at: www. uptodate.com/contents/viral-encephalitis-in-adults?source=search_result&; search=encephalitis&selectedTitle=1%7E150. Accessed April 1, 2013.

56. Torre D, Mancuso R, Ferrante P. Pathogenic mechanisms of meningitis/encephalitis caused by human herpesvirus-6 in immunocompetent adult patients. Clin Infect Dis 2005;41(3):422–3.

57. Isaacson E, Glaser CA, Forghani B, et al. Evidence of human herpesvirus 6 infection in 4 immunocompetent patients with encephalitis. Clin Infect Dis 2005;40(6):890–3.

58. Weinberg A, Li S, Palmer M, et al. Quantitative CSF PCR in Epstein-Barr virus infections of the central nervous system. Ann Neurol 2002;52(5):543–8.

59. Nash D, Mostashari F, Fine A, et al. The outbreak of West Nile virus infection in the New York City area in 1999. N Engl J Med 2001;344(24):1807–14.

60. Koskiniemi M, Piiparinen H, Rantalaiho T, et al. Acute central nervous system complications in varicella zoster virus infections. J Clin Virol 2002;25(3): 293–301.

61. van de Beek D, de Gans J, Tunkel AR, et al. Community-acquired bacterial meningitis in adults. N Engl J Med 2006;354(1):44–53.

62. Sáez-Llorens X, McCracken GH. Bacterial meningitis in children. Lancet 2003; 361(9375):2139–48.

63. Hlavin ML, Kaminski HJ, Ross JS, et al. Spinal epidural abscess: a 10-year perspective. Neurosurgery 1990;27:177–84.

64. Riddell J, Shuman EK. Epidemiology of central nervous system infection. Neuroimaging Clin N Am 2012;22:543–56.

65. Corwell BN. The emergency department evaluation, management, and treatment of back pain. Emerg Med Clin North Am 2010;28:811–39.

66. Pradilla G, Nagahama Y, Spivak AM, et al. Spinal epidural abscess: current diagnosis and management. Curr Infect Dis Rep 2010;12:484–91.

67. Ziai WC, Lewin JJ. Update in the diagnosis and management of central nervous system infections. Neurol Clin 2008;26:427–68.

68. Winters ME, Kluetz P, Zilberstein J. Back pain emergencies. Med Clin North Am 2006;90:505–23.

69. Perron AD, Huff JS. Spinal cord disorders. In: Marx JA, Hockberger RS, Walls RM, et al, editors. Rosen's emergency medicine: concepts and clinical practice. 7th edition. Philadelphia: Mosby Elsevier; 2009. p. 1389–97.

70. Tompkins M, Panuncialman I, Lucas P, et al. Spinal epidural abscess. J Emerg Med 2010;39:384–90.

71. Gladstone J, Bigal ME. Headaches attributable to infectious diseases. Curr Pain Headache Rep 2010;14:299–308.

72. Nathoo N, Narotam PK, Nadvi S, et al. Taming an old enemy: a profile of intracranial suppuration. World Neurosurg 2012;77:484–90.

73. Loring KE, Tintinalli JE. Central nervous system and spinal infections. In: Tintinalli JE, Stapczynski JS, Cline DM, et al, editors. Tintinalli's emergency medicine: a comprehensive study guide. 7th edition. New York: McGraw-Hill; 2011. p. 1172–8.

74. Mace SE. Central nervous system infections as a cause of altered mental status? What is the pathogen growing in your central nervous system? Emerg Med Clin North Am 2010;28:535–70.

75. Hoxworth JM, Glastonbury CM. Orbital and intracranial complications of acute sinusitis. Neuroimaging Clin N Am 2010;20:511–26.

76. Osborn MK, Steinberg JP. Subdural empyema and other suppurative complications of paranasal sinusitis. Lancet Infect Dis 2007;7:62–7.

77. Bannon PD, McCormack RF. Pott's puffy tumor and epidural abscess arising from pansinusitis. J Emerg Med 2011;41:616–22.

78. Waseem M, Khan S, Bomann S. Subdural empyema complicating sinusitis. J Emerg Med 2008;35:277–81.

79. Bayonne E, Kania R, Tran P, et al. Intracranial complications of rhinosinusitis: a review, typical imaging data and algorithm of management. Rhinology 2009;47: 59–65.

80. DeMuri GP, Wald ER. Complications of acute bacterial sinusitis in children. Pediatr Infect Dis J 2011;30:701–2.

81. Calik M, Iscan A, Abuhandan M, et al. Masked subdural empyema secondary to frontal sinusitis. Am J Emerg Med 2012;30:1657.e1–4.

82. Hicks CW, Weber JG, Reid JR, et al. Identifying and managing intracranial complications of sinusitis in children. Pediatr Infect Dis J 2011;30:222–6.

83. Kanu OO, Ukponmwan E, Bankole O, et al. Intracranial epidural abscess of odontogenic origin. J Neurosurg Pediatr 2011;7:311–5.

84. Desai BK, Walls T. "Case files from the University of Florida: when an earache is more than an earache": a case report. Int J Emerg Med 2011;4:33.

85. Leskinen K, Jero J. Acute complications of otitis media in adults. Clin Otolaryngol 2005;30:511–6.

86. Gelalis ID, Christoforou G, Motsis E, et al. Brain abscess and generalized seizure caused by halo pin intracranial penetration: case report and review of the literature. Eur Spine J 2009;18:S172–5.

87. Derber CJ, Troy SB. Head and neck emergencies: bacterial meningitis, encephalitis, brain abscess, upper airway obstruction, and jugular septic thrombophlebitis. Med Clin North Am 2012;96:1107–26.

88. Rath TJ, Hughes M, Arabi M, et al. Imaging of cerebritis, encephalitis, and brain abscesses. Neuroimaging Clin N Am 2012;22:585–607.

89. Pruitt AA. Neurologic infectious disease emergencies. Neurol Clin 2012;30:129–59.

90. Beckham JD, Tyler KL. Neuro-intensive care of patients with acute CNS infections. Neurotherapeutics 2012;9:124–38.

91. Centers for Disease Control and Prevention. Botulism. Available at: www.cdc.gov/nczved/divisions/dfbmd/diseases/botulism. Accessed April 2, 2013.

92. Sobel J. Botulism. Clin Infect Dis 2005;41(8):1167–73.

93. Shearer P, Jagoda A. Neuromuscular disorders. In: Marx J, Hockberger R, Walls R, editors. Rosen's emergency medicine: concepts and clinical practice. Philadelphia: Mosby; 2009. p. 1415.

94. Fernandez-Frackelton M. Bacteria. In: Marx J, Hockberger R, Walls R, editors. Rosen's emergency medicine: concepts and clinical practice. Philadelphia: Mosby; 2009. p. 1686–9.

95. Asimos AW. Weakness: a systematic approach to acute, non-traumatic, neurologic and neuromuscular causes. Emerg Med Pract 2002;4(12):1–28.

96. Della-Giustina D, Knutson T. Peripheral neuropathies. Crit Decisions Emerg Med 2010;24(10):12–8.

97. Arnon SS, Schechter R, Inglesby TV, et al. Botulinum toxin as a biological weapon: medical and public health management. JAMA 2001;285(8):1059–70.

98. Bodour JM, Flynn PM, Fekete T. Infections of central nervous system shunts and other devices. Available at: www.uptodate.com/contents/infections-of-central-nervous-system-shunts-and-other-devices?source=search_result&;search=fever+and+shunts&selectedTitle=2%7E150. Accessed April 1, 2013.

99. McGirt MJ, Zaas A, Fuchs HE, et al. Risk factors for pediatric ventriculoperitoneal shunt infection and predictors of infectious pathogens. Clin Infect Dis 2003;36(7):858–62.

100. Meredith FT, Phillips HK, Reller LB. Clinical utility of broth cultures of cerebrospinal fluid from patients at risk for shunt infections. J Clin Microbiol 1997;35(12):3109–11.

101. Lan CC, Wong TT, Chen SJ, et al. Early diagnosis of ventriculoperitoneal shunt infections and malfunctions in children with hydrocephalus. J Microbiol Immunol Infect 2003;36(1):47–50.

102. McClinton D, Carraccio C, Englander R. Predictors of ventriculoperitoneal shunt pathology. Pediatr Infect Dis J 2001;20(6):593–7.

103. Forward KR, Fewer HD, Stiver HG. Cerebrospinal fluid shunt infections: a review of 35 infections in 32 patients. J Neurosurg 1983;59(3):389–94.

104. Schoenbaum SC, Gardner P, Shillito J. Infections of cerebrospinal fluid shunts: epidemiology, clinical manifestations, and therapy. J Infect Dis 1975;131(5):543–52.

105. Gombert ME, Landesman SH, Corrado ML, et al. Vancomycin and rifampin therapy for *Staphylococcus epidermidis* meningitis associated with CSF shunts: report of three cases. J Neurosurg 1981;55(4):633–6.
106. Liferidge AT, et al. Ventriculoperitoneal shunt infections. In: GEMSoft emergency medicine electronic textbook. Neurology Section. 2012.

Drug-Induced Hyperthermic Syndromes
Part I. Hyperthermia in Overdose

Bryan D. Hayes, PharmD[a,b,*], Joseph P. Martinez, MD[a],
Fermin Barrueto Jr, MD[a,c]

KEYWORDS

- Hyperthermia • Thermoregulatory system • Hypermetabolism • Sympathomimetics
- Cocaine • Methlenedioxymethamphetamine • Anticholinergics • Salicylates

KEY POINTS

- Drugs and natural compounds that affect the thermoregulatory system can induce or contribute to hyperthermia when used in excess.
- Hyperthermia associated with drug overdose is dangerous and potentially lethal.
- Appropriate treatment strategies such as cooling and the administration of counteractive medications are discussed.

Emergency physicians frequently manage patients with drug overdoses. When the ingested drug induces reactions that cause hyperthermia, the diagnostic process and treatment become particularly challenging. Although the terms fever and hyperthermia are commonly used interchangeably, they are not equivalent. Fever is the normal physiologic response to an inflammatory pyrogen, and hyperthermia is an elevated core body temperature.

Drugs and toxins that affect the thermoregulatory system can cause or contribute to hyperthermia through one of two mechanisms: increased production of heat or impaired ability to dissipate heat. The body is sensitive to temperature changes. Severe or prolonged hyperthermia can result in disseminated intravascular coagulopathy (DIC), delirium, rhabdomyolysis, and death.[1] This article discusses sympathomimetics,

Funding Sources: Nothing to disclose.
Conflict of Interest: Nothing to disclose.
[a] Department of Emergency Medicine, University of Maryland School of Medicine, 110 South Paca Street, Sixth Floor, Suite 200, Baltimore, MD 21201, USA; [b] Department of Pharmacy, University of Maryland Medical Center, 22 South Greene Street, Baltimore, MD 21201, USA; [c] Department of Emergency Medicine, Upper Chesapeake Health Systems, 500 Upper Chesapeake Drive, Bel Air, MD 21015, USA
* Corresponding author. Department of Pharmacy, University of Maryland Medical Center, 22 South Greene Street, Baltimore, MD 21201.
E-mail address: bhayes@umem.org

anticholinergics, uncouplers of oxidative phosphorylation, hypermetabolism caused by levothyroxine, and overdoses that induce seizure.

THE THERMOREGULATORY SYSTEM

Changes in thermoregulation are initiated in the brain and hypothalamus, and an expansive network of neurons feeds information back to the hypothalamus.[2] Heat-sensitive and cold-sensitive neurons are located in the hypothalamus, spinal cord, skin, vessels, and even viscera.[3] The human body's intrinsic core body temperature is typically maintained at 37°C (98.6°F), with a standard deviation of 0.4°C (0.8°F).[4] Core body temperature fluctuates in most people during a 24-hour period, and in women of child-bearing age depending on their point in the menstrual cycle.

The body's normal response to heat stress includes vasodilation in the skin in an attempt to dissipate heat. To increase blood flow to the skin, cardiac output must increase. Blood flow to the skin is increased by the diversion of cardiac output from the renal and splanchnic vessels.[5]

The anatomic physiology of thermoregulation is well understood, but the mechanism by which neurotransmitters assist with action potential propagation is not as clear. Neurotransmitters such as serotonin, acetylcholine, norepinephrine, dopamine, prostaglandins, and adrenocorticotropic hormone are all involved, but studies on the effects of individual neurotransmitters have not elucidated precise pathways. In the autonomic nervous system, for example, the postsynaptic neuron and the neurotransmitter that it secretes determine whether the neuron is part of the sympathetic or parasympathetic system. Norepinephrine is generally the sympathetic neurotransmitter and acetylcholine the parasympathetic neurotransmitter. One of the most notable exceptions to this rule is the sympathetic postganglionic neurons controlling the sweat glands that secrete acetylcholine,[6] which explains why a person perspires during a fight-or-flight (sympathetic or adrenergic) response. The perspiration dissipates the heat produced by increased motor movement and helps maintain temperature equilibrium.

Drugs and toxins that affect any part of this thermoregulatory system can cause or contribute to hyperthermia through one of two mechanisms: increased production of heat (eg, sympathomimetics) or impaired ability to dissipate heat (eg, anticholinergics). Heat can also be produced by uncouplers of oxidative phosphorylation, such as salicylates,[7] and drugs that induce a hypermetabolic state, such as levothyroxine.[8] A physical increase in musculoskeletal activity, as in psychomotor agitation[9] and seizures, can also increase heat production. Some of the most profound cases of hyperthermia are seen in syndromes and disease states that affect specific neuronal or metabolic pathways. For example, in malignant hyperthermia, a genetic disease, the defective ryanodine receptor[10] within the sarcoplasmic reticulum does not resequester intracellular calcium after the calcium-mediated actin-myosin filament contraction mechanism has been initiated.[11] This irregularity causes continued contractions of skeletal muscle, increased heat production, and severe hyperthermia, usually after the administration of succinylcholine and/or inhaled volatile anesthetics such as halothane or sevoflurane. Serotonin syndrome and neuroleptic malignant syndrome involve serotonergic and dopaminergic pathways, respectively, which lead to severe hyperthermia.[12]

SYMPATHOMIMETICS
Mechanisms of Hyperthermia

The adrenergic, or sympathetic, nervous system consists of neurons that secrete neurotransmitters that are agonists of α and/or β receptors. The α receptors are contained in the peripheral vasculature, typically inducing vasoconstriction when an agonist binds with them. Presynaptic α_2 receptors mediate a negative feedback inhibition loop, but peripheral α_2 receptors still cause vasoconstriction.[13] The β receptors have subtypes β_1, β_2, and β_3.[14] The β_1 receptors are generally located within the myocardium along with some β_2 receptors. The β_2 receptors are contained mainly in peripheral vasculature as well as smooth muscle. β_3 Receptors are contained within adipose.

Sympathomimetics are agonists at α and/or β receptors, or mimic these effects on the adrenergic system. This discussion focuses primarily on drugs that are agonists, with peripheral mention of other drugs that mimic positive adrenergic stimulation. These agonist drugs can stimulate the receptor either directly or indirectly. Some sympathomimetics have a mix of direct and indirect effects (**Table 1**). The mechanism by which they cause hyperthermia is multifactorial and depends, at least in part, on the type of sympathomimetic as well as its behavioral/psychotropic effects. Direct-acting α-receptor agents such as ergot alkaloids[15] cause hyperthermia through vasoconstriction and impaired cutaneous heat loss. Direct-acting β-specific agents such as albuterol typically do not cause hyperthermia, because they dilate the vessels. The indirect-acting and mixed agents have adrenergic effects and other effects related to behavioral response. Euphoria, psychomotor agitation, hallucinations, and blunted response to pain are seen with amphetamines,[16] cocaine,[17] phencyclidine,[18] methylenedioxymethamphetamine (MDMA),[19] and other amphetamine derivatives. The combination of adrenergic surge, response to external stimuli (hallucinations), and lack of pain perception can cause excessive psychomotor agitation, which leads to increased heat production and is often a contributing factor in the clinical presentation of these overdoses.

Agents that Produce Sympathomimetic Toxicity

Illicit sympathomimetic drugs can cause severe toxicity. Hyperthermia is one of the major effects that correlate with mortality. In a study from a medical examiner's office, Bohnert and colleagues[20] found that the number of deaths related to cocaine increased dramatically when the ambient temperature was higher than 24°C. The relationship between drug overdose and ambient temperature was most pronounced among cocaine users, suggesting a heightened deleterious effect of the sympathomimetic hyperthermic response when combined with elevated ambient temperature.

Table 1
Sympathomimetics that cause hyperthermia

Drug	Direct/Indirect/Mixed Sympathomimetic
Amphetamines	Indirect
Caffeine	Mixed
Cocaine	Indirect
Ephedrine	Mixed
Ergot alkaloids	Direct α
Midodrine	Direct α
MDMA (Ecstasy)	Mixed
MDPV (bath salts)	Mixed
Phencyclidine	Indirect
Phenylephrine	Mixed
Phenylpropanolamine	Mixed
Pseudoephedrine	Mixed

Abbreviations: MDMA, methylenedioxymethamphetamine; MDPV, methylenedioxypyrovalerone.

Although no study has extrapolated this association to other sympathomimetics, the biological mechanism of the other drugs is similar. Classified as a prototypical indirect sympathomimetic, cocaine works via noncompetitive reuptake inhibition of biogenic amines, and causes profound hypertension, tachycardia, diaphoresis, and psychomotor agitation.[17]

MDMA, an amphetamine derivative, has serotonergic effects that induce tactile hallucinations.[19] Abusers of MDMA also experience hypertension and tachycardia, but usually not to the extremes that cocaine can induce. Secondary to its serotonergic effect, MDMA can cause syndrome of inappropriate antidiuretic hormone secretion (SIADH), leading to confusion, headaches, and even death if hyponatremia and the resulting cerebral edema are severe.[21] Many amphetamines and other sympathomimetics have serotonergic effects and thus have the potential to cause SIADH, but MDMA has a larger propensity to cause this imbalance. Methamphetamine, or "Ice," is known for its sympathomimetic effects and prolonged psychotropic effects that lead to psychosis. Prolonged use over several days, known as "tweaking," can lead to a prolonged psychotic presentation.[22]

New designer drugs such as "bath salts" have been implicated in many visits to emergency departments. The producers of "bath salts" use this marketing term on labeling to avoid legal prosecution, and some packaging states that the product is "not for human consumption."[23] Most "bath salts" contain a cathinone-derived molecule, such as methylenedioxypyrovalerone (MDPV) or mephedrone, which acts like an amphetamine. The drug can be insufflated, taken orally, injected, or smoked. It is easily accessible through "head shops" and the Internet. Hyperthermia, psychomotor agitation, psychosis, and death have been reported after use of such agents.[23]

Clinical Presentation

The clinical presentation of sympathomimetic overdose is the adrenergic response of hypertension, tachycardia, psychomotor agitation, and subsequent hyperthermia. The hyperthermia is a consequence of impaired heat dissipation through α-mediated vasoconstriction and increased heat production resulting from psychomotor agitation and impaired pain response. The sympathomimetic toxidrome also includes dilated but reactive pupils (unlike anticholinergic effects, which cause nonreactive dilated pupils). The patient can deteriorate to tremors, psychosis, and seizures. Death is attributable to hyperthermia, seizure, or end-organ damage caused by the hyperadrenergic stimulation.[20]

Treatment

The cornerstone of the treatment of hyperthermia and the sympathomimetic toxidrome is the control of psychomotor agitation and adrenergic stimulation. Gaining control of the psychomotor agitation usually begins to normalize the hypertension, hyperthermia, and tachycardia. Medications that increase the central nervous system inhibitory tone, such as benzodiazepines, will calm the psychomotor agitation; these drugs must be titrated to the desired effect. The normalization of vital signs should be attempted first with a benzodiazepine. No single benzodiazepine has been found to be clinically more effective than another for a patient who is sympathomimetic; however, midazolam or diazepam will provide the desired pharmacokinetics, rapid onset, and ability to titrate to the clinical end point of controlling psychomotor agitation and normalizing vital signs.[23] In the specific case of sympathomimetic-induced myocardial infarction, cessation of chest pain should be another clinical end point.[24] If benzodiazepines and nitroglycerin fail, reversal of the vasoconstriction through the use of an α-receptor antagonist such as phentolamine might be necessary.[24] In severe cases, paralysis with a nondepolarizing agent such as vecuronium may be required to prevent further heat production and to control the psychomotor agitation. Care must be taken, because paralysis can mask seizure activity. Benzodiazepines should be given concurrently, as the patient might still be sympathomimetic and require further treatment despite being paralyzed.

Depending on the degree of hyperthermia and ability to control the agitation, if the initial treatment modalities are not effective, plans for passive and active cooling must be implemented. Hyperthermia can lead to permanent neuronal damage,[25] so the cooling process is time dependent. The placement of ice packs on the groin and axilla, and the use of cooling fans and misting are often attempted and are easy to perform, but are not typically effective. Because of more routine use of therapeutic induction of hypothermia following cardiac arrest,[26] many emergency departments now have access to other methods of actively cooling patients. Administration of cooled intravenous saline through a peripheral or central venous catheter is an easy and practical intervention. Cooling mattresses have become standard issue in the maintenance of therapeutic hypothermia.[26] A new device uses convection-immersion by rapidly circulating ice water from a perforated topsheet and an underblanket.[27] Complete submersion of the patient in a tub filled with chilled water and ice is highly effective though less practical. During the treatment of hyperthermia, clinical suspicion for occult trauma must be heightened because of its possible masking by agitation, behavioral changes, and impulsivity.

Nonsteroidal anti-inflammatory drugs (NSAIDs) and acetaminophen are not effective in managing toxin-induced hyperthermia, because sympathomimetic-induced hyperthermia is not prostaglandin mediated. Treatment options that should be avoided include medications that can further impair the thermoregulatory system. Agents used routinely to suppress agitation (eg, haloperidol and other antipsychotics) have anticholinergic effects, which can worsen hyperthermia.[28] In fact, haloperidol and many antipsychotics can independently induce another hyperthermic state known as neuroleptic malignant syndrome. Finally, the sympathomimetic effect is mediated through a mix of α- and β-agonism. If a β-blocker is administered in an attempt to normalize hypertension and tachycardia, an unopposed α effect could worsen vasoconstriction.[29] This response has been reported to worsen cardiac hemodynamic indices and to exacerbate the risk of myocardial infarction.[30]

In summary, the classic clinical presentation of a sympathomimetic overdose is the amplified sympathomimetic toxidrome. Hyperthermia and psychomotor agitation resulting from this type of overdose are treated with benzodiazepines, passive and active cooling, and paralysis if needed. Normalization of vital signs is the clinical end point. The combination of hyperthermia and a hyperadrenergic state can lead to end-organ damage, including intracerebral hemorrhage, myocardial infarction, rhabdomyolysis, DIC, and cerebrovascular ischemia. One must also be wary of occult trauma in these patients. A clinical challenge and toxicologic emergency, hyperthermia resulting from sympathomimetic overdose is a potentially lethal condition if not aggressively treated in the emergency department.

ANTICHOLINERGICS
Mechanisms of Hyperthermia

Anticholinergic toxicity is commonly associated with hyperthermia. Anticholinergics cause hyperthermia primarily through impaired dissipation of heat from the body. Muscle activity can be increased, as seen during central muscarinic acetylcholine receptor blockade, and leads to restlessness, agitation, and seizures, all of which greatly increase heat production. Peripheral blockade of acetylcholine-mediated muscarinic receptors in exocrine sweat glands produces anhidrosis and impaired heat dissipation. Antipyretic agents that function via prostaglandin suppression (eg, acetaminophen) are ineffective, because the hyperthermia is not a result of resetting the hypothalamic thermostat.

Agents that Produce Anticholinergic Toxicity

Both pharmacologic and nonpharmacologic agents have anticholinergic properties (**Table 2**). Toxicity from naturally occurring anticholinergics has been reported since the advent of the written word. *Datura stramonium* was reportedly the drug that was consumed by Mark Anthony's troops in 38 AD as they were leaving Parthia. This ingestion caused the troops to become stuporous and confused, ultimately contributing to their defeat.[31] In more contemporary history, British soldiers attempting to suppress Bacon's Rebellion in 1676 in Jamestown, Virginia, inadvertently ate a salad containing *Datura* and "turned [into] natural fools" for 11 days.[32] "Jamestown weed," now referred to as jimson weed, remains a natural drug of abuse. Numerous other plants and mushrooms also have anticholinergic properties.

Multiple classes of pharmaceuticals possess anticholinergic properties. Antihistamines are a leading cause of anticholinergic toxicity. In 2010, the American Association of Poison Control Centers reported 69,291 single presentations attributable to antihistamines, with more than 28,000 being associated with diphenhydramine alone.[33] Other classes include antipsychotics, antiparkinsonian medications, antispasmodics, and ocular medications.

Cyclic antidepressants deserve special mention because of their intrinsic anticholinergic properties. Overdoses of these drugs can present with the classic anticholinergic syndrome. However, they also have fast sodium-channel–blocking properties that slow the propagation of depolarization across the myocardium, leading to widening of the QRS complex on the electrocardiogram. This effect has implications for the use of antidotal therapy for anticholinergic toxicity in these cases (see later discussion).

Clinical Presentation

The clinical presentation of a patient with anticholinergic toxicity reflects the blockade of muscarinic and acetylcholine receptors both centrally and peripherally. Central blockade leads to agitation, confusion, hallucinations, delirium, and even seizures or coma. Peripheral manifestations include dilated pupils, dry, flushed skin, urinary retention, adynamic ileus, and dry mucous membranes. Vital-sign abnormalities may include tachycardia, mild hyperthermia, and hypertension. The hyperthermia is not typically of the magnitude of that induced by sympathomimetics. The mnemonic commonly used to remember the anticholinergic toxidrome is "mad as a hatter, hot as a hare, dry as a bone, red as a beet, blind as a bat, full as a flask."

The anticholinergic and sympathomimetic toxidromes have significant overlap, but important differences are found in the skin, gastrointestinal tract, and reactivity of the mydriatic pupils (typically unreactive in anticholinergic overdose but reactive in sympathomimetic overdose) (**Table 3**). Elderly patients and those with brain injury can present with more of the central manifestations and fewer of the peripheral manifestations, making the diagnosis more challenging in these groups, and emphasizing an enhanced index of suspicion.

Treatment

The goals of treatment in anticholinergic toxicity are to restore hemodynamic stability, manage agitation, and prevent secondary injury such as rhabdomyolysis. Many

Table 2
Selected agents that can lead to anticholinergic toxicity

Antihistamines	Antiparkinsonian Agents	Antipsychotics	Ocular Agents	Antispasmodics	Plants	Mushrooms
Diphenhydramine	Benztropine	Phenothiazines	Homatropine	Oxybutynin	*Atropa belladonna* (deadly nightshade)	*Amanita muscaria*
Dimenhydrinate	Trihexyphenidyl	Butyrophenones	Cyclopentolate	Cyclobenzaprine	*Datura stramonium* (jimson weed)	*Amanita pantherina*
Hydroxyzine		Clozapine	Tropicamide	Dicyclomine	*Cestrum nocturnum* (angel's trumpet)	
Promethazine		Olanzapine			*Mandragora officinarum* (mandrake)	

Table 3
Differences between sympathomimetic and anticholinergic toxidromes on physical examination

Organ System	Sympathomimetic	Anticholinergic
Eyes	Dilated and reactive	Dilated and nonreactive
Oral mucosa	Moist	Dry
Lungs	Bronchodilator	Bronchodilator
Cardiovascular	Hypertension and tachycardia	Hypertension and tachycardia
Gastrointestinal	Bowel sounds unchanged	Decreased/absent bowel sounds
Genitourinary	Urination unchanged, occasional urinary retention	Urinary retention
Skin	Diaphoretic	Dry flushed skin
Neurologic	Euphoria, psychomotor agitation	Hallucinations

patients with anticholinergic toxicity can be managed with supportive care alone. Airway management may be needed, depending on the patient's mental status and sedation requirements. Gastric decontamination with activated charcoal can be considered, depending on the time since ingestion and the patient's mental status. As already noted, drug-induced hyperthermia does not respond to antipyretics, because it is caused by impaired heat dissipation rather than the resetting of the hypothalamic thermostat. Sedation should be accomplished with benzodiazepines. Aggressive management of agitation is recommended to prevent worsening hyperthermia and other sequelae such as trauma and rhabdomyolysis. Patients should be managed with cooling mists and ice packs over the major arteries after adequate sedation has been achieved. Although it may be tempting to administer an antipsychotic from the phenothiazine or butyrophenone class (eg, haloperidol) in combination with the benzodiazepine, these agents possess anticholinergic properties and can lower the seizure threshold.[34] In a patient with elevated body temperature and altered mental status, standard medical practice is to perform a lumbar puncture. If the patient has ingested an anticholinergic and the clinician can completely reverse the delirium, hallucination, and agitation, the lumbar puncture could reasonably be omitted, as confidence in a noninfectious cause has been bolstered.

Physostigmine is a reversible inhibitor of acetylcholinesterase, the enzyme that breaks down acetylcholine. The resultant increase in acetylcholine levels overcomes the effects of the anticholinergic drug at both nicotinic and muscarinic acetylcholine receptors. Physostigmine can be used as specific antidotal therapy in cases of anticholinergic toxicity. Routine use in all cases of anticholinergic toxicity is not recommended, because this drug has several potentially serious side effects. The use of physostigmine is typically reserved for treating severe agitation, tachycardia with hemodynamic instability, and severe hyperthermia with impaired sweating.[35]

The administration of physostigmine to a patient with an anticholinergic overdose can lead to bradycardia or heart block, especially in someone who is not anticholinergic; therefore cardiac monitoring is essential with the use of this drug. Atropine should be available at the bedside. An electrocardiogram should be obtained before administering physostigmine. Prolongation of the PR, QRS, or QTc interval precludes administration of this drug.[36] Physostigmine lowers the seizure threshold and may lead to status epilepticus. In addition, symptoms of cholinergic excess can occur with physostigmine treatment, especially in patients who are not anticholinergic or have ingested low doses of anticholinergic drugs. A cholinergic crisis is characterized by increased secretions with possible airway compromise, nausea, vomiting, diarrhea, and bronchospasm. Seizures and bradycardia can occur when physostigmine is given rapidly or in excessive doses, although the link between rate of administration and seizures is mere speculation.[36]

The use of physostigmine in patients exhibiting anticholinergic toxicity from cyclic antidepressant overdose remains controversial. A well-publicized article from the 1980s described complications of physostigmine treatment in cyclic antidepressant overdose, which ultimately led to asystole and death.[37] These cases led to the virtual abandonment of the use of physostigmine in any patient suspected of cyclic antidepressant use. This blanket moratorium has come under some scrutiny in more recent studies. Burns and colleagues[38] studied patients who had ingested cyclic antidepressants and were treated with physostigmine unless changes on their electrocardiograms were evident (PR interval >200 milliseconds or QRS interval >100 milliseconds). No patients experienced significant cardiac side effects. The investigators concluded that physostigmine is safe in cyclic antidepressant overdose in patients with normal electrocardiograms. In a review article published in 2003, Suchard[39] hypothesized that patients without electrocardiographic changes may have less severe cyclic antidepressant toxicity, suggesting that Burns' findings might have been influenced by selection bias. Suchard proposed that in less severe cyclic antidepressant toxicity the anticholinergic effects predominate, so that physostigmine can be used safely, whereas in more severe poisonings the cardiotoxicity may be more pronounced than the anticholinergic toxicity, meaning physostigmine might be dangerous.[39]

Clinically, physostigmine is not the agent of choice for patients with cyclic antidepressant overdoses even if they have central anticholinergic symptoms. Management centers around treatment of the sodium-channel blockade and administration of sodium bicarbonate. The presentation of a patient with undifferentiated overdose and anticholinergic symptoms should prompt an immediate electrocardiogram to evaluate for sodium-channel–blocking effects of possible cyclic antidepressants. Classic electrocardiographic changes include a prominent R wave in lead AvR, an S wave in leads I and AvL, and a QRS interval duration of greater than 100 milliseconds. Physostigmine, when used, should be administered in doses of 0.5 to 2 mg intravenously, given slowly over 1 to 2 minutes while the patient is under continuous cardiac monitoring.

OTHER XENOBIOTICS AS A CAUSE OF HYPERTHERMIA
Uncouplers of Oxidative Phosphorylation

The electron-transport chain is located in the inner membrane of the mitochondria. This chain of cytochrome and enzyme complexes is vital for energy production during aerobic metabolism. Oxidative phosphorylation is accomplished by the electron-transport chain in a multistep process. The 2 central steps in this chain are the transfer of electrons from reduced coenzymes to oxygen (oxidation/reduction) and the formation of energy-rich adenosine triphosphate (ATP) from its precursor adenosine diphosphate (phosphorylation). These 2 components are coupled together to maximize energy production and efficiency.[40]

If a xenobiotic uncouples oxidative phosphorylation, cells quickly exhaust their accessible energy supplies because ATP is not being produced. During this time other metabolic processes continue. The uninhibited pumps still push protons into the intermembrane space while electrons continue their path down the electron-transport chain in an attempt to reduce oxygen. Uncoupling of oxidative phosphorylation significantly compromises the established proton gradient that is necessary for mitochondrial function. When the electron-transport energy is uncoupled from ATP production it is released as heat, causing potentially harmful increases in body temperature.[41]

The most commonly used salicylate, aspirin (acetylsalicylic acid), has been in existence since the late 1800s. A myriad of available products containing salicylates are available in oral and topical formulations. Choosing (and using) a product is complicated by the various names and strengths available, and the similarity to acetaminophen with respect to dosing. Hyperthermia is just one of the many signs and symptoms associated with acute or chronic salicylate poisoning. Salicylate toxicity is characterized by hyperthermia, respiratory alkalosis, metabolic acidosis, tachypnea, altered mental status, and abdominal complaints. Mild hyperthermia is common,[42–47] and severe hyperthermia, with temperatures higher than 40°C (104°F), has been reported.[48–50] This particularly deadly toxidrome should be considered when hyperthermia is present. A review of the treatment of salicylate overdose is beyond the scope of this article.

Dinitrophenol was introduced in the 1930s as an agent for weight loss.[51] Its mechanism of action is to increase energy expenditure via uncoupling oxidative phosphorylation. Dieters reported weight loss of up to 2 lb (0.9 kg) per week.[52] The chemical is now used in herbicides, dyes, wood preservatives, and explosives, but people still experiment with its weight-loss properties.[53–55] The hyperthermia associated with this drug can be severe, with core body temperatures as high as 42°C (108°F).[56–59] The treatment of patients with salicylate or dinitrophenol poisoning should include aggressive cooling measures. Acetaminophen and other centrally acting antipyretics will not be effective, because the hyperthermia is a peripherally induced problem. Adjunctive therapy should include the administration of a benzodiazepine.

Thyroid Replacement Therapy

Overt hypothyroidism is prevalent, occurring in up to 2% of the general population.[60] Subclinical hypothyroidism may be even more common. Consequently, thyroid replacement therapy is common. To appreciate the clinical course of a thyroid replacement therapy overdose, it is important to have a basic understanding of the prescribed hormones. Thyroid hormone exists in 2 active forms: T_3 and T_4. Although the majority of circulating thyroid hormone is T_4 ($\sim$95%), T_3 is more biologically active. Once in the nucleus of the cell, most T_4 is deiodinated to T_3 by deiodinase enzymes.[61]

In the past, thyroid supplementation products were derived from porcine thyroid (Armour), which contained both T_3 and T_4. These products lacked stability and posed an increased risk of allergic reaction. The predominant form prescribed today, levothyroxine (T_4), is synthetically derived and much safer. Liothyronine (T_3) and liotrix (T_3/T_4) are also available but are rarely used. Levothyroxine's half-life is about 6 to 7 days and that of liothyronine is more on the order of 1 or 2 days.

Identifying a thyroid replacement therapy overdose can be challenging because the presentation can mimic other clinical entities, such as sympathomimetic poisoning or sepsis, and develops generally over 7 to 10 days (but has been reported as early as 2 or 3 days) as free T_4 is converted to T_3. Thyroid function tests, including measurement of the levels of thyroid-stimulating hormone (TSH), free T_4, and T_3, can facilitate the diagnosis. However, observed symptoms following ingestion of thyroid hormone do not correlate well with either the measured concentrations or the amount of levothyroxine ingested.[62]

Thyroid medications cause hyperthermia via the hormone's thermogenic effect, in addition to adrenergic stimulation and psychomotor agitation.[8,63–68] Hyperthermia can be extreme (>41°C or 106°F), but in an overdose setting will not emerge for more than 24 hours.[69] Treatment should involve the external cooling measures previously described as well as the intravenous administration of β-blockers such as propranolol to blunt the adrenergic response. Sodium ipodate, where available, is another option that inhibits peripheral conversion of T_4 to T_3, but its onset of action is 6 hours.[67] Seizures should be treated with benzodiazepines, which are also synergistic for reducing adrenergic stimulation and motor activity.

HYPERTHERMIA AS A RESULT OF TOXIN-INDUCED SEIZURES

Through alterations in inhibitory and excitatory neurotransmission or direct neurotoxic mechanisms, many xenobiotic overdoses manifest as seizures. The increased muscle activity associated with generalized convulsive seizures can predispose patients to hyperthermia. Most of the drugs previously discussed (sympathomimetics, anticholinergics, salicylates, and thyroid replacement preparations) have the potential to induce seizures. It is beyond the scope of this article to list every drug that carries the potential to cause seizures, but it is important to discuss a few commonly used xenobiotics that lower the seizure threshold in overdose and have been associated with hyperthermia.

Caffeine and theophylline, both in the methylxanthine class, have the potential to induce severe seizures that are refractory to treatment.[70–72] Temperatures of 39.5°C (103°F) have resulted from caffeine ingestion.[73] Isoniazid, an antituberculosis agent, causes a functional deficiency of pyridoxine, a cofactor in the synthesis of γ-aminobutyric acid (GABA).[74,75] Strychnine, used as a pesticide, causes loss of glycine inhibition in the central nervous system and spinal cord.[76–79] Temperatures as high as 43°C (109°F) have been reported.[80] Not surprisingly, these medications all have a propensity to cause true convulsive status epilepticus and, thus, severe hyperthermia.

In general, benzodiazepines should be considered first-line therapy, followed by barbiturates, propofol, or other sedative hypnotics. Rapid and timely treatment is necessary to prevent further seizure and the subsequent hyperthermia. Medications with GABA-agonist activity help control seizure activity and thereby reduce heat production generated by muscle contraction. Phenytoin rarely has a role in the management of toxin-induced seizures. Specifically for isoniazid, pyridoxine should be administered immediately with a benzodiazepine. An empiric intravenous pyridoxine dose of 5 g is recommended if the quantity of isoniazid ingested is unknown.

SUMMARY

Hyperthermia from drug overdose results from several mechanisms, including increased motor activity, decreased heat dissipation, and uncoupling of oxidative phosphorylation. Because sustained core body temperatures above 42°C (108°F) quickly lead to brain dysfunction, disseminated coagulopathy, rhabdomyolysis, and death, aggressive external and internal cooling measures are paramount. Although some xenobiotics have specific antidotes directed to halt the harmful processes, sedative agents with GABA-agonist activity serve as important adjuncts to promote cooling. Benzodiazepines are effective in almost all cases of toxin-induced hyperthermia, and should be used liberally.

REFERENCES

1. Sithinamsuwan P, Piyavechviratana K, Kitthaweesin T, et al. Exertional heatstroke: early recognition and outcome with aggressive combined cooling: a 12 year experience. Mil Med 2009;174:496–502.
2. Clapham JC. Central control of thermogenesis. Neuropharmacology 2012;63: 111–23.

3. Boulant JA. Hypothalamic neurons: mechanisms of sensitivity to temperature. Ann N Y Acad Sci 1998;856:108–15.
4. Dinarello CA, Porat R. Harrison's principles of internal medicine. 18th edition. New York: McGraw-Hill; 2011. p. 142.
5. Rowell LB. Cardiovascular aspects of human thermoregulation. Circ Res 1983; 52:367–79.
6. Hensel H. Neural processes in thermoregulation. Physiol Rev 1973;53: 948–1017.
7. Durnas C, Cusack BJ. Salicylate intoxication in the elderly: recognition and recommendations on how to prevent it. Drugs Aging 1992;2:20–34.
8. Majlesi N, Greller HA, McGuigan MA. Thyroid storm after pediatric levothyroxine ingestion. Pediatrics 2010;126(2):e470–3.
9. Marom T, Itskoviz D, Lavon H, et al. Acute care for exercise-induced hyperthermia to avoid adverse outcome from exertional heat stroke. J Sport Rehabil 2011; 20:219–27.
10. Lanner JT. Ryanodine receptor physiology and its role in disease. Adv Exp Med Biol 2012;740:217–34.
11. Hirshey Dirksen SJ, Larach MG, Rosenber H, et al. Special article: future directions in malignant hyperthermia research and patient care. Anesth Analg 2011; 113:1108–19.
12. Perry PJ, Wilborn CA. Serotonin syndrome vs neuroleptic malignant syndrome: a contrast of causes, diagnoses and management. Ann Clin Psychiatry 2012;24: 155–62.
13. Docherty JR. Subtypes of functional alpha1- and alpha2-adrenoceptors. Eur J Pharmacol 1998;361:1–15.
14. Insel PA. Seminars in medicine of the Beth Israel Hospital, Boston. Adrenergic receptors—evolving concepts and clinical implications. N Engl J Med 1996; 334:580–5.
15. Meggs WJ. Epidemics of mold poisoning past and present. Toxicol Ind Health 2009;25:571–6.
16. Kiyatkin EA, Sharma HS. Acute methamphetamine intoxication: brain hyperthermia, blood-brain barrier, brain edema and morphological cell abnormalities. Int Rev Neurobiol 2009;88:65–100.
17. Sharma HS, Muresanu D, Sharma A, et al. Cocaine induced breakdown of the blood-brain barrier and neurotoxcity. Int Rev Neurobiol 2009;88:297–334.
18. Armen R, Kanel G, Reynolds T. Phencyclidine-induced malignant hyperthermia causing submassive liver necrosis. Am J Med 1984;77:167–72.
19. Parrott AC. MDMA and temperature: a review of the thermal effects of 'Ecstasy' in humans. Drug Alcohol Depend 2012;121:1–9.
20. Bohnert AS, Prescott MR, Vlahov D, et al. Ambient temperature and risk of death from accidental drug overdose in New York City, 1990-2006. Addiction 2010; 105:1049–54.
21. Traub SJ, Hoffman RS, Nelson LS. The "ecstasy" hangover: hyponatremia due to 3,4-methylenedioxymethamphetamine. J Urban Health 2002;79(4):549–55.
22. Sexton RL, Carlson RG, Leukefeld CG, et al. "Tweaking and geeking, just having some fun": an analysis of methamphetamine poems. J Psychoactive Drugs 2010;42:377–83.
23. Ross EA, Watson M, Goldberger B. "Bath salts" intoxication. N Engl J Med 2011; 365:967–8.
24. Hoffman RS. Treatment of patients with cocaine-induced arrhythmias: bringing the bench to the bedside. Br J Clin Pharmacol 2010;69:448–57.

25. Burke S, Hanani M. The actions of hyperthermia on the autonomic nervous: central and peripheral mechanisms and clinical implications. Auton Neurosci 2012; 168:4–13.

26. Holzer M. Targeted temperature management for comatose survivors of cardiac arrest. N Engl J Med 2010;363:1256–64.

27. Howes D, Ohley W, Dorian P, et al. Rapid induction of therapeutic hypothermia using convective-immersion surface cooling: safety, efficacy and outcomes. Resuscitation 2010;81:388–92.

28. Lazarus A. Heatstroke in a chronic schizophrenic patient treated with high-potency neuroleptics. Gen Hosp Psychiatry 1985;7:361–3.

29. Pitts WR, Vongpatanasin W, Cigarroa JE, et al. Effects of intracoronary infusion of cocaine on left ventricular systolic and diastolic function in humans. Circulation 1998;97:1270–3.

30. De Giorgi A, Fabbian F, Pala M, et al. Cocaine and acute vascular disease. Curr Drug Abuse Rev 2012;5:129–34.

31. Lewin L. Phantastica: narcotic and stimulating drugs. New York: Dutton; 1964.

32. Beverley R. Book II: of the natural product and conveniencies in its Unimprov'd state, before the English went thither. The History and Present State of Virginia, In Four Parts. Chapel Hill (NC): University of North Carolina; 2006. p. 24.

33. Bronstein AC, Spyker DA, Cantilena LR Jr, et al. 2010 annual report of the American Association of Poison Control Centers' national poison data system (NPDS): 28th annual report. Clin Toxicol 2011;49:910–41.

34. Dubin WR, Feld JA. Rapid tranquilization of the violent patient. Am J Emerg Med 1989;7:313.

35. Weiner AL, Bayer MJ, McKay CA, et al. Anticholinergic poisoning with adulterated intranasal cocaine. Am J Emerg Med 1998;16:517–20.

36. Schneir AB, Offerman SR, Ly BT, et al. Complications of diagnostic physostigmine administration to emergency department patients. Ann Emerg Med 2003;42:14–9.

37. Pentel P, Peterson CD. Asystole complicating physostigmine treatment of tricyclic antidepressant overdose. Ann Emerg Med 1980;9:588–90.

38. Burns MJ, Linden CH, Graudins A, et al. A comparison of physostigmine and benzodiazepines for the treatment of anticholinergic poisoning. Ann Emerg Med 2000;35:374–81.

39. Suchard J. Assessing physostigmine's contraindication in cyclic antidepressant ingestions. J Emerg Med 2003;25:185–91.

40. Wallace KB, Starkov AA. Mitochondrial targets of drug toxicity. Annu Rev Pharmacol Toxicol 2000;40:353–88.

41. Brody TM. The uncoupling of oxidative phosphorylation as a mechanism of drug action. Pharmacol Rev 1955;7:335–63.

42. Pec J, Strmenova M, Palencarova E. Salicylate intoxication after use of topical salicylic acid ointment by a patient with psoriasis. Cutis 1992;50:307–9.

43. Pei YP, Thompson DA. Severe salicylate intoxication mimicking septic shock [letter]. Am J Med 1987;82:381–2.

44. Leatherman JW, Schmitz PG. Fever, hyperdynamic shock, and multiple-system organ failure: a pseudo-sepsis syndrome associated with chronic salicylate intoxication. Chest 1991;100:1391–6.

45. Thisted B, Krantz T, Strom J. Acute salicylate self-poisoning in 177 consecutive patients treated in ICU. Acta Anaesthesiol Scand 1987;31:312–6.

46. Fisher CJ Jr, Albertson TE, Foulke GE. Salicylate-induced pulmonary edema: clinical characteristics in children. Am J Emerg Med 1985;3:33–7.

47. Schlegel RJ, Altstatt LB, Canales L. Peritoneal dialysis for severe salicylism: an evaluation of indications and results. J Pediatr 1966;69:553–62.

48. Levy RI. Overwhelming salicylate intoxication in an adult. Arch Intern Med 1967; 119:399–402.

49. Robin ED, Davis RP, Rees SB. Salicylate intoxication with special reference to the development of hypokalemia. Am J Med 1959;26:869–82.

50. Candy JM, Morrison C, Paton RD. Salicylate toxicity masquerading as malignant hyperthermia. Paediatr Anaesth 1998;8:421–3.

51. Tainter ML, Stockton AB, Cutting WC. Dinitrophenol in the treatment of obesity. JAMA 1935;105:332–7.

52. Cutting WC, Mehrtens HG, Tainter ML. Actions and uses of dinitrophenol. JAMA 1933;101:195.

53. Grundlingh J, Dargan PI, El-Zanfaly M, et al. 2,4-Dinitrophenol (DNP): a weight loss agent with significant acute toxicity and risk of death. J Med Toxicol 2011; 7(3):205–12.

54. Miranda EJ, McIntyre IM, Parker DR, et al. Two deaths attributed to the use of 2,4-dinitrophenol. J Anal Toxicol 2006;30:219–22.

55. McFee RB, Caraccio TR, McGuigan MA, et al. Dying to be thin: a dinitrophenol related fatality. Vet Hum Toxicol 2004;46:251–4.

56. Macnab AJ, Fielden SJ. Successful treatment of dinitrophenol poisoning in a child. Pediatr Emerg Care 1998;14:136–8.

57. Bidstrup PL, Payne DJ. Dinitro-ortho-cresol: report of eight fatal cases occurring in Great Britain. Br Med J 1951;2:16–9.

58. MacBryde CM, Taussig BL. Functional changes in liver, heart and muscles, and loss of dextrose tolerance. JAMA 1935;105:13–7.

59. Barker K, Seger D, Kumar S. Comment on "Pediatric fatality following ingestion of Dinitrophenol: postmortem identification of a 'dietary supplement'". Clin Toxicol (Phila) 2006;44:351.

60. Vanderpump MP, Tunbridge WM, French JM, et al. The incidence of thyroid disorders in the community: a twenty-year follow-up of the Whickham Survey. Clin Endocrinol (Oxf) 1995;43:55–68.

61. Leonard JL, Visser TJ. Biochemistry of iodination. In: Hennemann G, editor. Thyroid hormone metabolism. New York: Marcel Dekker; 1986. p. 189–230.

62. Hack JB, John AL, Nelson LS, et al. Severe symptoms following massive intentional L-thyroxine ingestion. Vet Hum Toxicol 1999;41:323–6.

63. Sola E, Gomez-Balaguer M, Morillas C. Massive triiodothyronine intoxication: efficacy of hemoperfusion? Thyroid 2002;12:637–40.

64. Jonare A, Munkhammar P, Persson H. A case of severe levothyroxine poisoning in a child [abstract]. Clin Toxicol 2001;39:304–5.

65. Brown RS, Cohen JH, Braverman LE. Successful treatment of massive acute thyroid hormone poisoning with iopanoic acid. J Pediatr 1998;132:903–5.

66. Tunget CL, Clark RF, Turchen SG. Raising the decontamination level for thyroid hormone ingestions. Am J Emerg Med 1995;13:9–13.

67. Berkner PD, Starkman H, Person N. Acute L-thyroxine overdose; therapy with sodium ipodate: evaluation of clinical and physiologic parameters. J Emerg Med 1991;9:129–31.

68. Funderburk SJ, Spaulding JS. Sodium levothyroxine (Synthroid(R)) intoxication in a child. Pediatrics 1970;45:298–301.

69. Botella de Maglia J, Torrero LC, Sanchez AR, et al. Intoxicacion por triyodotironina. Estudio clinco y farmacocinetico. An Med Interna 2003;20:627–9.

70. Perrin C, Debruyne D, Lacotte J. Treatment of caffeine intoxication by exchange transfusion in a newborn. Acta Paediatr Scand 1987;76:679–81.
71. Higgins RM, Hearing S, Goldsmith DJ. Severe theophylline poisoning: charcoal haemoperfusion or haemodialysis? Postgrad Med J 1995;71:224–6.
72. Parr MJ, Willatts SM. Fatal theophylline poisoning with rhabdomyolysis. Anaesthesia 1991;46:557–9.
73. Rivenes SM, Bakerman PR, Miller MB. Intentional caffeine poisoning in an infant. Pediatrics 1997;99:736–8.
74. Lopez-Contreras J, Ruiz D, Domingo P. Isoniazid-induced toxic fever [letter]. Rev Infect Dis 1991;13:775.
75. Shah BR, Santucci K, Sinert R. Acute isoniazid neurotoxicity in an urban hospital. Pediatrics 1995;95:700–4.
76. Makarovsky I, Markel G, Hoffman A, et al. Strychnine—a killer from the past. Isr Med Assoc J 2008;10:142–5.
77. Oberpaur B, Donoso A, Claveria C. Strychnine poisoning: an uncommon intoxication in children. Pediatr Emerg Care 1999;15:264–5.
78. Dittrich K, Bayer MJ, Wanke LA. A case of fatal strychnine poisoning. J Emerg Med 1984;1:327–30.
79. Edmunds M, Sheehan TM, Van't Hoff W. Strychnine poisoning: clinical and toxicological observations on a non-fatal case. J Toxicol Clin Toxicol 1986;24:245–55.
80. Boyd RE, Brennan PT, Deng JF, et al. Strychnine poisoning: recovery from profound lactic acidosis, hyperthermia, and rhabdomyolysis. Am J Med 1983;74:507–12.

Hyperthermia Caused by Drug Interactions and Adverse Reactions

Mary S. Paden, MD, Lucy Franjic, MD, S. Eliza Halcomb, MD*

KEYWORDS

- Neuroleptic malignant syndrome • Serotonin syndrome • Malignant hyperthermia
- Drug-induced heat illness

KEY POINTS

- Three of the primary drug-induced manifestations of hyperthermia are neuroleptic malignant syndrome, serotonin syndrome, and malignant hyperthermia.
- Neuroleptic malignant syndrome, an uncommon but potentially fatal complication of the use of antipsychotic medications, is characterized by a gradual onset of rigidity, confusion, and, eventually, hyperpyrexia.
- Serotonin syndrome, which can result from the administration of serotonergic agents, is a potentially fatal hyperpyrexic syndrome.
- Malignant hyperthermia, a rare pharmacogenetic autosomal-dominant channelopathy of the sarcoplasmic reticulum of skeletal muscle, is rarely encountered in the emergency department.

NEUROLEPTIC MALIGNANT SYNDROME
Definition

By 1960, the scientific community had discovered chlorpromazine and haloperidol, known today as typical or classic antipsychotics.[1] Physicians began using these drugs in the treatment of schizophrenia, which worked well to temper the so-called positive signs of the disease, such as delusions, hallucinations, and disorganized thought. It is thought that these symptoms are caused by the overactivity of dopamine at the dopamine receptors (particularly the D2 receptors) in the brain.[2] Antipsychotics/neuroleptics work by manipulating dopamine pathways in the central nervous system. As the typical antipsychotics became more widely used, side effects began to emerge.

Disclosures: The authors have no disclosures to report.
Division of Emergency Medicine, Washington University School of Medicine, 660 South Euclid, Box 8072, St Louis, MO 63110, USA
* Corresponding author.
E-mail address: halcombs@wusm.wustl.edu

Emerg Med Clin N Am 31 (2013) 1035–1044
http://dx.doi.org/10.1016/j.emc.2013.07.003

Jean Delay and Pierre Deniker were French psychiatrists who first described a constellation of symptoms in their patients who were being treated with chlorpromazine. Chlorpromazine was being used, mainly in France at the time, as an antiemetic. They noted some of their patients acutely developed altered mental status, fever, rigidity, and other psychomotor changes.[3] These symptoms were referred to as *syndrome malin des neuroleptiques*.[4] Approximately a decade later in the United States, Herbert Meltzer described the same symptom constellation in a patient he was treating with fluphenazine.[3] We now refer to this as *neuroleptic malignant syndrome* (NMS).

Among patients being treated with dopamine antagonists, 0.5% to 3.0% will develop NMS. Among cases of NMS, morality ranges from 4% to 30%.[5–10] The true frequency of cases is difficult to establish because actual clinical presentations can manifest varying degrees of severity. For this reason, some patients never seek clinical attention and go unreported.

NMS occurs more frequently in young men, most likely because this population has a higher incidence of schizophrenia and, therefore, is more frequently treated with neuroleptic medication. Other factors, such as concomitant infection, dehydration, depot preparations of neuroleptics, potent neuroleptics, cotreatment with lithium, and rapid administration of neuroleptics, increase the likelihood of NMS.[8,11–13]

Pathogenesis

The underlying mechanism of the development of NMS is not completely understood. Two basic theories have been posited to explain this syndrome: (1) the antipsychotic-induced disruption of neurotransmitters in the central nervous system (namely dopamine) and (2) a direct effect on skeletal muscle through disruption of calcium transport in genetically predisposed individuals.[12,14–19] Three major pathways in the brain use dopamine: the nigrostriatal, mesocorticolimbic, and tuberoinfundibular circuits. These pathways are key in modulating motor activities, rewarding behavior, and prolactin regulation, respectively. Dopamine is also important in hypothalamic temperature regulation.[15] Patients treated with antipsychotics experience an abrupt reduction in dopaminergic transmission in the these pathways, mainly the striatum and hypothalamus, which leads to an altered core temperature and impaired thermoregulation as well as other manifestations of autonomic dysfunction.[20] The hypothalamus is unable to control mechanisms for heat dissipation, and dopamine blockade in the striatum may lead to muscular rigidity that generates heat. Both factors in combination contribute to the hyperthermia seen in NMS.[11,14] Altered mental status is often seen with NMS and possibly stems from multiple factors, including the blockade of dopamine receptors in the brain, genetic predisposition, sequelae of hyperthermia, or cross-reactivity/blockade of other neurotransmitters in the central nervous system.

A variety of dopamine receptors are located in the brain (D1–D5). Each antipsychotic will induce different effects with different degrees of severity based on their activity on distinct dopamine receptor subtypes as well as on other neurotransmitter receptors.[21] For example, atypical antipsychotics that block serotonin at the 5-hydroxytryptamine receptor 2A (5-HT2A) receptors and seem to have a lower incidence of NMS.[6] It is probable that multiple neurotransmitters play a role in the full clinical picture of NMS, so the syndrome cannot be attributed to the blockade of dopamine alone.[22]

NMS is an uncommon but potentially fatal complication of treatment with antipsychotic medications. The development of NMS is an emergency requiring immediate attention.[5,23] Of note, NMS can occur with typical *and* atypical antipsychotics as well as other drugs that modulate dopamine in the brain, such as metoclopramide, but are not classically used to treat schizophrenia. NMS can also be seen after the abrupt withdrawal of a dopamine agonist. This occurrence has been reported in patients with Parkinson disease who suddenly stop taking levodopa/carbidopa, amantadine, or bromocriptine.[24] The medications thought to cause NMS are listed in **Table 1**.

Clinical Presentation

The typical features of NMS include altered mental status, hyperthermia, muscular rigidity, and autonomic dysfunction. The rigidity and altered mentation usually precede other symptoms but not always. Atypical cases may present with only one or two of these features. It is advisable to maintain a high level of clinical suspicion for NMS in patients who have been taking antipsychotics or have had recent adjustments to their medication regimen and then present with any of the aforementioned symptoms. Mental status changes include agitation, lethargy, and even coma. Temperatures are typically quite elevated. The mean temperature is 103°F; even higher values have been reported. Muscular rigidity is the classic lead pipe or cogwheel rigidity that is often described in patients with Parkinson disease.[6,14] Other noted abnormalities include tachycardia, labile blood pressure, tremors, diaphoresis, incontinence, dysphagia, and sialorrhea.

The evaluation of patients presenting with the triad of fever, rigidity, and altered mental status should include complete blood count, total creatinine kinase, complete metabolic profile, coagulation profile, lithium level, urine drug screen, an electrocardiogram, computed tomography of the head, and possibly an electroencephalogram and lumbar puncture. Common laboratory test abnormalities include elevated levels of creatine kinase, myoglobin, hepatic transaminases, blood urea nitrogen, and creatinine. Patients can also display myoglobinuria, leukocytosis, metabolic acidosis, hypernatremia, or hyponatremia.

Diagnosis

Several diagnostic criteria have been set forth for the diagnosis of NMS but none is universally accepted. It is a diagnosis of exclusion.[9,11,22,25] Generally speaking, however, a combination of rigidity, altered mental status, pyrexia, and elevation of the creatine kinase level fulfill the case definition for NMS. Patients with this clinical constellation of symptoms should be treated presumptively.

The differential diagnosis for NMS includes other hyperthermic syndromes induced by toxins. These syndromes include anticholinergic syndrome and serotonin syndrome, which display the symptoms of elevated temperature, altered mentation, and neuromuscular dysfunction. However, these two syndromes usually have a

Table 1	
Typical and atypical antipsychotics that can cause NMS	
Neuroleptics	Phenothiazines: chlorpromazine, fluphenazine, prochlorperazine, thioridazine, promethazine, pimozide Butyrophenones: haloperidol, droperidol Thioxanthenes: thiothixene, chlorprothixene, clopenthixol Dibenzepines: olanzapine, clozapine Benzisoxazoles: risperidone
Dopamine antagonists	Metoclopramide hydrochloride, hydroxyzine, reserpine
Dopamine agonists Antiparkinsonian agents (sudden withdrawal)	Amantadine, levodopa, lithium, bromocriptine

more rapid onset than NMS. NMS usually occurs between 1 and 3 days after treatment with a neuroleptic. Other conditions to consider include rhabdomyolysis from other causes, meningitis, encephalitis, neuroleptic-related heat stroke, drug interactions with monoamine oxidase inhibitors, tetanus, intracranial masses, and exposure to other drugs/toxins.[22]

Timely diagnosis of NMS is imperative because it is a life-threatening condition. Death can result from respiratory failure, cardiovascular collapse, renal failure, arrhythmias, or disseminated intravascular coagulation (DIC). Morbidity from NMS is caused by rhabdomyolysis, which results in acute kidney injury, pneumonia secondary to aspiration, seizures, and cardiac arrhythmias.

Treatment Considerations

The treatment of NMS begins by recognizing the syndrome and stopping the dopamine antagonist that is responsible. If the syndrome was brought on by abruptly stopping a dopamine agonist, then that drug should be restarted. Early diagnosis and supportive care are the mainstays of successful outcomes.[14] Antipsychotics are metabolized and removed from the body slowly and cannot be filtered by dialysis, so patients might require supportive care for several days to weeks. These patients should be admitted to an intensive care unit for close monitoring. Supportive care includes aggressive hydration with crystalloid, oxygen administration, fever reduction with aggressive cooling maneuvers (ice packs, ice baths, cooling blankets), nutritional support, and cardiorespiratory support if necessary.[26] Early intubation should be considered in these patients. For induction of muscle relaxation/paralysis in these patients, a nondepolarizing agent, such as rocuronium, should be used as opposed to a depolarizing agent, such as succinylcholine.[22] Benzodiazepines are a mainstay of treatment of patients with NMS and help decrease agitation/sympathetic hyperactivity. All patients should also be started on low-molecular-weight heparin because venous thromboembolism is a significant cause of morbidity and mortality in this patient population. Some efficacy has been reported in using dopamine agonists, such as bromocriptine, levodopa, and amantadine, to reverse the symptoms of NMS more quickly than with supportive therapy alone.[10,27–31] Most toxicologists recommend the use of bromocriptine (2.5 mg 3 times a day) until symptoms resolve. The dose should then be tapered over a week to avoid the recrudescence of symptoms.

Dantrolene has also been evaluated in the treatment of NMS. It inhibits the release of calcium by the sarcoplasmic reticulum in skeletal muscle, thereby reducing the prolonged contractions that lead to muscle breakdown and eventual rhabdomyolysis. This medication is occasionally useful in the management of the rigidity associated with NMS. However, it is important to note that dantrolene acts peripherally, whereas NMS is a disease of the central nervous system. Therefore, dantrolene should not be used as the sole agent in the management of this disease. The fever associated with NMS is not prostaglandin mediated; therefore, there is no reason to use antipyretics, such as acetaminophen, ibuprofen, or aspirin, in the management of this disorder.

SEROTONIN SYNDROME
Definition

Serotonin syndrome (SS) is a potentially fatal syndrome of rigidity and hyperpyrexia that results from the administration of serotonergic agents. It is thought to be a spectrum disorder that ranges from mild symptoms of gastrointestinal distress to full-blown hyperthermia and rigidity.

Pathogenesis

The 5-HT2A receptors are the primary postsynaptic serotonin receptors thought to be responsible for the development of SS. SS is thought to occur when the concentration of serotonin (or serotonin agonist) at the postsynaptic receptor increases. Such conditions commonly result when exogenous agonists are administered or when reuptake or oxidation is inhibited.[32]

SS typically occurs shortly after an increase in the dose of a potent serotonin agonist, a monoamine oxidase inhibitor (MAOI), or a serotonin reuptake inhibitor (SRI) or after the addition of a second serotonergic agent, such as tramadol or dextromethorphan.[32] Tramadol is an analgesic with partial mu agonist activity and affects serotonin and norepinephrine activity with toxicity related to monoamine uptake inhibition.[33]

In addition to tramadol, other phenylpiperidine opioids (eg, meperidine, methadone, dextromethorphan, and propoxyphene) have a weak SRI effect, whereas drugs such as linezolid and isoniazid have MAOI properties.[34] Triptans (eg, sumatriptan) are a class of drugs used in the treatment of migraine headaches by acting as selective 5-hydroxy-tryptamine receptor 1B (5-HT1B) and 5-hydroxytryptamine receptor 1D (5-HT1D) receptor agonists.

Other classes of drugs that have an association with SS include herbal and dietary supplements, such as ginseng and St. John's wort; the anticonvulsant valproic acid; and antiemetics, such as ondansetron and metoclopramide, because they all affect serotonin concentration.[35]

The compound 3,4-methylenedioxymethamphetamine (Ecstasy) causes the release of serotonin, dopamine, and norepinephrine in the central nervous system and binds to their transporters, inhibiting their reuptake, especially serotonin. Other illicit drugs known to cause SS include cocaine and amphetamines. Cocaine, like MAOIs, inhibits serotonin metabolism.[34]

Clinical Presentation

SS presents with altered mental status and heightened neuromuscular and autonomic activity. Myoclonus is the most common finding in SS and is unique to it. Muscle rigidity can be seen in both SS and NMS. In patients with SS, muscle rigidity is most prominent in the lower extremities and is symmetric. Other neurologic manifestations seen in SS include seizures that are generalized and short lived, hyperreflexia, clonus, nystagmus, tremor, shivering, and gait ataxia. Dysfunction of the autonomic nervous system manifests as hyperthermia, diaphoresis, sinus tachycardia, hypertension, tachypnea, and mydriasis.[32,36] Hyperthermia in SS results from increased muscle tone and rigidity. The subsequent increase in muscle contraction leads to an increase in heat production that exceeds the body's ability to dissipate it.[34] Abnormalities in cognition and behavior include disorientation and confusion, agitation, and anxiety; in severe cases, patients can present in a coma.[32,36]

Diagnosis

The goal for emergency medicine physicians is to make this challenging diagnosis early. No confirmatory laboratory test exists, so the diagnosis rests entirely on the clinical presentation and is one of exclusion. Mild cases of SS can be misinterpreted as psychiatric or medical disorders, whereas severe cases can be inadvertently diagnosed as NMS.[32] It is important to exclude infection, such as septicemia or meningitis, and overdose of drugs, such as cocaine, Ecstasy, lithium, or anticholinergics.[34] In addition, without a proper diagnosis, emergency physicians might unknowingly precipitate SS by administering another serotonergic agent, such as meperidine, dextromethorphan, or tramadol.[32]

It is important to differentiate SS from NMS, which have many similarities. In general, in SS, patients are agitated with significant myoclonus and incoherent speech. Those presenting with NMS are usually mute, stare with a flat affect, and are immobile.[32,37]

Complications from SS include DIC, seizures, severe hypotension, respiratory distress syndrome, renal or hepatic failure, ventricular tachycardia, and death. Approximately 25% of patients require endotracheal intubation and ventilatory support, and most patients show dramatic improvement in the first 24 hours after the onset of symptoms. The mortality rate related to SS ranges between 2% and 12%, with the most common cause of death being related to severe hyperthermia.[32,36,38]

Treatment Considerations

The key to treatment is to discontinue all serotonergic medications and administer supportive care, such as intravenous fluids and benzodiazepines (which are nonspecific serotonin antagonists). Patients should be treated in an inpatient setting until their symptoms have resolved. Hyperthermia should be treated with aggressive cooling measures, including external cooling and hydration through intravenous fluids. Neurologic effects, including myoclonus, hyperreflexia, and seizures, can be treated with benzodiazepines. These drugs can also be used to treat patients with cognitive and behavior disturbances (eg, agitation and delirium). Patients with core temperatures of 41°C or greater require induction with neuromuscular paralytics and intubation with monitoring in an intensive care unit.[38] They have a worse prognosis and an increased risk of death.

The administration of the antihistamine cyproheptadine, a 5-HT2A inhibitor, should be considered in moderate cases and is recommended in severe cases because it is the most effective antiserotoninergic agent in humans. Its disadvantage is that it is available only as an oral preparation, to be given in an initial dose of 4 to 12 mg, with repeated dosing in 2 hours if no response is noted after the initial dose. Cyproheptadine therapy should be discontinued if patients do not respond after a total of 32 mg. If patients do respond, administration should continue at 4 mg of cyproheptadine every 6 hours for 48 hours to prevent relapse and recurrence.

Traditional antipyretics have limited use in the treatment of SS because the mechanism of hyperthermia involves increased muscle tone and not central thermoregulation.[32,34] Physical restraints should not be used because they exacerbate patients' agitation and, thus, escalate hyperthermia, lactic acidosis, and rhabdomyolysis.

Chlorpromazine, a 5-HT2A receptor antagonist, is another agent that has been studied in the treatment of SS. One of its advantages is that it is available in a parenteral form, but there are not enough data to support its routine use as a primary treatment of SS. It blocks dopamine receptors, which could potentiate muscle rigidity. It also could lower seizure threshold and exacerbate NMS.[32,34,36,37]

Dantrolene is a muscle relaxant used primarily to treat malignant hyperthermia (MH). It can be used in the treatment of SS, with the understanding that it largely provides muscle relaxation and does not address the underlying cause of the disease. After recovery from SS, it is best to avoid future exposures to serotonergic drugs (the risk of recurrence is unknown).[32]

MH
Definition

MH is an extraordinarily rare pharmacogenetic autosomal-dominant channelopathy of the sarcoplasmic reticulum of skeletal muscle. The disorder was first described by an

Australian anesthesiologist who was asked to evaluate a patient with a family history of 10 deaths during anesthesia.[39] The disorder is thought to occur in 1 per 5000 to 1 per 100,000 operative cases involving general anesthesia.[40] However, the prevalence of genetic polymorphisms associated with this disorder is thought to be as high as 1 per 3000.[40] Patients at risk for MH include family members of affected individuals as well as those who have underlying myopathic disorders, including muscular dystrophies, central cord disease, and hypokalemic periodic paralysis.[41]

Pathogenesis

Between 50% and 70% of cases of MH are associated with mutations of the ryanodine receptor (RYR_1). Several other calcium channel mutations are also causally associated with the precipitation of this illness.[42,43] In the normal state, the RYR_1 receptor regulates calcium flow from the sarcoplasmic reticulum (SR) of skeletal muscle. Depolarization of the plasma membrane causes the membrane-bound dihydropyridine receptor to initiate a conformational change in the ryanodine receptor, leading to channel opening and efflux of calcium from the SR, leading to an increase in intracellular calcium concentrations and muscle contraction.[44]

Mutations in the receptor lead to uncontrolled calcium release and sustained muscle contraction. Sarcoplasmic Ca^{2+}ATPase continuously takes up the excess calcium, reducing the concentration of intracellular ATP. This reduced concentration, in turn, leads to a hypermetabolic syndrome of increased oxygen consumption, decreased venous oxygen saturation, and hypercarbia; lactic acid production; and rhabdomyolysis with resulting hyperkalemia, hyperthermia, and DIC.[45] Pharmaceuticals associated with the development of MH include volatile inhalational anesthetics, such as halothane, isoflurane, sevoflurane, and desflurane, and the depolarizing muscle relaxant, succinylcholine.[40]

Clinical Presentation, Evaluation, Diagnosis

Typically, the earliest signs of MH include masseter spasm and a subtle increase in end-tidal carbon dioxide concentrations after the administration of an anesthetic agent. Tachypnea may ensue in spontaneously breathing patients in an attempt to compensate for increasing metabolic acidosis. Generalized rigidity leads to rhabdomyolysis, hyperkalemia, and hyperthermia, which is a late feature of the disease.[40] Death results from cardiac dysrhythmias, multiorgan failure, and bleeding diathesis.

MH is diagnosed largely on clinical grounds. A high index of suspicion facilitates early recognition and treatment of this disease.

Treatment Considerations

Early recognition, volume resuscitation, active cooling, and treatment of hyperkalemia in combination with early administration of dantrolene decrease the mortality associated with MH from 80% to 5%.[40] Dantrolene was first described to reverse the effects of MH in 1975 and has subsequently become the mainstay of treatment of this disorder.[46] Dantrolene reverses the effects of MH by partially blocking calcium efflux from the ryanodine receptor. The initial bolus dose is 2 to 3 mg/kg intravenously, repeated every 15 minutes until a total dose of 10 mg/kg has been reached. Subsequent dosing of 1 mg/kg should be given every 4 hours over the next 2 days to prevent recurrence.

MH is a hyperpyrexia rather than a fever. As such, it is not associated with hypothalamic regulation of temperature. Therefore, antipyretics, such as acetaminophen, are not useful in the management of this disease. Although it might seem reasonable to administer calcium channel blockers to patients with malignant dysrhythmias, these agents have been associated with cardiovascular collapse and severe hyperkalemia in animal studies.[47] Therefore, this treatment cannot be recommended.

SUMMARY

Three of the primary drug-induced manifestations of hyperthermia are NMS, SS, and MH. NMS, an uncommon but potentially fatal complication of the use of antipsychotic medications, is characterized by a gradual onset of rigidity, confusion, and, eventually, hyperpyrexia. The mainstay of treatment is aggressive cooling, sedation with benzodiazepines, and administration of bromocriptine. SS, which can result from the administration of serotonergic agents, is a potentially fatal hyperpyrexic syndrome. Cooling measures should be instituted for patients who present with confusion, fever, and rigidity. Cyproheptadine is useful in the management of mild to moderate cases of this syndrome; intensive care with intubation and paralytics is required for severe cases. MH, a rare pharmacogenetic autosomal dominant channelopathy of the sarcoplasmic reticulum of skeletal muscle, is rarely encountered in the emergency department. However, it can develop as long as 12 hours after surgery, so it is possible that someone who has undergone an outpatient procedure could seek help in an urgent-care setting. It can be seen shortly after the administration of succinylcholine, so a high index of suspicion should be maintained after intubation. Early use of dantrolene and aggressive supportive care are the mainstays of treatment and significantly reduce the mortality.

REFERENCES

1. The numbers count: mental disorders in America. Bethesda (MD): National Institute of Mental Health; 2013. Available at: www.nimh.nih.gov/health/publications/the-numbers-count-mental-disorders-in-america/index.shtml. Accessed March 13, 2013.
2. Seeman P, Kapur S. Schizophrenia: more dopamine, more D2 receptors. Proc Natl Acad Sci U S A 2000;97:7673–5.
3. Mann SC, Caroff SN, Keck PE, et al. Neuroleptic malignant syndrome and related conditions. 2nd edition. Washington, DC: American Psychiatric Publishing; 2003.
4. Delay J, Pichot P, Lempiere T, et al. Un neuroleptique majeur non phenothiazinique et non réserpinique, l'halopéridol, dans le traitement des psychoses. Ann Med Psychol 1960;18:145–52.
5. Susman VL. Clinical management of neuroleptic malignant syndrome. Psychiatr Q 2001;72:325–36.
6. Ananth J, Parameswaran S, Gunatilake S, et al. Neuroleptic malignant syndrome and atypical antipsychotic drugs. J Clin Psychiatry 2004;65:464–70.
7. Bottoni TN. Neuroleptic malignant syndrome: a brief review. Hospital Physician 2002;15(3):58–63.
8. Addonizio G, Susman VL, Roth SD. Neuroleptic malignant syndrome: review and analysis of 115 cases. Biol Psychiatry 1987;22:1004–20.
9. Caroff SN, Mann SC. Neuroleptic malignant syndrome. Med Clin North Am 1993; 77:184–202.
10. Strawn JR, Keck PE Jr, Caroff SN. Neuroleptic malignant syndrome. Am J Psychiatry 2007;164:870–6.
11. Levenson JL. Neuroleptic malignant syndrome. Am J Psychiatry 1985;142:1137–45.

12. Henderson VW, Wooten GF. Neuroleptic malignant syndrome: a pathogenetic role for dopamine receptor blockade? Neurology 1981;31:132–7.
13. Caroff SN, Mann SC. Neuroleptic malignant syndrome and malignant hyperthermia. Anaesth Intensive Care 1993;21:477–8.
14. Caroff SN. The neuroleptic malignant syndrome. J Clin Psychiatry 1980;41:79–83.
15. Cox B, Kerwin R, Lee TE. Dopamine receptors in the central thermoregulatory pathways of the rat. J Physiol 1978;282:471–83.
16. Burke RE, Fahn S, Mayeux R. Neuroleptic malignant syndrome caused by dopamine depleting drugs in a patient with Huntington's chorea. Neurology 1981;31:1022–6.
17. Toru M, Matsuda O, Makaguchi K. Neuroleptic malignant syndrome-like state following a withdrawal of antiparkinsonian drug. J Nerv Ment Dis 1981;169:324–7.
18. Bond WS. Detection and management of the neuroleptic malignant syndrome. Clin Pharm 1984;3:302–7.
19. McCarron MM, Boettger ML, Peck JI. A case of neuroleptic malignant syndrome successfully treated with amantadine. J Clin Psychiatry 1982;43:381–2.
20. Gurrera RJ, Chang SS. Thermoregulatory dysfunction in neuroleptic malignant syndrome. Biol Psychiatry 1992;32:334–43.
21. Addonizio G, Susman VL. Neuroleptic malignant syndrome: a clinical approach. St Louis (MO): Mosby; 1991.
22. Adnet P, Lestavel P, Krivosic-Horber R. Neuroleptic malignant syndrome. Br J Anaesth 2000;85:129–35.
23. Waldorf S. Update for nurse anesthetists: neuroleptic malignant syndrome. AANA J 2003;71:389–94.
24. Banushali MJ, Tuite PJ. The evaluation and management of patients with neuroleptic malignant syndrome. Neurol Clin 2004;22:389–411.
25. American Psychiatric Association: Diagnostic and statistical manual of mental disorders (DSM-IV). 4th edition. Washington, DC: American Psychiatric Press; 1994. p. 739–42.
26. Weiner JS, Khogali M. A physiological body-cooling unit for treatment of heat stroke. Lancet 1980;1:507–9.
27. Gangadhar BN, Desai NG, Channabasavanna SM. Amantadine in the neuroleptic malignant syndrome. J Clin Psychiatry 1984;45:526.
28. Nisijima K, Noguti M, Ishiguro T. Intravenous injection of levodopa is more effective than dantrolene as a therapy for neuroleptic malignant syndrome. Biol Psychiatry 1997;41:913–4.
29. Rosenberg MR, Green M. Neuroleptic malignant syndrome: review of response to therapy. Arch Intern Med 1989;149:1927–31.
30. Shoop SA, Cernek PK. Carbidopa/levodopa in treatment of neuroleptic malignant syndrome. Ann Pharmacother 1997;31:119.
31. Reulbach U, Dutsch C, Biermann T, et al. Managing an effective treatment for neuroleptic malignant syndrome. Crit Care 2007;11:R4.
32. Tintinalli J. Tintinalli's emergency medicine: a comprehensive study guide. 7th edition. New York: McGraw Hill Medical; 2011. p. 1202–3.
33. Takeshita J, Litzinger M. Serotonin syndrome associated with tramadol. Prim Care Companion J Clin Psychiatry 2009;11(5):273.
34. Hall AP, Henry JA. Acute toxic effects of 'Ecstasy' (MDMA) and related compounds: overview of pathophysiology and clinical management [review]. Br J Anaesth 2006;96(6):278–85.
35. Wooltorton E. Health and drug alerts: triptan migraine treatments and antidepressants: risk of serotonin syndrome. Can Med Assoc J 2006;175(8):874–5.

36. Mills KC. Serotonin syndrome: a clinical update. Crit Care Clin 1997;13:763.
37. Christensen RC. Identifying serotonin syndrome in the emergency department [letter]. Am J Emerg Med 2005;23:406–8.
38. Frank C. Recognition and treatment of serotonin syndrome. Can Fam Physician 2008;54(7):988–92.
39. Denborough MA, Forster JF, Lovell RR, et al. Anaesthetic deaths in a family. Br J Anaesth 1962;34(6):395–6.
40. Rosenberg H, Davis M, James D, et al. Malignant hyperthermia. Orphanet J Rare Dis 2007;2:21.
41. Marchant CL, Ellis FR, Halsall PJ, et al. Mutation analysis of two patients with hypokalemic periodic paralysis and suspected malignant hyperthermia. Muscle Nerve 2004;30(1):114–7.
42. Iles DE, Lehmann-Horn F, Scherer SW, et al. Localization of the gene encoding the alpha 2/delta-subunits of the L-type voltage-dependent calcium channel to chromosome 7q and analysis of the segregation of flanking markers in malignant hyperthermia susceptible families. Hum Mol Genet 1994;3:969–75.
43. Protasi F, Paolini C, Dainese M. Calsequestrin-1: a new candidate gene for malignant hyperthermia and exertional/environmental heat stroke. J Physiol 2009;587: 3095–100.
44. Zissimopoulos S, Lai FA. Ryanodine receptor structure, function and pathophysiology. In: Krebs J, Michalak M, editors. New comprehensive biochemistry, vol. 41. Philadelphia: Elsevier; 2007. p. 287–342.
45. Heffron JJ. Malignant hyperthermia: biochemical aspects of the acute episode. Br J Anaesth 1988;60(3):274–8.
46. Harrison GG. Control of the malignant hyperpyrexic syndrome in MHS swine by dantrolene sodium. Br J Anaesth 1975;47(1):62–5.
47. Saltzman LS, Kates RA, Corke BC, et al. Hyperkalemia and cardiovascular collapse after verapamil and dantrolene administration in swine. Anesth Analg 1984;63(5):473–8.

Fever in the Postoperative Patient

Mayur Narayan, MD, MPH, MBA[a,b,]*, Sandra P. Medinilla, MD, MPH[c]

KEYWORDS

- Fever • Inflammation • Atelectasis • Urinary tract infection • Pneumonia
- Necrotizing soft-tissue infection • Intra-abdominal abscess • *Clostridium difficile*

KEY POINTS

- Postprocedure fevers vary in the timing of their occurrence, duration, and severity.
- Such fevers do not all have an infectious cause, but they all require thorough investigation to rule out life-threatening conditions.
- This article summarizes the principles of diagnosis and management of postprocedure fevers for the emergency care provider.

INTRODUCTION

The emergence of fever, defined as a temperature greater than 38°C (100.4°F), during the perioperative time course can present a diagnostic and management challenge for the emergency medical care provider.[1] Infectious and noninfectious causes of the fever must be distinguished. Infectious causes should be considered mainly for fever presenting later than 48 hours after surgery, whereas early postoperative fever is most commonly attributed to noninfectious causes.[2] Others have stated that noninfectious causes appear to cause lower-temperature fevers (<38.9°C [102°F]), whereas a higher temperature should raise concern for an infectious cause.[3] Despite these claims, the cause of postprocedure fever is often not identified despite the rigorous efforts of clinicians. The classic "Ws" of postoperative fever (**Table 1**), long taught to medical students as mantra, have been challenged recently.[4]

The authors have no financial interests to disclose.

[a] Department of Surgery, Center for Injury Prevention & Policy, R Adams Cowley Shock Trauma Center, University of Maryland School of Medicine, 22 South Greene Street, Baltimore, MD 21201, USA; [b] Program in Trauma, Center for Injury Prevention & Policy, R Adams Cowley Shock Trauma Center, University of Maryland School of Medicine, 22 South Greene Street, Baltimore, MD 21201, USA; [c] Department of Surgery, Christiana Care Health Services, 4735 Ogletown-Stanton Road, Medical Arts Pavilion II, Suite 3301, Newark, DE 19713, USA
* Corresponding author. Department of Surgery, Center for Injury Prevention & Policy, R Adams Cowley Shock Trauma Center, University of Maryland School of Medicine, 22 South Greene Street, Baltimore, MD 21201.
E-mail address: mnarayan@umm.edu

Emerg Med Clin N Am 31 (2013) 1045–1058
http://dx.doi.org/10.1016/j.emc.2013.07.011
0733-8627/13/$ – see front matter © 2013 Elsevier Inc. All rights reserved.

Table 1
Classic "Ws" of postoperative fever

W	Cause	Timing
Wind	Atelectasis	POD 1–2
Water	Urinary tract infection	POD 2–3
Wound	Wound infection	POD 3–7
Walking	Deep vein thrombosis/thrombophlebitis	POD 5–7
Wonder drug	Drug fever	POD >7

Abbreviation: POD, postoperative day.
Data from Cline D, Stead LG. Abdominal emergencies. New York: McGraw Hill; 2007.

The causes of postprocedural fever range from inflammation or drug reaction to life-threatening necrotizing soft-tissue infection (NSTI). As with all medical diagnoses, a thorough history and physical examination should serve as the diagnostic starting point in ascertaining relevant information in terms of exposure to infectious pathogens. In addition, the timing of fever after a procedure can help differentiate potential causes. It is therefore useful to divide the time frame of postprocedure fever into 4 categories: immediate, acute, subacute, and delayed. Fevers that occur in the first 4 days after surgery are less likely to represent infectious complications than are fevers occurring on the fifth and subsequent days (**Fig. 1**). Fever can also accompany the continuum of systemic inflammatory response, sepsis, severe sepsis, and septic shock (**Table 2**).

The time of emergence of postprocedure fever can guide the provider's differential diagnosis and, thus, management decisions. In a prospective study of 81 patients with idiopathic postoperative fever, Garibaldi and colleagues[2] found that 80% of those with fever on the first postoperative day had no infection. Within the group in whom fever developed by the fifth postoperative day, 90% had an identifiable source such as wound infection (42%), urinary tract infection (UTI) (29%), or pneumonia (12%).[2,5] Dellinger[6,7] showed that early fevers (ie, emerging between days 1 and 4) rarely represent an infection. However, a fever that begins on or after postprocedure day 5 is much more likely to represent a clinically significant infection, so appropriate diagnostics to look for an infectious source may be useful. These tests can include laboratory investigations (blood culture, urine cultures, complete blood counts) and images (plain

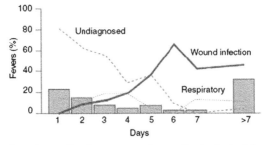

Fig. 1. Percentage of postoperative fevers occurring on the indicated day following an operative procedure. Lines indicate the percentage of fevers occurring on each day attributable to the cause indicated. (*From* Dellinger EP. Approach to the patient with postoperative fever. In: Gorbach S, Bartlett J, Blacklow N, editors. Infectious diseases. Philadelphia: Lippincott Williams & Wilkins; 2004. p. 817–23; with permission.)

Table 2
Definition of sepsis

Term	Definition
SIRS[a]	Body temperature $\geq$38 C or <36 C Heart rate >90 beats/min Respirations >20/min or $Paco_2$ <32 mm Hg White blood cell count >12.0 $\times$ 10^9/L or <4.0 $\times$ 10^9/L
Sepsis	SIRS plus infection
Severe sepsis	Sepsis associated with organ dysfunction, systemic hypoperfusion, or hypotension
Septic shock	Sepsis with arterial hypotension despite adequate fluid replacement

[a] At least 2 parameters are needed to meet the criteria for the systemic inflammatory response syndrome (SIRS).

Adapted from Bone RC, Balk RA, Cerra FB, et al. Definitions for sepsis and organ failure and guidelines for the use of innovative therapies in sepsis. The ACCP/SCCM Consensus Conference Committee. American College of Chest Physicians/Society of Critical Care Medicine. Chest 1992; 101:1644–55.

films, computed tomography [CT]). In this period, vigilance for occult infection should be maintained.[5]

INFLAMMATION AND HEALING

Immediate postoperative fever (occurring during the procedure or up to 1 hour following it) is most commonly caused by inflammatory changes from the release of pyrogenic cytokines, primarily interleukin (IL)-1, IL-6, tumor necrosis factor, and interferon-γ. These mediators increase capillary permeability and are central elements of the inflammatory response and, thus, healing.[8] The cytokines act directly on the anterior hypothalamus and cause a release of prostaglandins, which mediate the febrile response.[5] Studies have shown that IL-6 levels correlate directly with the magnitude of fever in patients undergoing a Whipple procedure (**Fig. 2**).[9]

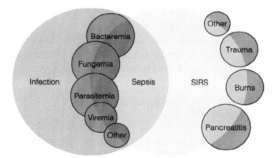

Fig. 2. Relationship of Infection, SIRS, Sepsis, Severe Sepsis, and Septic Shock. The diagram depicts the relationships between SIRS and infection. Note that only when SIRS occurs with an infection does sepsis or septic shock occur. For definitions of SIRS, Sepsis, Severe Sepsis, and Septic Shock, please see **Table 2**. (Data from Wheeler AP, Bernard GD. Treating patients with severe sepsis. N Engl J Med 1999;340(3):207–14; and Bone RC, Balk RA, Cerra FB, et al. Definitions for sepsis and organ failure and guidelines for the use of innovative therapies in sepsis. The ACCP/SCCM Consensus Conference Committee. American College of Chest Physicians/Society of Critical Care Medicine. Chest 1992;101(6):1644–55.)

Frank and colleagues[10] found that the mean time to maximum temperature elevation in patients who underwent vascular, abdominal, and thoracic surgeries was 11 hours. Blood concentrations of IL-6 correlated with fever elevation. The severity of the procedure, in terms of the extent of tissue trauma, can also influence the fever curve. For example, laparoscopic cholecystectomy is associated with fewer episodes of postoperative fever than an open approach.[11] The amount of tissue trauma seems to have a causal relationship with the release of IL-6 and thus to the development of fever. Inflammation secondary to cytokine release is now thought to be the most common cause of immediate postprocedure fever. For most patients, the fever resolves and a benign course can be expected.[2,5,12–14]

In the immediate postprocedure period, routine measurement of temperature followed by a detailed laboratory or diagnostic workup is not warranted as long as the patient is hemodynamically stable. Diagnostic tests, such as blood or urine cultures, should not be ordered routinely during this period. Patient physiology should drive diagnostic decision making in this phase. A prospective triple-blind study involving 308 consecutive patients found that measuring postoperative body temperature was of limited value in the detection of infection after elective surgery for noninfectious conditions.[15]

In the past, atelectasis was thought to be a common cause of postprocedure fever; however, numerous studies have shown that it is not clearly related to fever. Roberts and colleagues[16] evaluated 270 patients who had undergone elective abdominal surgery, and reported the presence of fever in 40%. When fever was defined as a temperature of 37.7°C (99.9°F) or higher, chest-film evidence of atelectasis was found in 57% of febrile patients. However, when the threshold for fever was raised to at least 38.0°C (100.4°F), only 47% of patients had atelectasis.

Engoren[17] showed that the incidence of atelectasis increased as the incidence of fever decreased with each successive postoperative day. Atelectasis was associated with neither the presence nor the severity of fever. Vermeulen and colleagues[15] reviewed the records of 284 general surgery patients, who had 2282 temperatures taken. Fever (temperature ≥38°C) was noted in 61 patients, and infection was found in 7 (11.5%). Infection was diagnosed in 12 of 223 patients (5.4%) without fever. As a predictor of infection, a temperature of 38°C had sensitivity of only 37% and specificity of 80%, a likelihood ratio of a positive test of 1.8, and a likelihood ratio of a negative test of 0.8. The positive predictive value of each individual temperature was only 8%.

Other common causes of immediate postprocedural fever include reactions to medication and transfusions, the presence of infection before the procedure, fulminant surgical-site infection, trauma, and adrenal insufficiency.

EMERGENT CAUSES OF EARLY POSTOPERATIVE FEVER

Several causes of early postoperative fever warrant special mention: NSTI/myonecrosis, pulmonary embolism, alcohol withdrawal, anastomotic leak, adrenal insufficiency, and malignant hyperthermia. These potentially life-threatening conditions mandate early diagnosis followed by prompt intervention.

Necrotizing Soft-Tissue Infections

NSTIs are invasive and potentially lethal if not evaluated, diagnosed, and treated promptly. NSTIs can manifest as necrotizing fasciitis, clostridial gas gangrene, Fournier gangrene, and invasive streptococcal cellulitis.[18] Although NSTIs are not common, they confer high risk; therefore, it is important to ensure that the diagnostic workup is adequate to exclude them. The time to presentation for NSTIs has significant variability. Presentations might occur particularly early, often within hours to days of the initial procedure.[18] Therefore, a posture of suspicion toward the classic clinical signs of NSTI is particularly important, that is, "dishwater drainage," erythema, edema, induration, bullae, and pain out of proportion to examination findings.

The pathogen can be introduced from hematogenous spread from distant sites of infection, minor trauma, or surgical incisions.[18,19] Fournier gangrene can be caused by colorectal or genitourinary surgical intervention. Other potential sources include intramuscular injections, odontogenic infections, or surgery.[20,21] Infection can be worsened by many risk factors such as vascular disease, impaired cellular immunity, diabetes mellitus, alcohol abuse, obesity, malnutrition, and the use of nonsteroidal anti-inflammatory drugs (NSAIDs).[18,22] All of these risk factors are very common among postoperative patients.

Commonly cultured organisms include Group A hemolytic streptococci, enterococci, coagulase-negative staphylococci, *Staphylococcus aureus*, *Staphylococcus epidermidis*, and clostridial species.[18] In the emergency setting, particularly severe cases can present with signs of systemic inflammation (tachycardia and fever) and even with evidence of end-organ dysfunction (eg, confusion, hypotension). Clinically the presence of subcutaneous gas on plain radiographs or CT should raise suspicion of NSTI and prompt early action. Early consultation with a surgical service is necessary, given that definitive diagnosis and treatment both require operative interventions (debridement, collection samples for pathologic evaluation, and confirmatory diagnosis). Clayton and colleagues[23] reported that the detection of gas on a radiograph had sensitivity of 39%, specificity of 95%, and a positive predictive value of 88% for NSTI. Scoring systems, such as the Laboratory Risk Indicator for Necrotizing Fasciitis (LRINEC) score (**Table 3**), have been developed to assist in diagnosis. Patients with an LRINEC score of greater than 6 on admission should be evaluated carefully; hospitalization, surgical assessment, and close monitoring are recommended.[24]

Prompt surgical consultation, in addition to administration of appropriate antibiotics and intravascular volume resuscitation, is imperative.[25,26] Broad antibiotic coverage should be initiated, covering gram-positive, gram-negative, and anaerobic organisms. Commonly used regimens include a penicillin (vancomycin in penicillin-allergic patients), clindamycin or metronidazole, and an aminoglycoside (or a third-generation cephalosporin or aztreonam).[18] Clindamycin should be administered to inhibit streptococcal toxins. Clinicians caring for these patients must remain watchful for signs of clinical deterioration. Patients who require large amounts of fluid resuscitation might develop pulmonary edema and subsequent respiratory failure requiring ventilatory support. Early surgical source control is the mainstay of management. When debridement begins early in the course of illness, defined as less than 24 hours after presentation, the morbidity and mortality rates are significantly diminished.[22,27]

Pulmonary Embolism

Murray and colleagues[28] found fever (temperature >38°C) attributed solely to acute pulmonary emboli in 57% of their series of 35 patients, whereas fever with no other definite or possible explanatory cause was observed in 14% of the 311 patients in the Prospective Investigation of Pulmonary Embolism Diagnosis (PIOPED) study. In general, fever associated with pulmonary embolism is of low grade (temperature rarely exceeding 38.3°C [101°F]) and short-lived, peaking the same day on which the pulmonary embolism occurs and gradually disappearing within 1 week. Septic thrombophlebitis can lead to septic pulmonary emboli, causing a high postprocedural temperature (**Fig. 3**).[29]

Table 3
Variables in the LRINEC score for diagnosing necrotizing soft-tissue infection

Laboratory Risk Indicator for Necrotizing Fasciitis (LRINEC) Score	
Variable	Score
C-reactive protein (mg/L)	
<150	0
≥150	4
Total white cell count (per mm³)	
<15	0
15–25	1
>25	2
Hemoglobin (g/dL)	
>13.5	0
11–13.5	1
<11	2
Sodium (mmol/L)	
≥135	0
<135	2
Creatinine (μmol/L)	
≤141	0
>41	2
Glucose (mmol/L)	
≤10	0
>10	1

Key: low risk (≤5 points), intermediate risk (6 or 7 points), and high risk (≥8 points). Internal validation revealed that a cutoff of ≥6 had a positive predictive value of 92% and a negative predictive value of 96%. Scores ≥8 were strongly suggestive of necrotizing soft-tissue infection (positive predictive value 93.4%).

Data from Wong CH, Khin LW, Heng KS, et al. The LRINEC (Laboratory Risk Indicator for Necrotizing Fasciitis) score: a tool for distinguishing necrotizing fasciitis from other soft tissue infections. Crit Care Med 2004;32:1535–41.

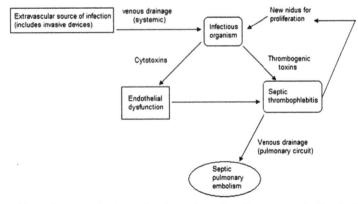

Fig. 3. Possible pathophysiologic mechanisms of septic pulmonary embolism in the setting of septic thrombophlebitis. (*From* Brenes JA, Goswami U, Williams DN. The association of septic thrombophlebitis with septic pulmonary embolism in adults. Open Respir Med J 2012;6:14–9; with permission.)

Anastomotic Leak/Intra-Abdominal Abscess

It is important to remember that abscesses can form after any type of surgical procedure. Patients presenting to the emergency department for evaluation of fever and abdominal pain after an intra-abdominal procedure should be presumed to have a surgical complication such as anastomotic leak. When the abdominal compartment is contaminated, an abscess may form. Patients can present with symptoms of frank peritonitis, including abdominal pain, nausea, and vomiting. The time lag between surgery and presentation can vary from 1 week to several months. Peritoneal contamination can occur during any interventional, endoscopic, laparoscopic, robotic, or open procedure. The bowel can be injured inadvertently when the peritoneum is entered; for example, with the trocar used during laparoscopy. Patients with prostatic and perinephric infections and abscesses can also present with fever and abdominal pain, but these are retroperitoneal abscesses. After diagnosis, prompt surgical consultation for source control should be obtained. Treatment with broad-spectrum antibiotics should be initiated after specimens for culture are obtained.[30]

Alcohol Withdrawal

Fever can be an occult sign of withdrawal symptoms in alcoholics. Manifestations of alcohol withdrawal vary from simple tremulousness to the most dramatic and severe form, delirium tremens, with its attendant fever, confusion, hallucinations, agitation, and overactivity of the autonomic nervous system. Patients who are in withdrawal from alcohol can present with simultaneous infections of the respiratory and urinary tracts. In some of them, no cause of infection is ever identified. Otero-Antón and colleagues[31] found no infectious cause of fever in one-third of patients with alcohol withdrawal syndrome. Febrile patients in withdrawal impose an especially difficult scenario on the emergency physician because of the vast array of potential causes of the fever and their typically unreliable and uncooperative manner (**Table 4**).[32]

Patients in alcohol withdrawal require aggressive medical treatment and observation. Benzodiazepines, such as diazepam or lorazepam, should be used liberally for sedation and delirium. The dosage should be based on validated tools, such as the Clinical Institute Withdrawal Assessment for Alcohol Scale (CIWA-Ar).[33] Patients at greater risk for adverse outcomes might require intubation and ventilatory support. Frequent assessment of the patient's progress is mandatory to determine whether medication doses should be adjusted.[34]

Table 4			
Causes of fever among the types of alcohol withdrawal syndrome			
	Anxiety and Tremor (n = 10)	Delirium (n = 38)	Seizures (n = 62)
Catheter-associated phlebitis	4 (40)	17 (45)	18 (29)
Urinary tract infection	0	6 (16)	5 (8)
Respiratory infection	1 (10)	8 (21)	6 (10)
Miscellaneous	0	1 (3)	2 (3)
Pyrexia of unknown cause	4 (40)	9 (24)	25 (40)

Data are presented as absolute numbers, with percentages in parentheses. Percentages have been approximated to the entire values.

From Otero-Antón E, González-Quintela A, Saborido J, et al. Fever during alcohol withdrawal syndrome. Eur J Intern Med 1999;10:112–6; with permission.

Adrenal Insufficiency

Acute adrenocortical insufficiency is a life-threatening condition that should always be in the early differential diagnosis of postprocedural fever. Undiagnosed or untreated, it can lead to severe rates of morbidity and mortality. The diagnosis can be challenging, because many of the presenting signs and symptoms are nonspecific. For instance, a postoperative fever might be treated presumptively as infection or systemic inflammatory response syndrome when it actually is a subtle indicator of adrenal insufficiency.[35]

Adrenal insufficiency is either primary or secondary. Primary adrenal insufficiency can result from glandular destruction or metabolic failure. Causes of glandular destruction include, but are not limited to idiopathic atrophy, hemorrhage, tuberculosis, fungal infection, and other diseases infiltrating the adrenal glands. Metabolic failure leads to insufficient hormone production, and usually results from either congenital adrenal hyperplasia, enzyme inhibitors, or autoimmune adrenal insufficiency caused by cytotoxic T lymphocytes. Secondary adrenal insufficiency, more common than the primary form, can result from hypopituitarism associated with hypothalamic-pituitary disease, or from suppression of the hypothalamic-pituitary axis by exogenous steroids or endogenous steroids, such as a tumor.[36,37]

Adrenal crisis can result from an acute exacerbation of chronic insufficiency, usually caused by sepsis or surgical stress. Acute adrenal insufficiency also can be caused by adrenal hemorrhage, classically from septicemia-induced Waterhouse-Friderichsen syndrome (fulminant meningococcemia) and anticoagulation complications. Steroid withdrawal is the most common cause of acute adrenocortical insufficiency, and almost always leads to a glucocorticoid deficiency. Aggressive supportive management should be initiated promptly, beginning with the ABCs of resuscitation (airway, breathing, circulation). Electrolyte abnormalities and hypoglycemia should be corrected. Hydrocortisone, 100 mg intravenously every 6 hours, and fludrocortisone acetate (mineralocorticoid), 0.1 mg daily, should be administered. The key management principle is treatment of the underlying problem that precipitates the crisis.[38]

Malignant Hyperthermia

Malignant hyperthermia, a life-threatening clinical syndrome of hypermetabolism, has been known to occur after the administration of inhalational anesthetic agents, muscle relaxants such as succinylcholine, and other drugs. It occurs in susceptible individuals who have abnormal regulation of calcium in skeletal muscle. This defect allows large quantities of calcium to be released from the sarcoplasmic reticulum of skeletal muscle, causing a hypermetabolic state. The hypermetabolic response leads to increased production of carbon dioxide, metabolic and respiratory acidosis, accelerated oxygen consumption, heat production, activation of the sympathetic nervous system, hyperkalemia, disseminated intravascular coagulation, and multiorgan dysfunction and failure.[39] Early clinical signs of malignant hyperthermia include a rapid, exponential increase in end-tidal carbon dioxide, muscle rigidity, tachypnea, tachycardia, hyperkalemia, and fever. Unrecognized, it can lead to myoglobinuria, subsequent multiorgan failure, and death. Early diagnosis, supportive care with ventilatory and circulatory support, and treatment with dantrolene can improve the outcome.[40]

OTHER CAUSES OF POSTOPERATIVE FEVER
Urinary Tract Infection

UTIs are the most common hospital-acquired infections, and are associated with indwelling catheters in 80% to 90% of cases.[30,41] Patients at highest risk are those with prostatic disease, those who have received spinal anesthesia, and those who have undergone anorectal surgery. Fever associated with UTI tends to emerge 3 to 5 days after surgery.[42] In addition to fever, patients can experience abdominal pain and sometimes ileus. Management typically includes evaluation of the urine (analysis and culture) and appropriate antibiotics when necessary. When presenting signs and symptoms are particularly severe, a diagnosis of pyelonephritis or intra-abdominal infectious complication should be considered.[30] Common infectious causes include *Escherichia coli*, *Klebsiella*, *Enterobacter*, *Pseudomonas*, and *Serratia*. When choosing the antibiotic to be administered for presumed postoperative UTI, these organisms determine the desired spectrum of coverage.[8]

Pneumonia

Almost all surgical patients are at increased risk for postoperative pneumonia. Pain limits their mobility, inspiratory effort, and ability to cough.[43] Exposure to mechanical ventilation, even for a short duration, increases the risk of pneumonia.[44] The depressed mental status induced by general anesthesia makes patients susceptible to aspiration if they vomit. Management of postprocedural pneumonia includes evaluation for leukocytosis, radiographic imaging, sputum culture, and, if appropriate, broad-spectrum antibiotics. The clinician should be mindful that, following laparotomy, radiography might reveal basilar atelectasis or pleural effusion below the diaphragm; in such cases, antibiotics are not required.[30] The decision to administer antibiotics should be based on culture and sensitivity information.[45]

Catheter-Related Bloodstream Infections

In the United States, patients in intensive care units log 15 million central vascular catheter days every year.[46,47] The use of peripheral, mid, and central catheters puts patients at increased risk for bloodstream infections and insertion-site–specific infections such as thrombophlebitis. Catheters become contaminated by 4 mechanisms (in decreasing order of frequency): (1) migration of organisms from the skin at the insertion site into the cutaneous catheter tract and along the surface of the catheter, with colonization of the catheter tip; (2) direct contamination of the catheter or its hub by contact with hands or contaminated fluids or devices; (3) hematogenous spread from anther focus of infection; and (4) contamination of infusate.[46] Patients with an indwelling catheter are at the highest risk for this type of infection.[46] During the assessment of a febrile patient with an indwelling catheter, the goal should be source control and identification of the offending organism through blood cultures. The clinician should have a low threshold for removing presumptively infected indwelling catheters early in the course of treatment, especially when disseminated infection is suspected. This removal is typically sufficient for source control. If the patient's temperature elevation and leukocytosis do not resolve within 24 hours after removal, antibiotics should be considered.[30] Coagulase-negative staphylococci are the most commonly implicated pathogens. Therefore, empiric therapy should include vancomycin (or other antibiotics that treat methicillin-resistant staphylococci).[30]

Infected Prosthetics

Procedures that involve placement of prosthetic material such as orthopedic hardware, neurosurgical ventriculoperitoneal shunts, abdominal mesh, or vascular grafting can all result in complicated surgical infections. The emergency medicine provider must recognize the prosthetic as a potential source of infection. A thorough history and physical examination, with particular attention to past procedures, should always be performed, as infections associated with prosthetics can be indolent and may not emerge for weeks to years after the procedure.[48] Graft infections can be caused by direct inoculation of the surgical site or hematogenous spread.[49] CT, magnetic resonance imaging, or white blood cell scintigraphy can be useful, but negative findings do not necessarily rule out infection.[50]

Infection from sternal wires or a surgical-site infection on the sternum can result in devastating complications such as mediastinitis. Sternal wound infections most often occur in the acute phase of fever (within a week after the procedure).[51] Meningitis can occur after neurosurgical procedures or after placement of an intracranial drain or monitor.[30] Prosthetics are frequent causes of infection; therefore, fever after neurosurgery should always mandate aggressive diagnostic and therapeutic measures.[52]

Clostridium difficile Infections

Enteric infections caused by Clostridium difficile are increasing in prevalence and resistance. Infection commonly occurs after the administration of an antibiotic that alters the normally protective bacterial flora of the colon. Transmission occurs via the fecal-oral route, primarily via contaminated environmental surfaces and the hands of health care workers. Twenty percent to 50% of hospitalized patients are colonized with the organism.[30,53] Risk factors for fulminant toxic megacolon or clinically significant infection include disruption of the normal colonic flora, exposure to an antibiotic, chemotherapy, and inflammatory bowel disease.[30] Toxic megacolon is a surgical emergency requiring emergent subtotal colectomy.

When C difficile infection is suspected, antibiotics and fluid resuscitation should be initiated immediately. Clinicians who have initiated antibiotic therapy to prevent surgical-site and catheter-related bloodstream infections might eventually witness the sequelae of the inappropriate use of antibiotics.[5] A patient with an acute abdomen who has received antibiotics within the past 2 months should be considered at high risk for C difficile colitis.[30] After a sample is obtained for detecting cytotoxin, empiric treatment with vancomycin (oral or per rectum as an enema) or intravenous or oral metronidazole should be initiated. Fecal transplantation and a new macrolide antibiotic, fidaxomicin (Dificid), are newer treatment modalities directed against more resistant strains.[54]

MANAGEMENT OF POSTPROCEDURE FEVER

Management strategies for patients with postprocedure fever should take into consideration the degree of fever and the timing of its onset. Routine laboratory studies, urinalysis and urine culture, blood cultures, wound cultures, and radiographic imaging should all be tailored to individual cases. Life-threatening or potentially life-threatening causes of the fever should be given diagnostic and treatment priority. Early consultation with the operative/procedure team can clarify the diagnostic approach and target management. A postprocedure fever algorithm can help emergency care providers through key decision making.

The definitive treatment of an identified focus of fever is source control; for example, drainage of an abscess, wide debridement of necrotizing infections, or removal of a foreign body such as an indwelling catheter. Timely use of broad-spectrum antibiotics can help prevent the patient from progressing on the continuum of fever to multisystem organ dysfunction. After culture results have been obtained, the antibiotic regimen should be reviewed to stem the development of resistant organisms.

Table 5 Causes of Postoperative Fever	
Non-Infectious	**Infectious**
Adrenal Insufficiency	Abscess
Alcohol Withdrawal	Bloodstream Infections
Atelectasis	Cholecystitis
Blood [Hematoma/CSF]	Clostridium difficile colitis
Dehydration	Endocarditis
Drug Fever	Infusion-related infections
Factitious	Intravascular device infections
Malignant Hyperthermia	Parotitis
Myocardial Infarction	Pneumonia
Neoplasms	Prostatitis
Pancreatitis	Sinusitis
Pheochromocytoma	Surgical Site Infections
Pericarditis/Dressler's syndrome	Transfusion related
Pulmonary Embolism	Urinary Tract infections
Thrombophlebitis	
Thyrotoxicosis	
Tissue Trauma	
Elsevier15Transfusion reaction	

Data from Steinberg JP, Zimmer S. Fever and Infection in the postoperative setting. In: Lubion MF, Smith RB, Dobson TF, et al, editors. Medical Management of the Surgical Patient: A textbook of Perioperative Medicine. 4th edition. Cambridge: Cambridge University Press; 2006.

SUMMARY

The diagnosis and management of postprocedure fever can be challenging. For emergency medicine providers, it is imperative that the evaluation take into consideration both noninfectious and infectious causes (**Table 5**). A clear understanding of the timing of the onset of fever in relation to the procedure (immediate, acute, subacute, or delayed) can differentiate likely diagnoses. A thorough history and physical examination are mandatory and will guide further diagnostic workup. Blood cultures, urinalysis, urine cultures, as well as routine laboratory studies can also aid in diagnosis. Imaging studies should be used judiciously, based on consideration of the procedure that has been performed. Source control remains the ultimate goal in patients found to have septic foci such as an abscess. Antibiotics should be administered promptly as an adjunct to source control.

REFERENCES

1. Perlino CA. Postoperative fever. Med Clin North Am 2001;85:1141–9.
2. Garibaldi RA, Brodine S, Matsumiya S, et al. Evidence for the non-infectious etiology of early postoperative fever. Infect Control 1985;6:273–7.
3. Cline D, Stead LG. Abdominal emergencies. New York: McGraw-Hill Professional; 2007. p. 146.
4. Cunha BA. Fever in the intensive care unit. Intensive Care Med 1999;25:648–51.
5. Pile JC. Evaluating postoperative fever: a focused approach. Cleve Clin J Med 2006;73(Suppl 1):S62–6.

6. Dellinger EP. Approach to the patient with postoperative fever. In: Gorbach S, Bartlett J, Blacklow N, editors. Infectious diseases. Philadelphia: Lippincott Williams & Wilkins; 2004. p. 817–23.

7. Dellinger EP. Should we measure body temperature for patients who have recently undergone surgery? Clin Infect Dis 2005;40:1411–2.

8. Fry D. Surgical infection. In: O'Leary J, editor. The physiologic basis of surgery. 3rd edition. Philadelphia: Lippincott Williams & Wilkins; 2002. p. 218–57.

9. Wortel CH, van Deventer SJ, Aarden LA, et al. Interleukin-6 mediates host defense responses induced by abdominal surgery. Surgery 1993;114:564–70.

10. Frank SM, Kluger MJ, Kunkel SL. Elevated thermostatic setpoint in postoperative patients. Anesthesiology 2000;93:1426–31.

11. Dauleh MI, Rahman S, Townell NH. Open versus laparoscopic cholecystectomy: a comparison of postoperative temperature. J R Coll Surg Edinb 1995;40:116–8.

12. Fanning J, Neuhoff RA, Brewer JE, et al. Frequency and yield of postoperative fever evaluation. Infect Dis Obstet Gynecol 1998;6:252–5.

13. Shaw JA, Chung R. Febrile response after knee and hip arthroplasty. Clin Orthop Relat Res 1999;367:181–9.

14. Livelli FD Jr, Johnson RA, McEnany MT, et al. Unexplained in-hospital fever following cardiac surgery. Natural history, relationship to postpericardiotomy syndrome, and a prospective study of therapy with indomethacin versus placebo. Circulation 1987;57:968–75.

15. Vermeulen H, Storm-Versloot MN, Goossens A. Diagnostic accuracy of routine postoperative body temperature measurements. Clin Infect Dis 2005;40:1404–10.

16. Roberts J, Barnes W, Pennock M, et al. Diagnostic accuracy of fever as a measure of postoperative pulmonary complications. Heart Lung 1988;17:166–70.

17. Engoren M. Lack of association between atelectasis and fever. Chest 1995;107: 81–4.

18. Kuncir EJ, Tillou A, St Hill CR, et al. Necrotizing soft-tissue infections. Emerg Med Clin North Am 2003;21:1075–87.

19. Forbes N, Rankin AP. Necrotizing fasciitis and nonsteroidal anti-inflammatory drugs: a case series and review of the literature. N Z Med J 2001;114:3–6.

20. Frick S, Cerny A. Necrotizing fasciitis due to *Streptococcus pneumoniae* after intramuscular injection of nonsteroidal anti-inflammatory drugs: report of 2 cases and review. Clin Infect Dis 2001;33:740–4.

21. Tung-Yiu W, Jehn-Shyun H, Ching-Hung C. Cervical necrotizing fasciitis of odontogenic origin: a report of 11 cases. J Oral Maxillofac Surg 2000;58:1347–52.

22. Kobayashi L, Konstantinidis A, Shackelford S, et al. Necrotizing soft tissue infections: delayed surgical treatment is associated with increased number of surgical debridements and morbidity. J Trauma 2011;71:1400–5.

23. Clayton MD, Fowler JE Jr, Sharifi R, et al. Causes, presentation and survival of fifty-seven patients with necrotizing fasciitis of the male genitalia. Surg Gynecol Obstet 1990;170:49–55.

24. Wong CH, Khin LW, Heng KS, et al. The LRINEC (Laboratory Risk Indicator for Necrotizing Fasciitis) score: a tool for distinguishing necrotizing fasciitis from other soft tissue infections. Crit Care Med 2004;32:1535–41.

25. Cunningham JD, Silver L, Rudikoff D. Necrotizing fasciitis: a plea for early diagnosis and treatment. Mt Sinai J Med 2001;68:253–61.

26. McHenry CR, Piotrowski JJ, Petrinic D, et al. Determinants of mortality for necrotizing soft-tissue infections. Ann Surg 1995;221:558–65.

27. Elliott DC, Kufera JA, Myers RA. Necrotizing soft tissue infections. Risk factors for mortality and strategies for management. Ann Surg 1996;224(5):672–83.

28. Murray HW, Ellis GC, Blumenthal DS, et al. Fever and pulmonary thromboembolism. Am J Med 1979;67:232–5.
29. Nucifora G, Badano L, Hysko F, et al. Pulmonary embolism and fever: when should right-sided infective endocarditis be considered? Circulation 2007;115: e173–6.
30. Dellinger EP. Nosocomial infections. In: Souba WW, Fink MP, Jurkovich GJ, et al, editors. ACS surgery: principles and practice. New York: WebMD Professional Publishing; 2005. p. 1423–40.
31. Otero-Antón E, González-Quintela A, Saborido J, et al. Fever during alcohol withdrawal syndrome. Eur J Intern Med 1999;10:112–6.
32. Wrenn KD, Larson S. The febrile alcoholic in the emergency department. Am J Emerg Med 1991;9:57–60.
33. Sullivan JT, Sykora K, Schneiderman J, et al. Assessment of alcohol withdrawal: the revised Clinical Institute Withdrawal Assessment of Alcohol Scale (CIWA-Ar). Br J Addict 1989;84:1353–7.
34. Kosten TR, O'Connor PG. Management of drug and alcohol withdrawal. N Engl J Med 2003;348:1786–95.
35. Omori K, Nomura K, Shimizu S, et al. Risk factors for adrenal crisis in patients with adrenal insufficiency. Endocr J 2003;50:745–52.
36. Williams GH, Dluhy RG. Disorders of the Adrenal Cortex. In: Fauci A, Braunwald E, Kasper D, editors. Harrison's Principles of Internal Medicine. New York: McGraw Hill; 2008. p. 2247–68.
37. Hall JE. Adrenocortical Hormones. In: John E, Hall JE, Guyton AC, editors. Guyton and Hall: a textbook of medical physiology. Philadephia: WB Saunders; 2011. p. 921–37.
38. Marik PE, Pastores SM, Annane D, et al. Recommendations for the diagnosis and management of corticosteroid insufficiency in critically ill adult patients: consensus statements from an international task force by the American College of Critical Care Medicine. Crit Care Med 2008;36:1937–49.
39. Gronert GA, Pessah IN, Muldoon SM, et al. Malignant hyperthermia. In: Miller RD, editor. Miller's anesthesia. 6th edition. Philadelphia: Elsevier Churchill Livingstone; 2005. p. 1169–90.
40. Larach MG, Gronert GA, Allen GC, et al. Clinical presentation, treatment, and complications of malignant hyperthermia in North America from 1987 to 2006. Anesth Analg 2010;110:498–507.
41. Garibaldi RA, Burke J, Dickman ML, et al. Factors predisposing to bacteriuria during indwelling urethral catheterization. N Engl J Med 1974;291: 215–9.
42. Ballestas HC. Postoperative fever: to what is the body really responding? AORN J 2007;86:983–92.
43. Smetana GW, Lawrence VA, Cornell JE. Preoperative pulmonary risk stratification for noncardiothoracic surgery: systematic review for the American College of Physicians. Ann Intern Med 2006;144:581–95.
44. Horan TC, Culver DH, Gaynes RP, et al. Nosocomial infections in surgical patients in the United States, January 1986-June 1992. Infect Control Hosp Epidemiol 1993;14:73–80.
45. Craven DE, Chroneou A, Zias N, et al. Ventilator-associated tracheobronchitis: the impact of targeted antibiotic therapy on patient outcomes. Chest 2009; 135:521–8.
46. O'Grady NP, Alexander M, Burns LA, et al. Guidelines for the prevention of intravascular catheter-related infections. Am J Infect Control 2011;39:S1–34.

47. Mermel LA. Prevention of intravascular catheter-related infections. Ann Intern Med 2000;132:391–402.

48. Cernohorsky P, Reijnen MM, Tielliu IF, et al. The relevance of aortic endograft prosthetic infection. J Vasc Surg 2011;54:327–33.

49. Phade SV, Keldahl ML, Morasch MD, et al. Late abdominal aortic endograft explants: indications and outcomes. Surgery 2011;150:788–95.

50. Vogel TR, Symons R, Flum DR. The incidence and factors associated with graft infection after aortic aneurysm repair. J Vasc Surg 2008;47:264–9.

51. Kohman LJ, Coleman MJ, Parker FB Jr. Bacteremia and sternal infection after coronary artery bypass grafting. Ann Thorac Surg 1990;49:454–7.

52. Kaufman BA, Tunkel AR, Pryor JC, et al. Meningitis in the neurosurgical patient. Infect Dis Clin North Am 1990;4:677–701.

53. McFarland LV, Mulligan ME, Kwok RY, et al. Nosocomial acquisition of Clostridium difficile infection. N Engl J Med 1989;320:204–10.

54. Novak-Weekley SM, Marlowe EM, Miller JM, et al. Clostridium difficile testing in the clinical laboratory by use of multiple testing algorithms. J Clin Microbiol 2010;48:889–93.

Fever in Immunocompromised Hosts

Devang M. Patel, MD*, David J. Riedel, MD

KEYWORDS

- Fever • HIV • AIDS • Neutropenic fever • Solid-organ transplant
- Tumor necrosis factor-α inhibitors • Hematopoietic stem cell transplant
- Emergency department

KEY POINTS

- A thorough history and physical examination are necessary to determine the type and severity of immunosuppression and elucidate patients' history of exposures to specific pathogens.
- Immunosuppressed patients are at risk for infections from many pathogens, including organisms commonly seen in normal hosts as well as rare and atypical organisms.
- Obtaining an early blood culture, before the introduction of antimicrobials, is critical to establishing a diagnosis in many patients.
- Prompt, empiric antimicrobial coverage should be given to patients at highest risk of systemic infection and to those showing signs or symptoms of clinical deterioration.
- Antimicrobial use in patients who are not systemically ill should be judicious so as not to compromise diagnostic procedures.
- Invasive diagnostic procedures might be required to establish the diagnosis.

Emergency department (ED) health care providers continue to see increasing numbers of immunocompromised patients; in many of these individuals, the immunocompromised state has an iatrogenic cause.[1,2] Since the 1980s, the human immunodeficiency virus (HIV) epidemic created one of the most important populations of immunocompromised hosts ever seen by physicians. The presentation of these patients has changed in the era of combined antiretroviral therapy (cART).[3,4] In addition, medicine has seen an increase in the number of solid-organ and hematologic transplantations, the use of chemotherapeutic agents for the treatment of malignancies, and the

Devang M. Patel and David J. Riedel contributed equally to this work.
Disclosure: The authors declare no conflicts of interest.
Division of Infectious Disease, Department of Medicine, Institute of Human Virology, University of Maryland School of Medicine, 725 West Lombard Street, Baltimore, MD 21201, USA
* Corresponding author. Division of Infectious Diseases, Institute of Human Virology, University of Maryland School of Medicine, 725 West Lombard Street, N559, Baltimore, MD 21201.
E-mail address: dpatel@ihv.umaryland.edu

Emerg Med Clin N Am 31 (2013) 1059–1071
http://dx.doi.org/10.1016/j.emc.2013.07.002
0733-8627/13/$ – see front matter © 2013 Elsevier Inc. All rights reserved.

administration of monoclonal antibodies for many autoimmune diseases, leading to an increase in the number of immunocompromised individuals living in communities.

When assessing immunocompromised patients, one of the most important first steps is to determine the type of immunosuppression the patients are experiencing. The type dictates what aspect of the immune system is affected, which in turn determines the types of pathogens most likely to cause disease in those patients. Some patients presenting to the ED with fever represent true emergencies (eg, neutropenic fever in patients with cancer) and must be treated empirically with antimicrobials immediately to avoid life-threatening complications. In most immunosuppressed patients, a fever represents a diagnostic dilemma requiring consultation by infectious diseases specialists and, in many cases, invasive diagnostic procedures to identify the infective organism. In the ED, empiric administration of antimicrobials should be used judiciously to treat the most likely infections suggested by the patients' clinical presentation. Overuse of antimicrobials can lead to unwanted side effects, drug-drug interactions, and difficulty in establishing a definitive diagnosis. This review focuses on the common febrile syndromes associated with the different types of immunosuppression and their importance in the ED setting.

HIV/AIDS

Most clinicians are aware of the decline in cell-mediated immunity that occurs during infection with HIV and leads to AIDS.[5] Just as important is the dysfunction in humoral immunity that predisposes patients to recurrent bacterial infections.[6] Over time, this immunosuppression puts patients at risk for opportunistic infections (OIs) (**Table 1**). In the era of cART, the number of hospitalizations for OIs has declined substantially, but infections (particularly bacterial pneumonia and cellulitis) are still the primary reason for the hospitalization of patients infected with HIV.[3,4] Rather than discuss the wide array of OIs described in the literature, the focus here is on the more common infections that ED health care providers are likely to encounter while caring for patients with HIV.

PULMONARY SYNDROMES

In the cART era, pulmonary syndromes, including chronic obstructive pulmonary disease and asthma, remain the top reason for hospitalization among patients with HIV.[4] Patients with pulmonary syndromes are at an increased risk of bacterial pneumonias

Table 1		
Primary prophylaxis in patients with HIV		
Opportunistic Infection	**Indications**	**Drug of Choice**
Pneumocystis pneumonia	CD4 count <200 cells/mm³ or thrush	Trimethoprim-sulfamethoxazole single or double strength daily
Coccidioides	CD4 count <250 cells/mm³ and positive IgM or IgG serology and live in endemic area (Southwest United States)	Fluconazole 400 mg daily or Itraconazole 200 mg BID
Toxoplasmosis	CD4 count <100 cells/mm³ and Toxo antibody positive	Trimethoprim-sulfamethoxazole double strength daily
Mycobacterium avium complex	CD4 count <50 cells/mm³	Azithromycin 1200 mg weekly

Abbreviation: Ig, immunoglobulin.

compared with the general population. They have a particular increase in invasive pneumococcal disease, which is related to a declining CD4 count.[7,8] Among OIs, *Pneumocystis jiroveci* pneumonia (PCP) remains the most common pulmonary infection, but its incidence has decreased dramatically with cART.[9] Worldwide, tuberculosis (TB) is the major pulmonary complication of HIV in TB-endemic areas.[10] Differentiating between these 3 syndromes remains the major challenge for clinicians caring for patients infected with HIV.

Clinical assessment with a careful history and physical examination often leads to the appropriate diagnosis. The duration of the illness is helpful in determining the type of pneumonia. Bacterial pneumonia is typically acute, whereas PCP tends to be subacute; TB is a chronic disease. The presentation of bacterial pneumonia in patients with HIV is similar to that in uninfected patients (ie, the abrupt onset of productive cough, dyspnea, pleuritic chest pain, fever, and myalgia).[11] Conversely, PCP has a more gradual onset with fever, progressive dyspnea, and nonproductive cough.[12] Tachypnea, severe dyspnea, and hypoxemia are the hallmarks of PCP and should make PCP the top consideration in patients with depressed CD4 counts (<200 cells per cubic millimeter) who are not taking prophylactic medication. If TB is suspected, patients should be asked about risk factors, such as travel to or immigration from endemic areas, incarceration, and homelessness. Symptoms classically associated with TB include fever, night sweats, weight loss, and cough; these symptoms might be less prominent in patients with lower CD4 counts. The examination findings might not be helpful in distinguishing between the 3 entities, but bacterial pneumonias typically have evidence of lobar consolidation, such as rales, egophony, or decreased breath sounds. Conversely, half of the patients with PCP have normal examination results. TB can present as lymphadenopathy and signs of lobar consolidation, and these signs are also less common with lower CD4 counts.

Chest radiography and laboratory studies can be helpful in determining the source of fever in patients with pulmonary syndromes. Radiographic findings in patients with HIV with bacterial pneumonias are similar to those in patients who are not carrying the virus. PCP is often characterized as a bilateral airspace disease that yields a ground-glass appearance on chest films. Lung cysts and pneumothorax are later findings. But many patients with PCP have normal chest imaging.[13] The typical findings of TB (ie, upper lobe disease with cavitation or intrathoracic adenopathy) are less common in patients with HIV, particularly those with lower CD4 counts, because they do not have the immune response necessary to elicit these changes.[14]

In terms of laboratory tests, sputum analysis is the most useful in determining the cause of disease. Sputum gram stains can be used to identify bacterial pneumonias even before patients have left the ED. Sputum evaluation for acid-fast bacilli (AFB) and PCP are less sensitive but diagnostic if positive.

Empiric therapy in the ED should include treatment of community-acquired pneumonia if patients present with evidence of pulmonary infection with lobar disease. Because of the decreased prevalence of PCP, attributable to cART in the United States, clinicians often prefer a definitive microbiologic or histopathologic diagnosis before committing patients to the full course of treatment. However, early empiric treatment of patients with possible or suspected PCP is still important given the high mortality rate associated with untreated PCP.[15] In the United States, TB typically requires definitive diagnosis before the initiation of treatment because of the toxicity of the drugs and the length of the treatment course.

Other pulmonary infections should also be considered, depending on the geographic setting and the patients' presentation. Pulmonary histoplasmosis is the most common endemic mycosis in patients with HIV in the United States and is seen in many areas, including the Ohio and Mississippi River valleys. In the pre-cART era, this infection occurred in as many as 27% of patients with AIDS in endemic areas.[16] The presentation of pulmonary histoplasmosis is similar to that of pulmonary TB, but disseminated histoplasmosis presents as a febrile wasting syndrome in patients with lower CD4 counts.[16] Another endemic fungus to consider is *Coccidioides*, which occurs primarily in the Southwestern United States. An analysis done in the pre-cART era showed symptomatic coccidioidomycosis to be a common disease in patients with CD4 counts less than 250 cells per cubic millimeter.[17] The presentation is easily confused with PCP and should be considered in patients with HIV from endemic areas who are not taking fluconazole prophylaxis.

NEUROLOGIC SYNDROMES

Several neurologic syndromes should be considered in patients with HIV presenting with fever. Cryptococcal meningoencephalitis is a major cause of HIV-related mortality worldwide.[18] The presentation consists of fever, headache, and malaise, which occur indolently over 1 to 2 weeks, generally in patients with CD4 counts less than 100 cells per cubic millimeter. Later presentations include confusion, vision loss, and hearing loss secondary to increased intracranial pressure. Some patients with cryptococcal meningoencephalitis present with pneumonia; cryptococcal pneumonia is an early manifestation preceding infection of the central nervous system. Skin lesions that mimic molluscum contagiosum serve as an additional clue of cryptococcal disease, but they are uncommon.[19] Cryptococcal antigen or culture from cerebrospinal fluid (CSF) provides the definitive diagnosis of cryptococcal meningoencephalitis. In patients with AIDS, serum cryptococcal antigen testing has similar sensitivity to CSF antigen testing.[20] Emergency physicians should attempt to measure opening pressure during the diagnostic lumbar puncture. An elevated opening pressure suggests cryptococcal disease. Treatment consists of antifungal therapy and therapeutic lumbar puncture to decrease intracranial pressure in patients who have elevated opening pressure.

Toxoplasma encephalitis is another major neurologic infection seen in patients with AIDS. *Toxoplasma* disease is a reactivation of the intracellular parasite in patients with CD4 counts less than 100 cells per cubic millimeter. Patients present with fever, headache, altered mental status, seizures, and focal neurologic signs. This diagnosis should be considered in patients with AIDS who have evidence of *Toxoplasma* antibodies and who are not taking prophylactic medication. Imaging shows ring-enhancing brain lesions, often with associated calcified lesions suggestive of old disease. Treatment is usually empiric based on clinical and radiographic findings because the only definitive way to diagnose *Toxoplasma* encephalitis requires brain biopsy. Patients' symptoms should recede within 2 weeks after starting empiric therapy.[21] If no improvement is seen in this period, other diagnoses should be entertained. The presentation of primary central nervous system lymphoma is similar to that of *Toxoplasma* encephalitis. The two can be indistinguishable without a brain biopsy. Up to 80% of patients with AIDS with this lymphoma have constitutional symptoms, including fever.[22]

OTHER FEBRILE SYNDROMES

Infections of the gastrointestinal (GI) tract typically induce diarrhea, but some cause only low-grade fever. Exceptions include cytomegalovirus (CMV) disease, which can affect any part of the GI tract. CMV disease occurs most frequently in patients with CD4 counts less than 50 cells per cubic millimeter. CMV esophagitis is characterized by fever, odynophagia, and nausea and, without endoscopy, can be difficult to differentiate from other causes of esophagitis. CMV colitis is associated with fever, weight loss, anorexia, abdominal pain, and diarrhea.[23] This disease requires biopsy for diagnosis, so it is unlikely to be diagnosed in the ED; but it should be included in the differential diagnosis for patients with AIDS with diarrhea. Treatment of CMV infections begins with ganciclovir even though drug resistance has been noted.[24]

Another febrile syndrome that was common in the pre-cART era is *Mycobacterium avium* complex (MAC). This disease is still seen in patients with advanced immunosuppression (CD4 count <50 cells per cubic millimeter) who are not on azithromycin prophylaxis. Localized disease can occur in immune-competent individuals, but this is usually a disseminated disease in patients with AIDS. Clinical manifestations of disseminated MAC include fever, night sweats, abdominal pain, diarrhea, and weight loss. If this disease is in the differential diagnosis during ED assessment, blood cultures for AFB should be sent early because this is a slow-growing organism requiring at least 1 week of incubation before identification.

SOLID-ORGAN TRANSPLANT RECIPIENTS

Organ transplant recipients have a significantly increased risk of infection in the posttransplant period. This risk correlates to the net state of immunosuppression and the patients' history of exposure to potential pathogens.[25] Fever following transplant must be addressed urgently, with a comprehensive search for microbiologic causes and early empiric or directed antimicrobial therapy, because unrecognized infections can progress rapidly. Three additional considerations are critical in the evaluation of fever in transplant recipients: (1) the usual signs and symptoms of infections might be muted by immunosuppression, making the identification of the source of infection difficult; (2) noninfectious causes of fever (eg, graft rejection and drug reactions) must be considered in the differential diagnosis; and (3) new antimicrobials should always be cross-checked against current immunosuppressive agents in order to avoid toxic drug-drug interactions.[25,26]

The types of infections encountered in transplant recipients are categorized as donor derived, recipient derived, community acquired, and nosocomial. Donor-derived infections are transported with the new organ and most commonly emerge within the initial weeks after the transplant.[26] Serologic screening of the donor reduces the risk of some but not all transmitted pathogens. The recipient could harbor latent pathogens that are activated during the period of most intensive immunosuppression, the first 6 months after the transplant.[27] Community-acquired infections are presenting with increasing severity in transplant recipients.[25] Donors and recipients have extensive interactions with the health care system in advance of the transplant procedure; some have prolonged hospitalizations, which heightens their risk of becoming colonized with drug-resistant pathogens.[25] Several recent reviews documented that abdominal pain and GI symptoms (27%–31%) and fever caused by infection (17%–28%) were the most common reasons for transplant recipients' presentations to EDs.[28–30]

The risk of infection after the transplant is driven by the degree of immunosuppression (**Table 2**). Because immunosuppressive agents are usually tapered over time, the risk is highest during the first 6 months after the transplant and gradually diminishes thereafter. Treating graft rejection with enhanced immunosuppression will reset the usual timeline of immune system recovery and prolong the period of increased risk.

In the early posttransplant period (within 1 month), nosocomial/resistant pathogens, donor-derived pathogens, and recipient colonizers are all common sources of

Table 2
Timing of transplant-related infections

First month	Donor-derived pathogens
	Bacteremia, candidemia from seeded allograft
	Health care–associated pathogens, including drug-resistant organisms
	Surgical site infections
	Clostridium difficile colitis
1–6 mo	Reactivation of herpes viruses (HSV, CMV, EBV, VZV)
	Hepatitis B and C
	TB
	Nocardia, Listeria
	Fungi
	Pneumocystis pneumonia
	Cryptococcosis
	Aspergillus
	Endemic fungi (eg, *Histoplasma*)
>6 mo	Community-Acquired Infections
	Respiratory viruses, community pneumonia, urinary infections
	With steroids or other enhanced immunosuppression for rejection
	CMV, *Aspergillus*
	Endemic fungi

Abbreviations: EBV, Epstein-Barr virus; HSV, herpes simplex virus; VZV, varicella zoster virus.

infection.[26,27] Technical complications from the surgical procedure (eg, wound infections, anastomotic leaks, and organ ischemia) are most common in the first few weeks after surgery.[27] Fortunately, with current prophylaxis protocols, opportunistic infections are uncommon.[26]

The period of 1 to 6 months after the transplant is characterized by the most intense immunosuppression and the highest likelihood for activation of opportunistic or latent infections, particularly viruses.[27] The pathogens commonly encountered during this period are herpes viruses (herpes simplex virus [HSV], CMV, Epstein-Barr virus [EBV], varicella zoster virus [VZV]), hepatitis B and C, *Mycobacterium tuberculosis*, *P jiroveci*, *Cryptococcus neoformans*, and BK virus. Less common pathogens are *Listeria, Nocardia, Toxoplasma, Strongyloides stercoralis, Leishmania*, and *Trypanosoma cruzi*.[26,27] With effective prophylaxis, the incidence of *Pneumocystis* infection, CMV, and hepatitis B can be reduced substantially.[26] Graft rejection commonly presents as fever during this period.

As the recipient gets further from the time of the transplant (beyond 6 months), the risk of infection is markedly reduced as immunosuppressants are tapered (assuming good graft function and no increased immunosuppression required by episodes of rejection). This period is characterized by community-acquired infections, such as pneumonia, respiratory virus infections, and urinary tract infections.[26,27] In patients whose immunosuppressive regimens are intensified for the treatment of graft rejection (particularly with corticosteroids), the risk for OIs (eg, CMV, *Aspergillus*) is increased.

The ED assessment of transplant patients with fever should include a detailed review of epidemiologic exposures and pretransplant serologies (both donor and recipient), notation of the time since the transplant, and the use of antimicrobial prophylaxis and immunosuppressive agents. The chart should be reviewed for any history of colonization with drug-resistant organisms. When all of this information has been gathered, the net state of immunosuppression can be estimated and a reasonable differential diagnosis of the potential causes of the fever can be formulated.

The physical examination must be meticulous because the usual signs and symptoms of infection can be attenuated and subtle findings could be easily overlooked. The surgical site should be examined carefully for signs of wound infection, dehiscence, or hematoma formation. Indwelling catheters, drains, and other hardware should be evaluated for signs of inflammation or purulent discharge. The skin, lungs, and neurologic system must be assessed carefully for subtle findings or new lesions.

In addition to basic laboratory tests, the initial laboratory evaluation for transplant recipients presenting with an isolated fever should include urinalysis, urine culture, at least 2 sets of blood cultures, and a quantitative CMV polymerase chain reaction (PCR). Imaging can begin with conventional radiography of a focal area of complaint, but computed tomography and magnetic resonance imaging (MRI) are often necessary because of their higher sensitivity and frequent lack of overt physical examination findings.[31] If concurrent or rare pathogens are suspected, invasive diagnostic procedures are usually indicated to make or confirm the diagnosis.[26] For example, bronchoscopy with bronchoalveolar lavage and biopsy should be performed in transplant patients with fever and new pulmonary infiltrates. Transplant patients presenting with altered mental status should undergo lumbar puncture and MRI. CSF should be sent for typical evaluation (cell count and differential, glucose, protein) along with cultures for bacteria, fungi, and AFB; cryptococcal antigen; and viral PCRs (HSV, CMV, EBV, VZV).

Most transplant patients with a new fever should probably be evaluated in the hospital, unless the cause is straightforward and easily managed on an outpatient basis.[32] If patients seem quite well with only an isolated fever without identifiable source, antibiotics could be withheld if patients can be monitored closely for signs of deterioration.[32] The management of transplant patients presenting with signs and symptoms of infection can be complicated by drug-drug interactions, so any new antimicrobial should be checked to ensure compatibility with the patients' current medications.[33] In any patient who seems unwell, empiric antimicrobials should be started promptly and provide broad coverage of suspected and potential organisms. Because transplant recipients can be colonized with drug-resistant organisms, extended-spectrum antibiotics that are effective against such organisms should be considered.[33] Aggressive surgical management of wound infections and other complications stemming from the procedure should be performed early in the course of care because antibiotics alone are inadequate in compromised hosts.[34,35]

NEUTROPENIC PATIENTS WITH CANCER

Infectious complications in patients undergoing cancer treatment are important causes of morbidity and mortality. Fever in the setting of neutropenia from cancer chemotherapy represents a true oncologic emergency and should never be discounted. Although a nonspecific finding, fever often represents the only outward sign of a serious infection in these immunocompromised hosts.[36] Most patients with chemotherapy-induced neutropenia experience fever at some point during their treatment, but a microbiologic source of infection is identifiable in only a minority (20%–30%) of febrile episodes.[37] The most common sites of infection are the GI tract, lung, sinuses, skin, and bloodstream. Central venous catheters are also important sources that should not be overlooked. This discussion focuses on neutropenic patients with cancer with fever who come to an ED from home, seeking evaluation and treatment.

The risk of infectious complications is directly related to the depth and duration of neutropenia. Neutropenia is generally defined as an absolute neutrophil count (ANC) of less than 500 cells per cubic millimeter and is characterized as profound when the ANC is less than 100 cells per cubic millimeter.[37] High-risk patients are those with profound neutropenia lasting a week or more and those with significant medical comorbidities.[37] Lower-risk patients have less severe ANC nadirs or a shorter duration (<1 week) of profoundly depressed ANCs.

The epidemiology of pathogens encountered in neutropenic patients with cancer reveals a pattern that depends primarily on the duration of neutropenia. Early in the course of neutropenia (ie, in the first 1 or 2 weeks), infections are most often caused by bacteria. As the duration of neutropenia increases over 2 weeks, the risk of yeast (mostly *Candida* species) and molds (eg, *Aspergillus* species) increases significantly.[36] Traditionally, gram-negative bacteria, such as *Pseudomonas aeruginosa*, *Escherichia coli*, and *Klebsiella pneumoniae*, have caused the bulk of infections and have been associated with a high mortality rate; however, as the use of long-term intravascular catheters and access devices and prophylactic antibiotics has increased, there has been a shift toward more gram-positive infections with *Staphylococcus aureus*, coagulase-negative staphylococci, viridans streptococci, and enterococcal species.[38,39] The bacterial flora can be altered substantially in patients taking prophylactic antibiotics at home, increasing the risk for drug-resistant pathogens. Other causes of fever in patients presenting from the community are viruses, including respiratory syncytial virus, parainfluenza, and influenza A and B. These common viruses should not be overlooked, particularly during the winter outbreak season.

The history should include a detailed review of any new site-specific symptoms and the patients' use of antimicrobial prophylaxis, sick contacts, and history of recent infections.[37] The medical history should be reviewed for colonization with multiresistant pathogens and recent exposures to noninfectious causes of fever (eg, blood transfusion).[37]

The physical examination should be performed carefully, with an awareness that outward signs (eg, erythema, induration) might be subtle because of the patients' lack of inflammatory cells. The focus should be on several critical areas: the skin (particularly around indwelling ports or catheters), sinuses, oropharynx, abdomen, lungs, and perineum/perirectal area.[1,37]

The initial laboratory evaluation should include a complete blood cell (CBC) count with differential and measurement of serum creatinine, blood urea nitrogen, electrolytes, hepatic transaminase enzymes, and total bilirubin.[37] At least 2 sets of blood cultures are recommended, with a set collected simultaneously from each lumen of a central venous catheter, if present, and from a peripheral vein site. Two blood culture sets from separate venipunctures should be sent if no central catheter is present.[37] Culture specimens from other sites of suspected infection should be obtained as clinically indicated.[7]

Empiric antibacterials should be started urgently (ie, within 2 hours) in neutropenic patients with cancer because they are at high risk for rapid progression of infection.[37] Delays in the initiation of antibiotics have been associated with mortality rates in excess of 50% at 24 hours.[40] Patients should be prepared for inpatient management with intravenous antibiotics. Initial antimicrobial therapy is empiric but focused on gram-negative bacteria (antipseudomonal coverage is essential). The Infectious Diseases Society of America (IDSA) recommends monotherapy with an antipseudomonal β-lactam agent, such as cefepime, a carbapenem (meropenem or imipenem-cilastatin), or piperacillin-tazobactam.[37] The long debate about combination versus monotherapy for severe gram-negative infections largely centered around this clinical scenario; current evidence supports the use of empiric monotherapy.[41] In general, additional antibiotics are necessary only if complications or antibacterial resistance is known or suspected. A hospital antibiogram might be helpful in understanding the typical rates of antibiotic resistance found in the local setting. Gram-positive coverage (eg, vancomycin) is *not* automatically included in the initial empiric regimen, although its addition is warranted in some instances. The IDSA's guidelines list several indications for adding gram-positive bacterial coverage to the empiric regimen: (1) hemodynamic instability or other evidence of severe sepsis; (2) pneumonia documented radiographically; (3) blood culture that is positive for gram-positive bacteria, before final identification and susceptibility testing are available; (4) clinically suspected serious catheter-related infection (eg, chills or rigors with infusion through the catheter and cellulitis or purulence around the catheter entry/exit site); (5) skin or soft tissue infection at any site; (6) colonization with methicillin-resistant *Staphylococcus aureus*, vancomycin-resistant enterococcus, or penicillin-resistant *Streptococcus pneumonia*; and (7) severe mucositis, if fluoroquinolone prophylaxis has been given and ceftazidime is used as empiric therapy. When these factors are absent, gram-positive coverage can be reserved. Antifungal or antiviral coverage is also not generally part of the initial empiric coverage regimens unless specific exposures or histories are known. For example, anti-influenza coverage might be added for a patient with classic flulike symptoms, in the appropriate season, after exposure to a sick contact with the flu.

HEMATOPOIETIC STEM CELL TRANSPLANT PATIENTS

Patients who undergo hematopoietic stem cell transplantation (HSCT) (also known as bone marrow transplantation) are at increased risk for numerous infectious complications, which are leading causes of morbidity and mortality in this population. Recent data show a trend toward a reduced incidence of infections among patients undergoing this procedure.[42] The immediate period after transplantation (pre-engraftment) is marked by severe neutropenia and always entails prolonged hospitalization at least until neutrophil recovery. The infectious complications that are common during this period are not the focus of this review; instead, the authors focus on the period after hospital discharge, during which HSCT patients are likely to come to the ED with a new fever. Infections occurring after the engraftment are generally divided into those that emerge within 3 weeks to 3 months (early postengraftment) and those that develop more than 3 months later (late postengraftment).[43]

The risk of infection after HSCT depends on the degree of immunosuppression and the patients' environmental or past exposures to possible pathogen sources. The early postengraftment period is characterized by progressive recovery in cell-mediated immunity.[43] The most important pathogens during this period are the herpes viruses, especially CMV. Typical bacterial infections associated with indwelling catheters (gram positive) and mucosal damage (gram negative) can invade the bloodstream.[44] Other infections during this period are *P jiroveci* and opportunistic mycoses, such as *Aspergillus* species, *Fusarium* species, and Zygomycetes.

After 3 months ($\sim$100 days), cellular and humoral immunity has largely recovered and OIs are uncommon.[43] However, in patients who had graft-versus-host disease (GVHD) and were treated with enhanced immunosuppression, viral infections (particularly CMV and VZV) become more common.[44] Bacteremia, especially with encapsulated organisms (eg, *Streptococcus pneumoniae*), is important in those with chronic GVHD. Community-acquired infections (especially seasonal respiratory viruses) are also important causes of fever later after the transplant.[44]

For HSCT patients presenting with fever, the history should emphasize the time after the transplant, the type of transplant (autologous vs allogeneic), the use of prophylactic antimicrobials, and previous infections (exposure history or serologies). The physical examination should concentrate on the skin (especially indwelling ports and catheters), sinuses, oropharynx, abdomen, and lungs.[37] The standard laboratory evaluation should include a CBC count with differential and measurement of serum creatinine, blood urea nitrogen, electrolytes, hepatic transaminase enzymes, and total bilirubin, along with at least 2 sets of blood cultures (at least one from each lumen of indwelling catheters).[37] Culture specimens from other sites of suspected infection should be obtained as clinically indicated. In solid-organ transplant recipients, invasive testing might be necessary to diagnose uncommon or multiple infections.[37]

Empiric treatment of febrile HSCT patients often includes broad antibacterial coverage after basic culture results have been obtained. The source of fever should be investigated thoroughly and antibiotic therapy should be adjusted based on suspicion for certain organisms or on the presenting clinical syndrome. Adjustments can be made after culture and diagnostic test results are finalized.

TUMOR NECROSIS FACTOR-α INHIBITORS

Tumor necrosis factor-α (TNF-α) inhibitors are biologic agents used to treat a variety of inflammatory diseases, ranging from spondyloarthropathies to inflammatory bowel disease. TNF-α is a cytokine produced by macrophages and other immune cells to mediate the inflammatory response to infections. It is responsible for production of chemokines that recruit inflammatory cells to form granulomas. TNF-α is also a major activator of macrophages, which are responsible for killing bacteria within granulomas; it also regulates the inflammatory response necessary to maintain granulomas.[45,46] Thus, the use of TNF-α blockers, such as etanercept, infliximab, and adalimumab, puts these patients at risk for a host of granulomatous infections.

Reactivation of TB is the best-known infectious complication of using TNF-α inhibitors. This risk can be up to 10 times higher than in the general population, depending on the agent being used.[45,47] The risk of TB seems to be higher with infliximab than with etanercept, and the time to disease is shorter (often within 90 days after the initiation of treatment).[47] The classic presentation of TB (fever, weight loss, night sweats, and cough) might not be seen in patients who are taking TNF-α inhibitors because of their higher likelihood of having disseminated disease as a result of their inability to form granulomas. This characteristic often leads to a delay in diagnosis. Therefore, the Centers for Disease Control and Prevention recommends the screening of all patients for TB before the initiation of TNF-α inhibitor therapy.[48] Patients with latent TB should be started on an isoniazid regimen before starting TNF-α inhibitors. ED care providers might see patients who were not treated for latent TB. In addition to being at risk for TB, these patients are also at risk for nontuberculous mycobacterial infections, which should be considered in the differential diagnosis.

The use of TNF-α inhibitors puts patients at risk for other granulomatous infections and uncommon bacterial infections. Endemic fungi cause granulomatous infection in much the same way as TB, and that risk is increased by the use of TNF-α inhibitors. Reactivation of latent fungal disease as well as the acquisition of new disease, such as histoplasmosis or coccidioides, has been described in association with the use of these agents.[49] As with TB, patients with these endemic fungi often present with disseminated disease rather than primary pulmonary disease, possibly delaying the diagnosis. In addition to endemic fungi, clinicians evaluating febrile patients taking TNF-α inhibitors should consider uncommon bacterial infections, such as *Legionella* pneumonia and listeriosis. Both of these entities are listed in the 2011 boxed warning from the US Food and Drug Administration for all TNF-α inhibitors. The risk of these diseases is higher among patients taking TNF-α inhibitors than in the general population.

An increased prevalence of viral infections has also been documented in association with the use of TNF-α inhibitors and should be in the differential diagnosis for this patient group.[50]

SUMMARY

Many immunocompromised patients with fever come to EDs for medical care. A thorough history and physical examination are critical to pinpoint potential sites of infection, elucidate epidemiologic exposures, and suggest possible causes. Immunocompromised patients are at risk for rare and unusual organisms as well as concurrent infections. Determining the type and severity of immunosuppression is critical for establishing the patients' risk of life-threatening illness and the need for urgent, empiric antimicrobials. Blood cultures and other diagnostic tests have the highest yield when performed before administering antimicrobials, but they should never be delayed for severely ill patients. Invasive diagnostic procedures are often the key step in the diagnosis. Patients should be admitted to the hospital when the ED care provider deems that further care is warranted. Immunocompromised patients with fever represent some of the most difficult challenges in medical practice today.

REFERENCES

1. Mendelson M. Fever in the immunocompromised host. Emerg Med Clin North Am 1998;16(4):761–79.
2. Pizzo PA. Fever in immunocompromised patients. N Engl J Med 1999;341(12): 893–900.
3. Buchacz K, Baker RK, Moorman AC, et al. Rates of hospitalizations and associated diagnoses in a large multisite cohort of HIV patients in the United States, 1994–2005. AIDS 2008;22(11):1345–54.
4. Berry SA, Fleishman JA, Moore RD, et al. Trends in reasons for hospitalization in a multisite United States cohort of persons living with HIV, 2001–2008. J Acquir Immune Defic Syndr 2012;59(4):368–75.
5. Stein DS, Korvick JA, Vermund SH. CD4+ lymphocyte cell enumeration for prediction of clinical course of human immunodeficiency virus disease: a review. J Infect Dis 1992;165(2):352–63.
6. Moir S, Malaspina A, Ogwaro KM, et al. HIV-1 induces phenotypic and functional perturbations of B cells in chronically infected individuals. Proc Natl Acad Sci USA 2001;98(18):10362–7.
7. Hirschtick RE, Glassroth J, Jordan MC, et al. Bacterial pneumonia in persons infected with the human immunodeficiency virus. Pulmonary Complications of HIV Infection Study Group. N Engl J Med 1995;333(13):845–51.
8. Klugman KP, Madhi SA, Feldman C. HIV and pneumococcal disease. Curr Opin Infect Dis 2007;20(1):11–5.
9. Kelley CF, Checkley W, Mannino DM, et al. Trends in hospitalizations for AIDS-associated *Pneumocystis jiroveci* pneumonia in the United States (1986 to 2005). Chest 2009;136(1):190–7.
10. Corbett EL, Watt CJ, Walker N, et al. The growing burden of tuberculosis: global trends and interactions with the HIV epidemic. Arch Intern Med 2003;163(9): 1009–21.
11. Janoff EN, Breiman RF, Daley CL, et al. Pneumococcal disease during HIV infection: epidemiologic, clinical, and immunologic perspectives. Ann Intern Med 1992;117(4):314–24.

12. Kales CP, Murren JR, Torres RA, et al. Early predictors of in-hospital mortality for *Pneumocystis carinii* pneumonia in the acquired immunodeficiency syndrome. Arch Intern Med 1987;147(8):1413–7.

13. Crans CA Jr, Boiselle PM. Imaging features of *Pneumocystis carinii* pneumonia. Crit Rev Diagn Imaging 1999;40(4):251–84.

14. Barnes PF, Bloch AB, Davidson PT, et al. Tuberculosis in patients with human immunodeficiency virus infection. N Engl J Med 1991;324(23):1644–50.

15. Horner RD, Bennett CL, Rodriguez D, et al. Relationship between procedures and health insurance for critically ill patients with *Pneumocystis carinii* pneumonia. Am J Respir Crit Care Med 1995;152(5 Pt 1):1435–42.

16. Wheat LJ, Connolly-Stringfield PA, Baker RL, et al. Disseminated histoplasmosis in the acquired immune deficiency syndrome: clinical findings, diagnosis and treatment, and review of the literature. Medicine 1990;69(6):361–74.

17. Ampel NM, Dols CL, Galgiani JN. Coccidioidomycosis during human immunodeficiency virus infection: results of a prospective study in a coccidioidal endemic area. Am J Med 1993;94(3):235–40.

18. Park BJ, Wannemuehler KA, Marston BJ, et al. Estimation of the current global burden of cryptococcal meningitis among persons living with HIV/AIDS. AIDS 2009;23(4):525–30.

19. Murakawa GJ, Kerschmann R, Berger T. Cutaneous *Cryptococcus* infection and AIDS: report of 12 cases and review of the literature. Arch Dermatol 1996; 132(5):545–8.

20. Asawavichienjinda T, Sitthi-Amorn C, Tanyanont V. Serum cryptococcal antigen: diagnostic value in the diagnosis of AIDS-related cryptococcal meningitis. J Med Assoc Thai 1999;82(1):65–71.

21. Porter SB, Sande MA. Toxoplasmosis of the central nervous system in the acquired immunodeficiency syndrome. N Engl J Med 1992;327(23):1643–8.

22. Baumgartner JE, Rachlin JR, Beckstead JH, et al. Primary central nervous system lymphomas: natural history and response to radiation therapy in 55 patients with acquired immunodeficiency syndrome. J Neurosurg 1990;73(2): 206–11.

23. Dieterich DT, Rahmin M. Cytomegalovirus colitis in AIDS: presentation in 44 patients and a review of the literature. J Acquir Immune Defic Syndr 1991;4(Suppl 1): S29–35.

24. Drew WL, Paya CV, Emery V. Cytomegalovirus (CMV) resistance to antivirals. Am J Transplant 2001;1:307–12.

25. Fishman JA, Issa NC. Infection in organ transplantation: risk factors and evolving patterns of infection. Infect Dis Clin North Am 2010;24(2):273–83.

26. Fishman JA. Infection in solid-organ transplant recipients. N Engl J Med 2007; 357(25):2601–14.

27. Fishman JA. Infections in immunocompromised hosts and organ transplant recipients: essentials. Liver Transpl 2011;17(Suppl 3):S34–7.

28. Savitsky EA, Votey SR, Mebust DP, et al. A descriptive analysis of 290 liver transplant patient visits to an emergency department. Acad Emerg Med 2000;7(8): 898–905.

29. Unterman S, Zimmerman M, Tyo C, et al. A descriptive analysis of 1251 solid organ transplant visits to the emergency department. West J Emerg Med 2009; 10(1):48–54.

30. Turtay MG, Oguzturk H, Aydin C, et al. A descriptive analysis of 188 liver transplant patient visits to an emergency department. Eur Rev Med Pharmacol Sci 2012;16(Suppl 1):3–7.

31. Fishman JE, Rabkin JM. Thoracic radiology in kidney and liver transplantation. J Thorac Imaging 2002;17(2):122–31.
32. Dummer JS, Thomas LD. Risk factors and approaches to infections in transplant recipients. In: Mandell GL, Bennett JE, Dolin R, editors. Mandell, Douglas, and Bennett's principles and practice of infectious diseases. 7th edition. Philadelphia: Elsevier; 2010. p. 3821–37.
33. Grim SA, Clark NM. Management of infectious complications in solid-organ transplant recipients. Clin Pharmacol Ther 2011;90(2):333–42.
34. Mehrabi A, Fonouni H, Wente M, et al. Wound complications following kidney and liver transplantation. Clin Transplant 2006;20(Suppl 17):97–110.
35. Zuckermann A, Barten MJ. Surgical wound complications after heart transplantation. Transpl Int 2011;24(7):627–36.
36. Baden LR, Bensinger W, Angarone M, et al. Prevention and treatment of cancer-related infections. J Natl Compr Canc Netw 2012;10(11):1412–45.
37. Freifeld AG, Bow EJ, Sepkowitz KA, et al. Clinical practice guideline for the use of antimicrobial agents in neutropenic patients with cancer: 2010 update by the Infectious Diseases Society of America. Clin Infect Dis 2011;52(4):e56–93.
38. Klastersky J, Ameye L, Maertens J, et al. Bacteraemia in febrile neutropenic cancer patients. Int J Antimicrob Agents 2007;30(Suppl 1):S51–9.
39. Klastersky J, Awada A, Paesmans M, et al. Febrile neutropenia: a critical review of the initial management. Crit Rev Oncol Hematol 2011;78(3):185–94.
40. Bodey GP, Jadeja L, Elting L. Pseudomonas bacteremia: retrospective analysis of 410 episodes. Arch Intern Med 1985;145(9):1621–9.
41. Paul M, Soares-Weiser K, Leibovici L. Beta lactam monotherapy versus beta lactam-aminoglycoside combination therapy for fever with neutropenia: systematic review and meta-analysis. BMJ 2003;326(7399):1111.
42. Gooley TA, Chien JW, Pergam SA, et al. Reduced mortality after allogeneic hematopoietic-cell transplantation. N Engl J Med 2010;363(22):2091–101.
43. Wingard JR, Hsu J, Hiemenz JW. Hematopoietic stem cell transplantation: an overview of infection risks and epidemiology. Infect Dis Clin North Am 2010;24(2):257–72.
44. Tomblyn M, Chiller T, Einsele H, et al. Guidelines for preventing infectious complications among hematopoietic cell transplant recipients: a global perspective. Bone Marrow Transplant 2009;44(8):453–5.
45. Koo S, Marty FM, Baden LR. Infectious complications associated with immuno-modulating biologic agents. Infect Dis Clin North Am 2010;24(2):285–306.
46. Salvana EM, Salata RA. Infectious complications associated with monoclonal antibodies and related small molecules. Clin Microbiol Rev 2009;22(2):274–90.
47. Wallis RS, Broder MS, Wong JY, et al. Granulomatous infectious diseases associated with tumor necrosis factor antagonists. Clin Infect Dis 2004;38(9):1261–5.
48. Centers for Disease Control and Prevention (CDC). Tuberculosis associated with blocking agents against tumor necrosis factor-alpha–California, 2002–2003. MMWR Morb Mortal Wkly Rep 2004;53(30):683–6.
49. Wallis RS, Broder M, Wong J, et al. Reactivation of latent granulomatous infections by infliximab. Clin Infect Dis 2005;41(Suppl 3):S194–8.
50. Domm S, Cinatl J, Mrowietz U. The impact of treatment with tumour necrosis factor-α antagonists on the course of chronic viral infections: a review of the literature. Br J Dermatol 2008;159:1217–28.

Fever in the Pediatric Patient

Robyn Wing, MD, Maya R. Dor, DO, Patricia A. McQuilkin, MD*

KEYWORDS

- Fever • Fever without source • Occult pneumonia • Urinary tract infection
- Febrile seizure • Meningococcemia • Sickle cell disease • Febrile neutropenia

KEY POINTS

- Fever is defined as a rectal temperature greater than 38.0°C (>100.4°F). A fever that was documented recently at home should be considered the same as a temperature documented in the emergency department.
- All febrile infants younger than 28 days should receive a 'full sepsis workup' and be admitted for parenteral antibiotic therapy. Clinical and laboratory criteria can be used to identify low-risk febrile infants aged 1 to 3 months, who can be treated on an outpatient basis with close follow-up.
- The PCV7 (7-valent conjugate pneumococcal vaccine) vaccine has markedly decreased the incidence of serious bacterial infection in vaccinated infants and children, but children who are unvaccinated or have received fewer than 2 doses of vaccine are still at risk for pneumococcal disease. The impact of the new PCV13 vaccine remains to be seen, but this new medication should decrease the risk even further.
- Occult urinary tract infections occur often in children with fever without a source (FWS); therefore, a catheterized urine specimen should be obtained for urine testing in girls and uncircumcised boys younger than 2 years and in circumcised boys younger than 6 months.
- Fever with petechiae below the nipples should lead to consideration of meningococcemia. Diagnosis and rapid initiation of treatment are critical to decrease mortality from this devastating illness.

Fever, defined as a rectal temperature greater than 38.0°C (100.4°F), is the most common complaint for children and infants who are brought to emergency departments (EDs).[1,2] The emergency physician must distinguish benign from life-threatening disease and educate families, as appropriate, about the causes and

---

Drs Wing and Dor have equally contributed to this article.

Funding Sources: None.

Conflict of Interest: None.

Department of Pediatrics, University of Massachusetts Medical School, 55 Lake Avenue North, Worcester, MA 01655, USA
* Corresponding author.

E-mail address: Patricia.McQuilkin@umassmemorial.org

Emerg Med Clin N Am 31 (2013) 1073–1096

http://dx.doi.org/10.1016/j.emc.2013.07.006
emed.theclinics.com

management of fevers. The approach to fevers in children is guided by the patient's age, immunization status, and immune status as well as the results of a careful physical examination. In this article, the approach to pediatric fever is discussed and significant causes of both common and dangerous fevers in children are highlighted.

Although fever is recognized by health care providers as a beneficial physiologic response that facilitates the fight of the immune system against pathogens, it evokes fear and anxiety in caregivers.[3] In 1980, Schmitt introduced the term fever phobia after finding, in a survey, that 52% of parents believed that a temperature of 40°C or even less can cause neurologic damage.[4] In an assessment of the incidence of fever phobia in an urban pediatric ED, Poirier and colleagues[5] found that 32% of caregivers named seizure as the main danger of fever, 18% named death, and 15% named brain damage. These results indicate that many caregivers seem to confuse the beneficial effects of fever with the harmful effects of hyperthermia.[6] This phobia prompts many ED visits for the management of fever in children.

APPROACH TO PEDIATRIC FEVER

The presence of fever in children and young people affects clinical management decisions and therefore must be recorded accurately. This documentation can be challenging, because measuring the temperature in children can be difficult, especially when they are uncooperative or restless. Also, parents use different methods to measure temperature. Rectal temperature measurement is more accurate than tympanometry and use of the axilla.[7,8] Wide fluctuations are noted with tympanometry, especially in young children, and axillary temperatures can vary by as much as 1°F (5/9°C).[9] A fever documented at home by measuring the temperature with a thermometer should be treated in the same manner as a fever documented in the ED.[10] Studies have found no correlation between fever reduction with antipyretic medication and the likelihood of a serious bacterial infection (SBI)[11–16]; therefore, this history should not influence patient management.

FEVER WITHOUT SOURCE IN CHILDREN YOUNGER THAN 3 YEARS

Most children younger than 3 years with fever have a clinically apparent source of infection. Sources include proven bacterial infections (including otitis media in infants older than 3 months) or named viral syndromes (croup, stomatitis, herpangina, varicella, and bronchiolitis) in infants older than 1 month.[17] However, in 20% of children, a source of infection cannot be elucidated even after a thorough history is obtained and a physical examination is performed.[18,19] Although most of these children harbor self-limiting viral illnesses, there should always be concern for the few infants and children in whom complications from invasive bacterial disease might develop.[20,21] It is important to screen and stratify neonates and infants at risk for occult bacteremia. The incidence of SBI is higher in febrile infants younger than 3 months than in older children. Fever without a source (FWS) in this age group raises the suspicion of a serious underlying disease.[22]

PNEUMOCOCCAL CONJUGATE VACCINE AND THE RISK OF OCCULT BACTEREMIA

Before the introduction of the 7-valent conjugate pneumococcal vaccine (PCV7; Prevnar, Lederle Laboratories/Wyeth-Ayerst, NY) in 2000, the incidence of occult bacteremia in well-appearing children younger than 3 years with FWS and a temperature 39.0°C or higher was 2% to 3%. Effective vaccination programs targeted against

Haemophilus influenzae and *Streptococcus pneumonia* have decreased the rate to between 0.25% and 0.91%.[23–29] Most neonates younger than 2 months have not yet received these vaccinations and therefore are vulnerable to infections caused *H influenzae* and *Streptococcus pneumoniae*. Recent retrospective studies found virtually no SBI caused by those 2 organisms in neonates younger than 3 months, which the investigators attributed to the herd immunity effect caused by the successful vaccination of older infants.[29–31] Occult bacteremia in well-appearing neonates with FWS was found to be caused by *Escherichia coli*, *Streptococcus hemolyticus*, group B streptococci, *Staphylococcus epidermitis*, and coagulase-negative staphylococci.[30]

At the time of its introduction, PCV7 contained isolates of 85% to 97% of the pneumococcal species that cause disease in children younger than 2 years.[32] However, after PCV7 was introduced in the United States, the distribution of pneumococcal pathogens shifted. Sixty-four percent of invasive pneumococcal disease (IPD) in children younger than 5 years was found to be caused by 6 additional serotypes, which are now included in the 13-valent pneumococcal conjugate vaccine (PCV13, Pfizer Vaccines, NY).[33] PCV13 was licensed in 2010 for infants older than 6 weeks and contains pneumococcal capsular polysaccharides corresponding to the 6 serotypes currently causing more than 70% of IPD worldwide.[34] Data from England suggest that the routine use of PCV13 has already decreased the incidence of IPD caused by serotypes not included in PCV7 but included in PCV13.[35]

FEVER IN THE NEONATE (YOUNGER THAN 28 DAYS)

Clinicians cannot rely on history and physical examination alone to exclude SBI in the febrile neonate. ED practice guidelines for the evaluation of febrile neonates younger than 28 days continue to call for a full sepsis workup, which includes complete blood count (CBC), blood culture, urinalysis and urine culture, lumbar puncture with evaluation of cerebrospinal fluid (CSF), and administration of antibiotics in the ED followed by hospitalization pending results of cultures.[1,36] Some investigators also advocate screening transaminases or obtaining a chest radiograph to evaluate for neonatal herpes simplex virus (HSV) infection, given its propensity to involve the liver and the lungs in this age group.[37,38] Studies of the applicability of low-risk criteria to infants between the ages of 1 and 28 days found that more SBIs were missed in these very young infants compared with older infants, validating the need for a full sepsis evaluation with hospital admission in this age group.[39–42] The decision to obtain CSF for HSV polymerase chain reaction (PCR) and to treat with acyclovir is discussed later. The decision to obtain a chest radiograph should be based on clinical symptoms.

Neonatal medications for treatment of presumed SBI include ampicillin (200–300 mg/kg/d intravenously [IV], divided every 8 hours [if the infant is <7 days old] or every 6 hours [if the infant is >7 days old]) plus a third-generation cephalosporin (cefotaxime, 150 mg/kg/d IV, divided every 8 hours). Ceftriaxone is contraindicated in neonates because of the risk of albumin displacement and the subsequent increased risk of hyperbilirubinemia and kernicterus. Vancomycin can be used instead of ampicillin if the neonate has gram-positive cocci on CSF Gram stain or is at risk for *Staphylococcus aureus* infection. Consider acyclovir (60 mg/kg/d IV divided every 8 hours) for ill-appearing infants; infants with seizures, skin lesions, or increased transaminase levels; and those with CSF pleocytosis and a negative Gram stain until an alternative diagnosis is established or the HSV PCR becomes negative.[43] Viral testing and treatment of influenza in neonates are discussed later. An algorithm for the evaluation and management of previously healthy infants younger than 28 days with a FWS is presented as **Fig. 1**.

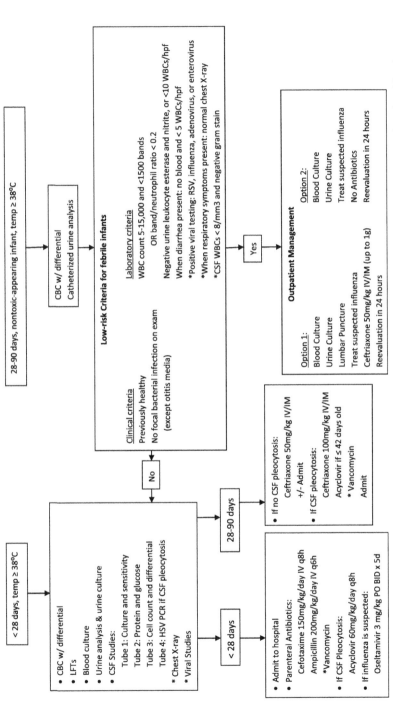

Fig. 1. Algorithm for management of a previously healthy infant 90 days of age or younger with a fever without source. This algorithm is a suggested, but not exhaustive, approach to management. hpf, high-power field. * optional; see text. (*Adapted from* Lee B, McCallin T. Microbiology and infectious disease. In: Tschudy MM, Arcara KM. The Harriet Lane handbook. 19th edition. St Louis (MO): Mosby; 2011; with permission. *Modified from* Baraff LJ. Management of fever without source in infants and children. Ann Emerg Med 2000;36(6):602–14; and Baraff LJ. Management of infants and young children with fever without source. Pediatr Ann 2008;37(10):673–9.)

NEONATAL HERPES

Neonatal herpes is an important consideration in the evaluation of a neonate with FWS. In recent years, the incidence of fetal and neonatal herpes has increased, concomitant with the increase in HSV infections among women of childbearing years.[37] Risk factors for neonatal HSV infection include maternal primary infection during pregnancy or delivery, exposure to cervical viral shedding, delivery before 38 weeks, fetal scalp monitoring, maternal age younger than 21 years, low birth weight, and rupture of membranes more than 4 to 6 hours before delivery.[44–46] It is therefore crucial to obtain a comprehensive medical and prenatal history from the mother, specifically about history and timing of HSV infection, for any neonate presenting with FWS. Only 20% to 30% of HSV-infected mothers provide a history of genital herpes,[47,48] but most of them (60%–80%) have subclinical infection with asymptomatic viral shedding at the time of delivery.[44,49–51] Infants born vaginally to mothers with a primary HSV infection are exposed to higher viral loads and fewer maternal antibodies than those born to mothers with secondary infections; the incidence of neonatal HSV is concomitantly higher (33%–50% vs 3%–5%, respectively).[45,48,52,53] HSV has an incubation period of 5 to 21 days. Infected neonates usually present with symptoms in the first 2 weeks of life, but symptoms can occur at any time during the first 6 weeks.[54,55] Clinicians must therefore have a high level of suspicion to make an early diagnosis of HSV infection in neonates and thereby improve the prognosis.[37]

HSV-2 causes 75% to 85% of neonatal HSV infections. Most of them (85%) are acquired vertically during the peripartum period, with the remainder (5%–10%) contracted before labor or after birth.[56] Neonatal HSV infections are divided into 3 clinical presentations: disseminated disease; disease localized to the skin, eyes, and mouth (SEM); and central nervous system (CNS) disease.

Disseminated disease presents during the first week of life, accounting for 35% of neonatal HSV cases, and has the highest mortality.[53] Any neonate presenting with signs of sepsis in the setting of negative bacterial cultures or severe liver dysfunction should raise concern for disseminated HSV infection. Mortality correlates with increases in aspartate transaminase level more than 10 times the upper limit of normal and neonatal lethargy at the time of acyclovir initiation.[37] Multiple organs can become involved, including the CNS, adrenal gland, SEM, with a predilection for the liver and lungs.[56]

SEM disease often presents late in the first week of life, accounts for 40% of disease, and has the lowest mortality of the 3 presentations.[37,57] Neonates with the SEM form of HSV infection present with vesicular skin lesions, keratitis, or chorioretinitis, with the face and scalp most commonly affected.[58]

CNS disease presents latest (between weeks 2 and 3 of life) and accounts for 35% of neonatal HSV infections. Neonates can present with cranial nerve abnormalities, irritability, a bulging fontanelle, seizures, encephalitis, apnea, bradycardia, and skin findings. Infant prematurity and seizures are risk factors for death.[56]

The presence of fever, irritability, abnormal CSF findings, increased transaminase levels, and skin lesions (especially in the setting of seizures) should raise concern for neonatal HSV infection.[53,56] Only 17% to 39% of neonates infected with HSV present with skin lesions, so their absence does not exclude the diagnosis.[56] Diagnostic evaluation includes HSV PCR, viral culture, electroencephalogram, and liver transaminases. Although viral culture of skin vesicles, mouth, eyes, urine, blood, stool, and CSF is the gold standard for diagnosis, PCR can confirm it with or without skin lesions in 24 hours, with a sensitivity of 71% to 100%.[56,59] Analysis of PCR results from blood and CSF samples increases the sensitivity of PCR testing for HSV DNA.[59] A negative CSF or serum PCR result does not exclude the presence of HSV infection. In addition to PCR and viral cultures, screening for increases in serum transaminase level and a chest radiograph to detect pneumonitis are recommended, given the propensity of HSV infection, especially the disseminated form, to involve the liver and lungs.[37]

Seventy percent of patients with untreated localized SEM disease progress to CNS and disseminated disease; therefore, early diagnosis and treatment with acyclovir are imperative to the prevention of morbidity and mortality in neonates infected with HSV.[60,61] The presence of CSF pleocytosis in the setting of a negative Gram stain necessitates HSV PCR of CSF and serum, with subsequent high-dose acyclovir administration. Acyclovir, given at 60 mg/kg/d in 3 divided doses, improves outcomes in patients with disseminated disease or CNS manifestations.[62]

FEVER IN INFANTS 1 TO 3 MONTHS OF AGE

Several protocols, based on the Boston, Philadelphia, and Rochester criteria, have been developed to help clinicians identify infants and children who are at low risk for SBI, so that they can be managed safely as outpatients, reducing the number of unnecessary hospitalizations.[41,63–65] For this reason, the evaluation of well-appearing infants between 1 and 3 months of age presenting with FWS varies in EDs. The most recent recommendations for low-risk criteria and management of fever in nontoxic appearing infants between 28 and 90 days of age are summarized in **Fig. 1.**

These protocols do not clarify the role of lumbar puncture in the stratification of low-risk and high-risk febrile infants. Lumbar puncture, therefore, remains optional in infants 1 to 3 months of age but should be performed if empirical antibiotics are to be started. If a child returns to the ED and a lumbar puncture performed at that time reveals pleocytosis, a negative culture indicates either aseptic meningitis or only partially treated bacterial meningitis, necessitating a full course of parenteral antibiotics.[66]

Similar to the decision to obtain a lumbar puncture, the decision to obtain a chest radiograph in infants and children presenting with FWS is not always a clear one. Occult pneumonia is present in up to 26% of children with FWS and a white blood cell (WBC) count greater than 20,000/mm^3 (most lower respiratory infections in children have a viral source).[67–72] Bacterial lower respiratory tract infections often occur as a secondary infection after an initial respiratory viral infection.[66] A meta-analysis that evaluated reports of febrile infants younger than 3 months[73] showed that 33.2% of all those presenting with at least 1 clinical finding of pulmonary disease (ie, tachypnea >50 breaths/min, cyanosis or O$_2$ saturation <95%, rales, rhonchi, retractions, wheezing, coryza, grunting, stridor, nasal flaring, or cough) had chest radiographs positive for pneumonia. This evidence supports obtaining a chest radiograph in febrile infants who are younger than 3 months, have a temperature greater than 38°C, and present with at least 1 clinical sign of pulmonary disease.[1]

The requirement for hospital admission and IV antibiotic administration in this age range depends on the laboratory findings. All infants 28 to 90 days of age with CSF pleocytosis should be admitted to the hospital for IV antibiotic administration while CSF cultures are followed. Infants 42 days of age or younger with CSF pleocytosis should also be treated with acyclovir.[38] For patients with urinary tract infections (UTIs) (discussed later), neonates younger than 1 month should be hospitalized for IV administration of antibiotics, and outpatient management could be appropriate for infants aged 28 to 60 days.[66] Hospital admission should also be considered for infants in families with social concerns such as transportation challenges, lack of resources, and unreliable follow-up. Cultures should be followed for 36 to 48 hours, because 90% of bacterial pathogens grow within the first 24 hours. All infants sent home must have follow-up within 24 hours by telephone or visit. Infants who received IV/intramuscular (IM) antibiotics need a second IM dose, pending culture results. Antibiotic management for infants aged 2 to 3 months includes a third-generation cephalosporin (ceftriaxone, 50 mg/kg IM/IV).

UTIS

In the postvaccination era, UTIs are now the most common occult bacterial infections in children. They occur in 2% of febrile children younger than 5 years and are present in 6% to 8% of febrile girls and 2% to 3% of febrile boys younger than 12 months.[74–77] Risk factors for occult UTI include female gender, uncircumcised male, temperature greater than 39.0°C, FWS in a child younger than 1 year, and FWS in females between 1 and 2 years of age.[1,76] Shaikh and colleagues[78] found UTI as the diagnosis in 7.5% of febrile infant girls between 0 and 3 months of age, 2.4% of circumcised boys, and 20.1% of uncircumcised boys. Among febrile children with UTIs, 60% to 65% have evidence of pyelonephritis.[79] Studies have also shown a 12.4% incidence of positive blood cultures from neonates admitted for UTI, emphasizing the importance of screening for and treating UTIs in febrile infants.[80,81]

Current guidelines for evaluation and management of UTI in children 2 to 24 months of age recommend obtaining a urine culture in conjunction with urinalysis before giving antibiotics when UTI is suspected. Because of the low specificity (70%) and high false-positive rate (85%) of urine culture from a bag collection, urethral catheterization (sensitivity 95%, specificity 99%) and suprapubic aspiration are the best methods for diagnosing UTIs in young children.[1] The diagnosis requires abnormal urinalysis results ($\geq$10 WBCs/high-powered field or bacteriuria) and 50,000 or more colony-forming units/mL of a single uropathogen on culture. Lower colony counts are often caused by colonization of the distal urethra and periurethral area and do not represent true UTI. Treatment with antibiotics for 7 to 14 days is recommended (ceftriaxone, cefixime, cephalexin, or bactrim, depending on local antibiotic sensitivity patterns). On follow-up, a renal and bladder ultrasonographic examination is indicated after the first febrile UTI, but routine voiding cystourethrography (VCUG) is no longer recommended. A VCUG might be indicated if an ultrasonographic image shows abnormalities or the patient has recurrent febrile UTIs. After a child's first febrile UTI, parents should be advised to seek medical care promptly (within 48 hours) for future febrile illnesses to ensure that recurrent infections can be diagnosed and treated quickly.[82]

VIRAL INFECTIONS

Although SBI testing is crucial in the 1-day to 90-day age group, most infants with FWS have an underlying viral illness as the cause of fever. As the ability to diagnose viral illnesses improves, the role of these tests in the management of febrile infants is being investigated. Many recent studies have investigated whether febrile infants with viral illnesses could have a concomitant SBI. Studies have shown significantly lower rates of SBI in infants presenting with FWS with proven viral syndromes, such as bronchiolitis, influenza, varicella, croup, stomatitis, and herpangina. One large prospective study[22] looked at rates of SBI in infants 1 to 90 days old presenting with FWS with and without viral syndromes. The incidence of SBI in infants with a viral syndrome was 4.2% versus 12.3% in febrile infants without a proven viral syndrome. This study also stratified infants into high and low risk according to Rochester criteria and found significantly lower rates of SBI in high-risk infants with viral infections (5.5%) compared with high-risk infants without viral infections (16.9%). The difference in SBI rates between infants with and without a proven virus in low-risk infants was not statistically significant (1.7% vs 3.1%).[22] Another study[83] looking at rates of SBI in febrile infants younger than 60 days found significantly lower rates of SBI in infants diagnosed with influenza virus infection (2.5%) than in infants presenting with FWS without influenza (11.7%). Other studies[84,85] found significantly lower rates of SBI in infants with bronchiolitis (2.2%–7%) compared with infants without bronchiolitis (9.6%–12.5%). Viral testing for respiratory syncytial virus, influenza, adenovirus, rotavirus, enterovirus, and herpesvirus has proved useful in predicting a low risk for SBI, but detection of rhinovirus alone has not been significant.[86,87]

The addition of rapid viral diagnostic testing to commonly used high-risk criteria, such as the Rochester criteria, could allow more careful categorization of infants with FWS at risk for SBI. Viral testing of nasal specimens using PCR, enzyme-linked immunosorbent assay, or direct-fluorescent assay detection (DFA) should be performed when a respiratory virus is suspected. Enteroviral testing with both blood and CSF PCR provides the best diagnostic yield for enterovirus infections.[87] The risk of SBI in infants with documented viral infections is comparable with that of a low-risk infant, so physicians should consider treating them as such. The results of viral testing can be combined with 24-hour bacterial culture results to optimize treatment plans for patients, decrease antibiotic use, and decrease length of stay in patients admitted for FWS.[38]

The American Academy of Pediatrics recommends antiviral therapy for any child at high risk of complications of influenza infection, which includes all children younger than 2 years. Treatment should be initiated as soon as possible after illness onset and should not be delayed while awaiting definitive influenza test results. Rapid antigen tests have a low sensitivity and should not be used to rule out influenza.[88] Dosing of oseltamivir in infants younger than 12 months is 3 mg/kg/dose by mouth twice a day for 5 days.[88]

FEVER IN CHILDREN 3 TO 36 MONTHS OF AGE

Previously healthy and well-appearing children aged 3 to 36 months who present with FWS account for approximately 6% of all pediatric ED visits.[18] Similar to younger infants, most febrile children in this age group have a self-limiting viral illness.[89,90] However, it is important to identify infants with occult bacteremia, because of the risk of subsequent complications, including pneumonia, septic arthritis, osteomyelitis, meningitis, sepsis, and death.[91] The prevalence of occult bacteremia among febrile children aged 3 to 36 months is between 0.5% and 2%; the lower rates are observed in populations with PCV7 vaccination coverage of approximately 80%.[1,27,92] The threshold for when to evaluate the age group for occult SBI is a rectal temperature 39°C or greater (102.2°F). Children at greatest risk for UTI are boys younger than 6 months, uncircumcised males, females younger than 24 months, and patients with known urinary tract abnormalities. Specimens for urinalysis and urine culture should be obtained by urethral catheterization in these patients.[43,82] If the results are positive (according to the aforementioned criteria), antibiotics and close follow-up are warranted.

The recommendation for evaluation of previously healthy, well-appearing children aged 3 to 36 months with temperature 39.5°C (103.1°F) or greater and FWS is to consider obtaining a CBC with manual differential in unvaccinated children and children who have received fewer than 2 doses of the pneumococcal vaccine (PCV7 or

PCV13). A blood culture with empirical antibiotic therapy for children with a peripheral WBC count of 15,000/mm^3 or greater or an absolute neutrophil count greater than or equal to 10,000 should be considered.[66] Guidelines for antibiotic treatment call for administration of ceftriaxone, 50 mg/kg IM/IV. Twenty-four-hour follow-up by telephone or visit is necessary if antibiotics are given in the ED. In this postvaccination era, with its changing epidemiology in the pathogens responsible for occult bacteremia, the decrease in the rate of *Streptococcus pneumoniae* bacteremia has led to questions about the necessity for traditionally recommended screening tests for occult bacteremia in children aged 3 to 36 months with FWS.[1,93] The newer multivalent vaccine, PCV13, should provide even more protection for infants and will likely further lower the risk of occult bacteremia. The most recent recommendations for management of fever in non-toxic appearing infants aged 3–36 months are summarized in **Fig. 2**.

OCCULT PNEUMONIA IN CHILDREN 3 TO 36 MONTHS OF AGE

Seven percent of children younger than 2 years with temperatures higher than 38°C have pneumonia.[94] Most children older than 3 months with pneumonia have clinical signs of infection (tachypnea, nasal flaring, grunting, oxygen saturation <95%, cyanosis, abnormal lung sounds), but approximately 3% of young patients without these symptoms have radiographic evidence of occult pneumonia.[93,95–97] Studies have also reported high rates of occult pneumonia (20%–30%) among highly febrile children older than 3 months with temperatures greater than 39°C and WBC counts greater than 20,000/mm^3, without clinical signs of pneumonia.[67] Blood cultures yield positive findings in only 3% to 5% of young children with pneumonia.[67,98] Recommendations for when to obtain a chest radiograph in a febrile infant without respiratory symptoms differ greatly among sources. The American College of Emergency Physicians recommends consideration of a chest radiograph in febrile children 3 months of age and older with temperatures greater than 39°C and a WBC count greater than 20,000/mm^3 without clinical evidence of a lower respiratory tract infection.[1] However, more recent guidelines recommend a chest radiograph in febrile children older than 3 months who have FWS, a temperature of 40°C or greater, or a WBC count greater than 20,000/mm^3.[43]

FIRST COMPLEX FEBRILE SEIZURE

There is a well-established association between seizures of any type (prolonged, focal, or recurrent) and acute bacterial meningitis.[99–102] A complex febrile seizure might be the sole presenting sign of acute bacterial meningitis.[99,100,103–110] Simple febrile seizures are described as self-limiting, lasting less than 15 minutes, with tonic-clonic features, no reoccurrences within the next 24 hours, and no postictal features. Complex febrile seizures are described as seizures lasting longer than 15 minutes; a series of seizures recurring within a 24-hour period; or focal seizures with tonic or clonic movements, loss of muscle tone, laterality with or without secondary generalization, head or eye deviation to 1 side, or subsequent transient unilateral paralysis (lasting minutes to occasionally days).[111]

The incidence of acute bacterial meningitis in children who present after their first simple febrile seizure seems to be low.[112] Between 12% and 27% of children diagnosed with acute bacterial meningitis have been reported to have had a seizure (of any type).[99,113] A retrospective cohort study looking at the incidence of acute bacterial meningitis in otherwise healthy children aged 6 to 60 months presenting to the ED after their first complex febrile seizure found that few of them who had a complex febrile

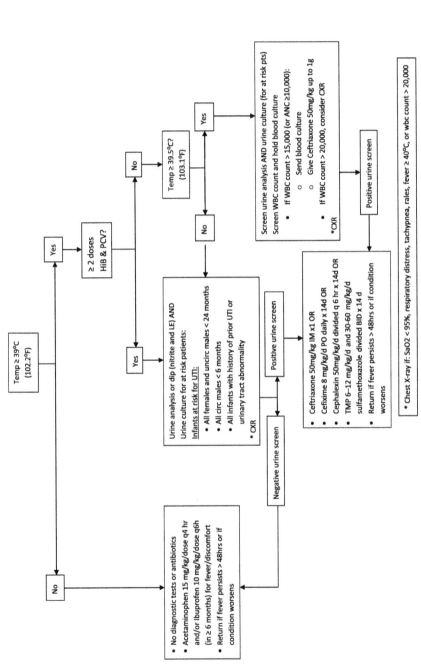

Fig. 2. Algorithm for management of a previously healthy, nontoxic appearing child, 3 to 36 months of age, with a fever without source. This algorithm is a suggested, but not exhaustive, approach to management. (*Adapted from* Lee B, McCallin T. Microbiology and infectious disease. In: Tschudy MM, Arcara KM. The Harriet Lane handbook. 19th edition. St Louis (MO): Mosby; 2011; with permission. *Modified from* Baraff LJ. Management of fever without source in infants and children. Ann Emerg Med 2000;36(6):602–14; and Baraff LJ. Management of infants and young children with fever without source. Pediatr Ann 2008;37(10):673–9.)

seizure had acute bacterial meningitis in the absence of other signs or symptoms. The investigators of that study concluded that patients whose only feature of a complex febrile seizure was 2 brief nonfocal seizures in 24 hours are at particularly low risk for acute bacterial meningitis.[111,112] Therefore, it is recommended that lumbar puncture be performed based on clinical suspicion and additional signs and symptoms that suggest meningitis, rather than a complex febrile seizure alone.

KAWASAKI DISEASE

Kawasaki disease (KD) is a systemic vasculitis of unknown cause, affecting small and medium vessels. The leading cause of acquired heart disease in North American and Japanese children, KD is believed to be an immune-mediated vasculitis that primarily affects children younger than 5 years.[36,114,115] In the United States, the incidence in 2006 was estimated to be 20.8/100,000 among children younger than 5 years.[116]

The diagnosis of KD is made clinically; there is no diagnostic test for this disease. The classic presentation of KD is fever for 5 days or more and the presence of at least 4 of the 5 following clinical criteria:

- Bilateral and nonexudative bulbar conjunctivitis
- Oropharyngeal changes: strawberry tongue; diffuse erythema of the oropharyngeal mucosa without exudate; erythema, cracking, fissuring, or bleeding of the lips
- Cervical lymphadenopathy (>1.5 cm diameter, usually unilateral)
- Polymorphous nonvesicular or bullous rash (most commonly a nonspecific, diffuse maculopapular eruption)
- Peripheral extremity changes with erythema or edema of the palms or soles (in the acute phase) or periungal desquamation in the subacute phase

The term incomplete KD is used when a child presents with fever lasting 5 days or more with only 2 or 3 of the clinical criteria listed earlier. Atypical KD is the term used for patients who fulfill the criteria for KD and have a clinical feature not usually associated with it (eg, renal impairment).[117]

Other clinical features that support the diagnosis of KD include severe irritability (a common finding), aseptic meningitis, mild acute iridocyclitis or anterior uveitis on slit lamp examination, and oligoarticular and polyarticular arthritis and arthralgias.[117–121] In 1 study,[122] 61% of patients had gastrointestinal complaints (diarrhea, vomiting, abdominal pain) and 35% had respiratory symptoms (rhinorrhea or cough). Otitis media or tympanitis secondary to inflammation can also be seen in KD.[118,123] Hydrops of the gallbladder occurs in approximately 15% of patients in the acute phase and can be seen on abdominal ultrasonography.[117,124] For patients who do not fulfill these diagnostic criteria, abdominal ultrasonography can be useful in supporting the diagnosis. The criteria can be applied once other diseases with similar presentations have been excluded.[117,118] It is not uncommon to document a concomitant infection in patients with KD.[125,126] In 1 study, 33% of children with typical KD had a confirmed concomitant infection.[125] Therefore, suspicion for KD needs to remain high, especially if an infection does not explain the clinical features.

The fever of KD is usually high and unresponsive to antibiotics and often to antipyretics as well.[118] The clinical features might not all be present at once, so it is important to inquire about all of the clinical features when obtaining the patient's history. It is important to reevaluate a child with a persistent fever or FWS and a child whose fever is not responding to antibiotics, because the diagnosis may become clear on reevaluation.

The results of laboratory investigations in the acute phase of KD are nonspecific but could support the diagnosis in children who do not fulfill diagnostic criteria. The acute-phase reactants (erythrocyte sedimentation rate and C-reactive protein [CRP]) are almost always increased either in the early febrile period or on later repeat testing. A high WBC count with a predominance of neutrophils is found frequently. Anemia might be present, especially with prolonged inflammation. A characteristic feature of KD is thrombocytosis; however, this finding usually occurs in the second week of the illness, during the subacute phase. Hypoalbuminemia is common, as are increased serum transaminase levels. Sterile pyuria might indicate urethritis or meatitis.[118]

Children suspected of having KD should be admitted to the hospital and treated with IV immunoglobulin (IVIG) to reduce the risk of cardiac complications, most notably, coronary artery aneurysm (CAA). CAA develops in approximately 20% of untreated children and is the most common cause of morbidity and mortality associated with this disease. The American Heart Association recommends that all children suspected of having KD be treated with a single dose of 2 g/kg of IVIG infused over 12 hours. It also recommends that high-dose aspirin be initiated at a dose of 80 to 100 mg/kg per day in 4 divided doses as long as the child is febrile, then switching to low-dose aspirin after the child has been afebrile for 48 to 72 hours.[117,127] Mortality as low as 0.026% has been achieved among children treated with this regimen.[128]

Although most children respond well to initial treatment, 11.6% to 38.3% have persistent or a recurrence of fever beyond 48 hours after completion of IVIG, which is a risk factor for CAA.[129–131] Children returning to the ED with fever persistence or recurrence 48 hours after finishing IVIG therapy for KD should be presumed to have a recurrence until proved otherwise and should be treated with a second infusion of 2 g/kg of IVIG over 12 hours.[117]

MENINGOCOCCEMIA

Neisseria meningitidis, also known as *Meningococcus,* is a gram-negative *Diplococcus* that colonizes the human upper respiratory tract and can cause life-threatening clinical syndromes. Upper respiratory tract infections and exposure to active and passive tobacco smoking damages nasopharyngeal cells, increasing susceptibility to invasive disease.[132,133] The incidence of invasive meningococcal disease in the United States is 1.1/100,000, with peak incidence in late winter and early spring.[134] Most cases occur in children, with 46% occurring in children younger than 2 years.[135] Individuals living in crowded living conditions, such as dormitories and military barracks, are at increased risk for invasive disease.[136] Two licensed vaccines are available to reduce the burden of invasive disease. However, the quadrivalent polysaccharide vaccine (Menomune, Sanofi Pasteur, Swiftwater, PA, USA; also referred to as MPSV4) and the quadrivalent conjugate vaccine (Menactra, Sanofi Pasteur, Swiftwater, PA, USA; also referred to as MCV4) do not cover serogroup B, which causes approximately 50% of cases of invasive disease worldwide and 30% in the United States.[137]

N meningitidis can cause a rapidly fatal illness. The 2 most common clinical syndromes (acute meningococcal meningitis and fulminant meningococcemia) must be recognized promptly for immediate diagnosis and treatment. Approximately 50% of patients with invasive disease present with acute purulent meningitis.[138] Its classic symptoms, like all presentations of bacterial meningitis, include headache, fever, photophobia, stiff neck, nausea, vomiting, altered mental status, and bulging fontanelle in infants. Meningococcemia, or meningococcal septicemia, without meningitis occurs in 5% to 20% of patients with invasive disease.[139] It can initially present with acute onset of fever, chills, arthralgia, and myalgia. Patients can experience a transient resolution of symptoms within the first 6 hours, and a maculopapular rash, resembling a viral exanthem, may appear.[140] Then the characteristic nonblanching hemorrhagic (petechial or purpuric) skin lesions may manifest, being more prominent on the extremities. Children with fever and petechial rash merit close examination and consideration by the emergency physician, because they have an 11% chance of having meningococcemia.[141] Patients with petechiae confined to the distribution of the superior vena cava are less likely to have meningococcal infection.[142] In addition, in meningococcemia, the hemorrhagic skin lesions generally progress and are larger and bluer than the pinpoint petechiae associated with thrombocytopenia or coughing.[138] Without prompt treatment, 15% to 20% progress to purpura fulminans, which may necessitate skin grafts or amputations.[143] Complications of meningococcemia include adrenal hemorrhage (Waterhouse-Friderichsen syndrome), stroke, disseminated intravascular coagulation, and acute respiratory distress syndrome.[136]

N meningitidis is diagnosed by Gram stain and culture from CSF or blood. Cultures might be negative if the patient has been pretreated with antibiotics, but PCR can detect *N meningitidis* in culture-negative patients.[144,145] Rapid bacterial antigen detection is not reliable, but newer bedside diagnostic tests are being developed.[146,147] *N meningitidis* should be considered in every patient with CSF pleocytosis and should be treated based on clinical suspicion.

The treatment of meningococcal disease includes aggressive fluid resuscitation and management of shock and early antibiotic therapy. The mortality associated with invasive disease has dropped from 70% to 90% to 10% as a result of rapid antibiotic treatment.[136] Empirical therapy for suspected meningococcal disease should include an extended-spectrum cephalosporin, such as ceftriaxone (100 mg/kg/d) or cefotaxime (200 mg/kg/d IV in 3 divided doses). Penicillin (300,000 U/kg/d IV every 4–6 hours) may be used for definitive treatment. Patients with a severe penicillin allergy should be treated with chloramphenicol, when available, or meropenem (but note 2%–3% cross-reactivity with penicillin).[148] For patients with unexplained petechial rash and fever without signs of meningitis or meningococcal septicemia, an increased WBC count or increased CRP level may indicate an increased risk of meningococcal disease and reason to treat empirically.[141,149]

Shock should be managed aggressively with fluids and vasopressor medications. Patients with meningitis should be monitored and treated for increased intracranial pressure. Although there is conflicting evidence about the benefit of adjuvant corticosteroid therapy in children with septic shock,[150,151] steroids are indicated in cases of adrenal insufficiency, which can occur in association with adrenal hemorrhage from meningococcemia.

In addition to standard precautions, patients with meningococcal infection require isolation with droplet precautions until 24 hours after initiation of effective antimicrobial therapy.[148] Chemoprophylaxis is warranted for household and close contacts, regardless of immunization status. These contacts include those who sleep in the same dwelling, those who could be exposed to oral secretions, and child-care or preschool contacts during the 7 days preceding the onset of disease in the patient. If possible, the following medications should be administered to contacts within 24 hours: ciprofloxacin (500 mg by mouth once for adults), rifampin (5 mg/kg every 12 hours for 2 days for infants <1 month old or 10 mg/kg every 12 hours for 2 days for children >1 month), or ceftriaxone (125 mg IM for children <12 years and 250 mg IM for children >12 years).[148] Postexposure immunoprophylaxis with the meningococcal vaccine should be considered when an outbreak occurs.[152]

SICKLE CELL DISEASE

In children with sickle cell disease (SCD), fever is frequently the first indication of serious and life-threatening infection. Infection is the leading cause of death in patients with SCD, and the approach to fever in these patients should be conservative. Children with SCD are at high risk of bacteremia, because of the early and predictable loss of splenic function. This condition increases the risk of invasive infection by encapsulated organisms such as *H influenzae*, *Streptococcus pneumoniae*, *E coli*, and *Salmonella*.[153] Before the availability of the *H influenzae* type b and pneumococcal conjugate vaccines, children with SCD had a 13% risk of developing bacterial sepsis. The PCV7 vaccine has decreased the incidence of IPD by more than 90%.[154]

The National Institutes of Health recommend the following workup for all children with SCD who present with FWS: CBC, blood culture, chest radiograph, oxygen saturation measurement, urinalysis, urine culture, and throat culture.[36] Children with SCD who are at particularly high risk for bacteremia include those who are younger than 1 year, those with a history of pneumococcal infection, those with an infiltrate on a chest film, and those with the following laboratory findings: WBC count greater than 30,000 or less than 5000, platelet count less than 100,000, and hemoglobin level less than 5 g/dL. Children with SCD and any of these findings should be admitted and placed on IV antibiotics while awaiting blood culture results. Children who do not meet these high-risk criteria but meet criteria for outpatient follow-up can be given a long-acting parenteral antibiotic, such as ceftriaxone, and then be seen on an outpatient basis.

Other sources of infection should also be considered when children with SCD present to the ED. Fever with cough, chest pain, or dyspnea can indicate acute chest syndrome (ACS). In the young child, ACS often presents as fever and cough without pain.[155] This life-threatening condition cannot be excluded by chest radiograph, and patients who raise a high index of suspicion should be admitted for IV fluid hydration, IV antibiotics, oxygen therapy when warranted, and close observation. Influenza is associated with significant morbidity and mortality in patients with SCD. Children with SCD and suspected influenza should be treated with antiviral medication and treated conservatively. Osteomyelitis, meningitis, and arthritis are all more commonly seen in patients with SCD.

Parvovirus infection in children with SCD can constitute an emergency because of its frequent association with aplastic crisis. Children with parvovirus present with fever, headache, nausea, and the slapped cheek rash that is the hallmark of this infection. Because parvovirus causes bone marrow suppression, it frequently can cause aplastic crisis in children with SCD. The first sign of crisis is a lowered reticulocyte count, which can be seen in the first 5 days of illness. The hemoglobin level then decreases accordingly. Children with SCD and suspected parvovirus should be admitted under isolation, and hemoglobin levels should be observed closely, because transfusion might be warranted.

FEBRILE NEUTROPENIA

Fever and neutropenia are the most frequent and potentially lethal complications of chemotherapy in children. Management with emergency hospitalization and empirical IV administration of broad-spectrum antibiotics has decreased mortality to less than 1%.[156]

Febrile neutropenia is defined as the persistence of a temperature 38.5°C or greater for more than 2 hours or a single temperature of 39°C in a patient with an absolute neutrophil count less than 500 cells/mm³.[157] Recent studies stratified neutropenic patients into risk groups. Neutropenic children at low risk of bacteremia and serious medical complications are those who present as outpatients, who have been neutropenic for less than 7 days, and who have no significant comorbidity. One study indicated that these children have a 4% risk of bacteremia or serious medical complication versus a 41% risk in children not meeting these criteria.[158] Neutropenic children are vulnerable to bacterial, fungal, and viral infections. Recent epidemiologic trends have shown an increase in gram-positive bacteria and fungi as causative agents of infection.[159]

Guidelines for management of children with febrile neutropenia were published in 2012.[160] On the patient's presentation in the ED, blood cultures should be obtained from all lumens of central venous catheters. If possible, blood specimens should also be obtained from peripheral sites. Urinalysis and urine culture should be performed if a clean-catch midstream specimen can be obtained. Chest radiographs should be obtained only in symptomatic patients.

Treatment of febrile neutropenia consists of monotherapy with an antipseudomonal β-lactam IV antibiotic or a carbapenem to provide empirical coverage. Addition of a second agent to provide gram-negative coverage should be reserved for patients who are clinically unstable or in centers where resistance exists. Studies have shown success with treating low-risk patients with oral outpatient regimens such as fluoroquinolones or amoxicillin/clavulinate.[161]

SUMMARY

Children and infants presenting to the ED with fever can pose a challenge to the emergency physician. Because fever in children provokes much anxiety among caregivers, it is important to identify children who are at risk for dangerous outcomes.

Important points regarding the management of febrile infants and children are summarized as follows:

- Fever is defined as a rectal temperature greater than 38.0°C (>100.4°F). A fever that was documented recently at home should be considered the same as a temperature documented in the ED.
- All febrile infants younger than 28 days should receive a full sepsis workup and be admitted for parenteral antibiotic therapy.
- Clinical and laboratory criteria can be used to identify low-risk febrile infants aged 1 to 3 months who can be treated on an outpatient basis with close follow-up.
- The PCV7 vaccine has markedly decreased the incidence of SBI in vaccinated infants and children, but children who are unvaccinated or have received fewer than 2 doses of vaccine are still at risk for pneumococcal disease. The impact of the new PCV13 vaccine remains to be seen, but this new medication should decrease the risk even further.
- Neonatal herpes is a potentially devastating illness. Early diagnosis and treatment are essential to reduce mortality. The diagnosis should be strongly considered in the presence of HSV risk factors, atypical sepsis, unexplained acute hepatitis, and focal seizure activity. Acyclovir therapy should be initiated before viral dissemination or significant CNS replication occurs.
- The use of rapid flu tests can distinguish influenza from other viral illnesses, assist in ruling out occult bacteremia in febrile infants, and direct the treatment of high-risk children with antiviral medications.
- Occult UTIs occur often in children with FWS; therefore, a catheterized urine specimen should be obtained for urine testing in girls and uncircumcised boys younger than 2 years and in circumcised boys younger than 6 months.

- Occult pneumonia should be considered in children with a temperature greater than 40°C and a WBC count greater than 20,000 or FWS with respiratory symptoms.
- Fever with petechiae below the nipples should lead to consideration of meningococcemia. Diagnosis and rapid initiation of treatment are critical to decrease mortality from this devastating illness.
- Children with SCD and neutropenia are at high risk for bacterial infections and require special evaluation.

ACKNOWLEDGMENTS

We thank Christina Hermos, MD, Pegeen Eslami, MD, Catherine James, MD, Falgun Wylie, and William (Jerry) Durbin, MD, for review of the fever algorithms.

REFERENCES

1. American College of Emergency Physicians Clinical Policies Committee, American College of Emergency Physicians Clinical Policies Subcommittee on Pediatric Fever. Clinical policy for children younger than three years presenting to the emergency department with fever. Ann Emerg Med 2003;42(4):530–45.
2. Slater M, Krug SE. Evaluation of the infant with fever without source: an evidence based approach. Emerg Med Clin North Am 1999;17(1):97–126.
3. Sherman JM, Sood SK. Current challenges in the diagnosis and management of fever. Curr Opin Pediatr 2012;24(3):400–6.
4. Schmitt BD. Fever phobia: misconceptions of parents about fevers. Am J Dis Child 1980;134(2):176–81.
5. Poirier MP, Collins EP, McGuire E. Fever phobia: a survey of caregivers of children seen in a pediatric emergency department. Clin Pediatr (Phila) 2010;49(6):530–4.
6. Betz MG, Grunfeld AF. 'Fever phobia' in the emergency department: a survey of children's caregivers. Eur J Emerg Med 2006;13(3):129–33.
7. Craig JV, Lancaster GA, Taylor S, et al. Infrared ear thermometry compared with rectal thermometry in children: a systematic review. Lancet 2002;360(9333):603–9.
8. Craig JV, Lancaster GA, Williamson PR, et al. Temperature measured at the axilla compared with rectum in children and young people: systematic review. BMJ 2000;320(7243):1174–8.
9. Hissink Muller PC, van Berkel LH, de Beaufort AJ. Axillary and rectal temperature measurements poorly agree in newborn infants. Neonatology 2008;94(1):31–4.
10. Anbar RD, Richardson-de Corral V, O'Malley PJ. Difficulties in universal application of criteria identifying infants at low risk for serious bacterial infection. J Pediatr 1986;109(3):483–5.
11. Torrey SB, Henretig F, Fleisher G, et al. Temperature response to antipyretic therapy in children: relationship to occult bacteremia. Am J Emerg Med 1985;3(3):190–2.
12. Weisse ME, Miller G, Brien JH. Fever response to acetaminophen in viral vs. bacterial infections. Pediatr Infect Dis J 1987;6(12):1091–4.
13. Baker MD, Fosarelli PD, Carpenter RO. Childhood fever: correlation of diagnosis with temperature response to acetaminophen. Pediatrics 1987;80(3):315–8.
14. Mazur LJ, Jones TM, Kozinetz CA. Temperature response to acetaminophen and risk of occult bacteremia: a case-control study. J Pediatr 1989;115(6):888–91.

15. Baker RC, Tiller T, Bausher JC, et al. Severity of disease correlated with fever reduction in febrile infants. Pediatrics 1989;83(6):1016–9.
16. Yamamoto LT, Wigder HN, Fligner DJ, et al. Relationship of bacteremia to antipyretic therapy in febrile children. Pediatr Emerg Care 1987;3(4):223–7.
17. Greenes DS, Harper MB. Low risk of bacteremia in febrile children with recognizable viral syndromes. Pediatr Infect Dis J 1999;18(3):258–61.
18. Lee GM, Harper MB. Risk of bacteremia for febrile young children in the post-*Haemophilus influenzae* type b era. Arch Pediatr Adolesc Med 1998;152(7): 624–8.
19. Soman M. Characteristics and management of febrile young children seen in a university family practice. J Fam Pract 1985;21(2):117–22.
20. Byington CL, Rittichier KK, Bassett KE, et al. Serious bacterial infections in febrile infants younger than 90 days of age: the importance of ampicillin-resistant pathogens. Pediatrics 2003;111(5 Pt 1):964–8.
21. Nizet V, Vinci RJ, Lovejoy FH Jr. Fever in children. Pediatr Rev 1994;15(4): 127–35.
22. Byington CL, Enriquez FR, Hoff C, et al. Serious bacterial infections in febrile infants 1 to 90 days old with and without viral infections. Pediatrics 2004;113(6): 1662–6.
23. Klein JO. Management of the febrile child without a focus of infection in the era of universal pneumococcal immunization. Pediatr Infect Dis J 2002;21(6):584–8.
24. Mintegi S, Benito J, Sanchez J, et al. Predictors of occult bacteremia in young febrile children in the era of heptavalent pneumococcal conjugated vaccine. Eur J Emerg Med 2009;16(4):199–205.
25. Sard B, Bailey MC, Vinci R. An analysis of pediatric blood cultures in the post-pneumococcal conjugate vaccine era in a community hospital emergency department. Pediatr Emerg Care 2006;22(5):295–300.
26. Whitney CG, Farley MM, Hadler J, et al. Decline in invasive pneumococcal disease after the introduction of protein-polysaccharide conjugate vaccine. N Engl J Med 2003;348(18):1737–46.
27. Wilkinson M, Bulloch B, Smith M. Prevalence of occult bacteremia in children aged 3 to 36 months presenting to the emergency department with fever in the postpneumococcal conjugate vaccine era. Acad Emerg Med 2009;16(3): 220–5.
28. Adams WG, Deaver KA, Cochi SL, et al. Decline of childhood *Haemophilus influenzae* type b (Hib) disease in the Hib vaccine era. JAMA 1993;269(2):221–6.
29. Poehling KA, Talbot TR, Griffin MR, et al. Invasive pneumococcal disease among infants before and after introduction of pneumococcal conjugate vaccine. JAMA 2006;295(14):1668–74.
30. Morley EJ, Lapoint JM, Roy LW, et al. Rates of positive blood, urine, and cerebrospinal fluid cultures in children younger than 60 days during the vaccination era. Pediatr Emerg Care 2012;28(2):125–30.
31. Bressan S, Berlese P, Mion T, et al. Bacteremia in feverish children presenting to the emergency department: a retrospective study and literature review. Acta Paediatr 2012;101(3):271–7.
32. Alpern ER, Alessandrini EA, McGowan KL, et al. Serotype prevalence of occult pneumococcal bacteremia. Pediatrics 2001;108(2):E23.
33. Johnson HL, Deloria-Knoll M, Levine OS, et al. Systematic evaluation of serotypes causing invasive pneumococcal disease among children under five: the pneumococcal global serotype project. PLoS Med 2010;7(10). http://dx.doi. org/10.1371/journal.pmed.1000348.

34. Webster J, Theodoratou E, Nair H, et al. An evaluation of emerging vaccines for childhood pneumococcal pneumonia. BMC Public Health 2011;11(Suppl 3):S26.

35. Miller E, Andrews NJ, Waight PA, et al. Effectiveness of the new serotypes in the 13-valent pneumococcal conjugate vaccine. Vaccine 2011;29(49):9127–31.

36. Claudius I, Baraff LJ. Pediatric emergencies associated with fever. Emerg Med Clin North Am 2010;28(1):67–84.

37. Colletti JE, Homme JL, Woodridge DP. Unsuspected neonatal killers in emergency medicine. Emerg Med Clin North Am 2004;22(4):929–60.

38. Byington CL, Reynolds CC, Korgenski K, et al. Costs and infant outcomes after implementation of a care process model for febrile infants. Pediatrics 2012; 130(1):e16–24.

39. Ferrera PC, Bartfield JM, Snyder HS. Neonatal fever: utility of the Rochester criteria in determining low risk for serious bacterial infections. Am J Emerg Med 1997;15(3):299–302.

40. Kadish HA, Loveridge B, Tobey J, et al. Applying outpatient protocols in febrile infants 1-28 days of age: can the threshold be lowered? Clin Pediatr (Phila) 2000;39(2):81–8.

41. Baker MD, Bell LM. Unpredictability of serious bacterial illness in febrile infants from birth to 1 month of age. Arch Pediatr Adolesc Med 1999;153(5):508–11.

42. Chiu CH, Lin TY, Bullard MJ. Application of criteria identifying febrile outpatient neonates at low risk for bacterial infections. Pediatr Infect Dis J 1994;13(11):946–9.

43. Baraff LJ. Management of infants and young children with fever without source. Pediatr Ann 2008;37(10):673–9.

44. Overall JC Jr. Herpes simplex virus infection of the fetus and newborn. Pediatr Ann 1994;23(3):131–6.

45. Brown ZA, Benedetti J, Ashley R, et al. Neonatal herpes simplex virus infection in relation to asymptomatic maternal infection at the time of labor. N Engl J Med 1991;324(18):1247–52.

46. Rudnick CM, Hoekzema GS. Neonatal herpes simplex virus infections. Am Fam Physician 2002;65(6):1138–42.

47. Brown ZA, Benedetti JK, Watts DH, et al. A comparison between detailed and simple histories in the diagnosis of genital herpes complicating pregnancy. Am J Obstet Gynecol 1995;172(4 Pt 1):1299–303.

48. Kesson AM. Management of neonatal herpes simplex virus infection. Paediatr Drugs 2001;3(2):81–90.

49. Diamond C, Mohan K, Hobson A, et al. Viremia in neonatal herpes simplex virus infections. Pediatr Infect Dis J 1999;18(6):487–9.

50. Prahlow JA, Linch CA. A baby, a virus, and a rat. Am J Forensic Med Pathol 2000;21(2):127–33.

51. Liesegang TJ. Herpes simplex virus epidemiology and ocular importance. Cornea 2001;20(1):1–13.

52. Carey BE. Neonatal herpes simplex: pulmonary and intracranial findings. Neonatal Netw 2002;21(6):63–7.

53. American Academy of Pediatrics. Herpes simplex. In: Pickering L, editor. Red book: 2012 report of the committee on infectious disease. Elk Grove Village (IL): American Academy of Pediatrics; 2000. p. 309–18.

54. Brown ZA. Genital herpes complicating pregnancy. Dermatol Clin 1998;16(4): 805–10.

55. American Academy of Pediatrics. Herpes simplex. In: Pickering L, editor. Red book: 2012 report of the committee on infectious disease. Elk Grove Village (IL): American Academy of Pediatrics; 2012. p. 398.

56. Kimberlin DW, Lin CY, Jacobs RF, et al. Natural history of neonatal herpes simplex virus infections in the acyclovir era. Pediatrics 2001;108(2):223–9.
57. Kohl S. The diagnosis and treatment of neonatal herpes simplex virus infection. Pediatr Ann 2002;31(11):726–32.
58. Dhar S, Dhar S. Disseminated neonatal herpes simplex: a rare entity. Pediatr Dermatol 2000;17(4):330–2.
59. Malm G, Forsgren M. Neonatal herpes simplex virus infections: HSV DNA in cerebrospinal fluid and serum. Arch Dis Child Fetal Neonatal Ed 1999;81(1): F24–9.
60. Whitley RJ, Nahmias AJ, Visintine AM, et al. The natural history of herpes simplex virus infection of mother and newborn. Pediatrics 1980;66(4):489–94.
61. Whitley RJ. Neonatal herpes simplex virus infections: pathogenesis and therapy. Pathol Biol (Paris) 1992;40(7):729–34.
62. Enright AM, Prober CG. Neonatal herpes infection: diagnosis, treatment and prevention. Semin Neonatol 2002;7(4):283–91.
63. Baker MD, Bell LM, Avner JR. Outpatient management without antibiotics of fever in selected infants. N Engl J Med 1993;329(20):1437–41.
64. Jaskiewicz JA, McCarthy CA, Richardson AC, et al. Febrile infants at low risk for serious bacterial infection–an appraisal of the Rochester criteria and implications for management. Febrile Infant Collaborative Study Group. Pediatrics 1994;94(3):390–6.
65. Baskin MN, O'Rourke EJ, Fleisher GR. Outpatient treatment of febrile infants 28 to 89 days of age with intramuscular administration of ceftriaxone. J Pediatr 1992;120(1):22–7.
66. Baraff LJ. Management of fever without source in infants and children. Ann Emerg Med 2000;36(6):602–14.
67. Bachur R, Perry H, Harper MB. Occult pneumonias: empiric chest radiographs in febrile children with leukocytosis. Ann Emerg Med 1999;33(2):166–73.
68. Claesson BA, Trollfors B, Brolin I, et al. Etiology of community-acquired pneumonia in children based on antibody responses to bacterial and viral antigens. Pediatr Infect Dis J 1989;8(12):856–62.
69. Bettenay FA, de Campo JF, McCrossin DB. Differentiating bacterial from viral pneumonias in children. Pediatr Radiol 1988;18(6):453–4.
70. Swingler GH. Radiologic differentiation between bacterial and viral lower respiratory infection in children: a systematic literature review. Clin Pediatr (Phila) 2000;39(11):627–33.
71. Boyer K, Cherry J. Nonbacterial pneumonia. In: Feigin R, Cherry J, editors. Textbook of pediatric infectious disease. Philadelphia: WB Saunders; 1992.
72. Turner RB. Epidemiology, pathogenesis, and treatment of the common cold. Ann Allergy Asthma Immunol 1997;78(6):531–40.
73. Bramson RT, Meyer TL, Silbiger ML, et al. The futility of the chest radiograph in the febrile infant without respiratory symptoms. Pediatrics 1993;92(4):524–6.
74. Shaw KN, Gorelick M, McGowan KL, et al. Prevalence of urinary tract infection in febrile young children in the emergency department. Pediatrics 1998;102(2): e16.
75. Hoberman A, Chao HP, Keller DM, et al. Prevalence of urinary tract infection in febrile infants. J Pediatr 1993;123(1):17–23.
76. Hoberman A, Wald ER. Urinary tract infections in young febrile children. Pediatr Infect Dis J 1997;16(1):11–7.
77. Bauchner H, Philipp B, Dashefsky B, et al. Prevalence of bacteriuria in febrile children. Pediatr Infect Dis J 1987;6(3):239–42.

78. Shaikh N, Morone NE, Bost JE, et al. Prevalence of urinary tract infection in childhood: a meta-analysis. Pediatr Infect Dis J 2008;27(4):302–8.

79. Hoberman A, Wald ER, Hickey RW, et al. Oral versus initial intravenous therapy for urinary tract infections in young febrile children. Pediatrics 1999;104(1 Pt 1): 79–86.

80. Magin EC, Garcia-Garcia JJ, Sert SZ, et al. Efficacy of short-term intravenous antibiotic in neonates with urinary tract infection. Pediatr Emerg Care 2007; 23(2):83–6.

81. Sastre JB, Aparicio AR, Cotallo GD, et al. Urinary tract infection in the newborn: clinical and radio imaging studies. Pediatr Nephrol 2007;22(10):1735–41.

82. Subcommittee on Urinary Tract Infection, Steering Committee on Quality Improvement and Management, Roberts KB. Urinary tract infection: clinical practice guideline for the diagnosis and management of the initial UTI in febrile infants and children 2 to 24 months. Pediatrics 2011;128(3):595–610.

83. Krief WI, Levine DA, Platt SL, et al. Influenza virus infection and the risk of serious bacterial infections in young febrile infants. Pediatrics 2009;124(1):30–9.

84. Levine DA, Platt SL, Dayan PS, et al. Risk of serious bacterial infection in young febrile infants with respiratory syncytial virus infections. Pediatrics 2004;113(6): 1728–34.

85. Bilavsky E, Shouval DS, Yarden-Bilavsky H, et al. A prospective study of the risk for serious bacterial infections in hospitalized febrile infants with or without bronchiolitis. Pediatr Infect Dis J 2008;27(3):269–70.

86. Doby B, Korgenski K, Reynolds C, et al. Detection of rhinovirus does not decrease the likelihood of serious bacterial infection in febrile infants younger than 90 days of age [poster]. Presented at the Annual Meeting of the Pediatric Academic Society. Denver (Colorado), May 1, 2011.

87. Rittichier KR, Bryan PA, Bassett KE, et al. Diagnosis and outcomes of enterovirus infections in young infants. Pediatr Infect Dis J 2005;24(6):546–50.

88. Committee on Infectious Diseases, American Academy of Pediatrics. Recommendations for prevention and control of influenza in children, 2012–2013. Pediatrics 2012;130(4):780–92.

89. Lee GM, Fleisher GR, Harper MB. Management of febrile children in the age of the conjugate pneumococcal vaccine: a cost-effectiveness analysis. Pediatrics 2001;108(4):835–44.

90. Jaffe DM, Tanz RR, Davis AT, et al. Antibiotic administration to treat possible occult bacteremia in febrile children. N Engl J Med 1987;317(19):1175–80.

91. Kuppermann N. Occult bacteremia in young febrile children. Pediatr Clin North Am 1999;46(6):1073–109.

92. Waddle E, Jhaveri R. Outcomes of febrile children without localising signs after pneumococcal conjugate vaccine. Arch Dis Child 2009;94(2):144–7.

93. Baraff LJ, Bass JW, Fleisher GR, et al. Practice guideline for the management of infants and children 0 to 36 months of age with fever without source. Agency for Health Care Policy and Research. Ann Emerg Med 1993;22(7):1198–210.

94. Taylor JA, Del Beccaro M, Done S, et al. Establishing clinically relevant standards for tachypnea in febrile children younger than 2 years. Arch Pediatr Adolesc Med 1995;149(3):283–7.

95. Leventhal JM. Clinical predictors of pneumonia as a guide to ordering chest roentgenograms. Clin Pediatr (Phila) 1982;21(12):730–4.

96. Zukin DD, Hoffman JR, Cleveland RH, et al. Correlation of pulmonary signs and symptoms with chest radiographs in the pediatric age group. Ann Emerg Med 1986;15(7):792–6.

97. Singal BM, Hedges JR, Radack KL. Decision rules and clinical prediction of pneumonia: evaluation of low-yield criteria. Ann Emerg Med 1989;18(1):13–20.
98. Hickey RW, Bowman MJ, Smith GA. Utility of blood cultures in pediatric patients found to have pneumonia in the emergency department. Ann Emerg Med 1996; 27(6):721–5.
99. Rosman NP, Peterson DB, Kaye EM, et al. Seizures in bacterial meningitis: prevalence, patterns, pathogenesis, and prognosis. Pediatr Neurol 1985;1(5): 278–85.
100. Rosman NP. Evaluation of the child who convulses with fever. Paediatr Drugs 2003;5(7):457–61.
101. Nigrovic LE, Kuppermann N, Malley R. Development and validation of a multivariable predictive model to distinguish bacterial from aseptic meningitis in children in the post-*Haemophilus influenzae* era. Pediatrics 2002;110(4): 712–9.
102. Nigrovic LE, Kuppermann N, Macias CG, et al. Clinical prediction rule for identifying children with cerebrospinal fluid pleocytosis at very low risk of bacterial meningitis. JAMA 2007;297(1):52–60.
103. Chin RF, Neville BG, Scott RC. Meningitis is a common cause of convulsive status epilepticus with fever. Arch Dis Child 2005;90(1):66–9.
104. Fetveit A. Assessment of febrile seizures in children. Eur J Pediatr 2008;167(1): 17–27.
105. Armon K, Stephenson T, MacFaul R, et al. An evidence and consensus based guideline for the management of a child after a seizure. Emerg Med J 2003; 20(1):13–20.
106. Green SM, Rothrock SG, Clem KJ, et al. Can seizures be the sole manifestation of meningitis in febrile children? Pediatrics 1993;92(4):527–34.
107. Kneen R, Appleton R. Status epilepticus with fever: how common is meningitis? Arch Dis Child 2005;90(1):3–4.
108. Offringa M, Moyer VA. Evidence based paediatrics: evidence based management of seizures associated with fever. BMJ 2001;323(7321):1111–4.
109. Warden CR, Zibulewsky J, Mace S, et al. Evaluation and management of febrile seizures in the out-of-hospital and emergency department settings. Ann Emerg Med 2003;41(2):215–22.
110. Akpede GO, Sykes RM. Convulsions with fever as a presenting feature of bacterial meningitis among preschool children in developing countries. Dev Med Child Neurol 1992;34(6):524–9.
111. Kimia A, Ben-Joseph EP, Rudloe T, et al. Yield of lumbar puncture among children who present with their first complex febrile seizure. Pediatrics 2010;126(1): 62–9.
112. Kimia AA, Capraro AJ, Hummel D, et al. Utility of lumbar puncture for first simple febrile seizure among children 6 to 18 months of age. Pediatrics 2009;123(1): 6–12.
113. Rosenberg NM, Meert K, Marino D, et al. Seizures associated with meningitis. Pediatr Emerg Care 1992;8(2):67–9.
114. Taubert KA, Rowley AH, Shulman ST. Nationwide survey of Kawasaki disease and acute rheumatic fever. J Pediatr 1991;119(2):279–82.
115. Yanagawa H, Nakamura Y, Ojima T, et al. Changes in epidemic patterns of Kawasaki disease in Japan. Pediatr Infect Dis J 1999;18(1):64–6.
116. Holman RC, Belay ED, Christensen KY, et al. Hospitalizations for Kawasaki syndrome among children in the United States, 1997–2007. Pediatr Infect Dis J 2010;29(6):483–8.

117. Newburger JW, Takahashi M, Gerber MA, et al. Diagnosis, treatment, and long-term management of Kawasaki disease: a statement for health professionals from the Committee on Rheumatic Fever, Endocarditis and Kawasaki Disease, Council on Cardiovascular Disease in the Young, American Heart Association. Circulation 2004;110(17):2747–71.

118. Lang B. Recognizing Kawasaki disease. Paediatr Child Health 2001;6(9): 638–43.

119. Ohno S, Miyajima T, Higuchi M, et al. Ocular manifestations of Kawasaki's disease (mucocutaneous lymph node syndrome). Am J Ophthalmol 1982;93(6):713–7.

120. Burns JC, Joffe L, Sargent RA, et al. Anterior uveitis associated with Kawasaki syndrome. Pediatr Infect Dis 1985;4(3):258–61.

121. Gong GW, McCrindle BW, Ching JC, et al. Arthritis presenting during the acute phase of Kawasaki disease. J Pediatr 2006;148(6):800–5.

122. Baker AL, Lu M, Minich LL, et al. Associated symptoms in the ten days before diagnosis of Kawasaki disease. J Pediatr 2009;154(4):592–5.

123. Yoskovitch A, Tewfik TL, Duffy CM, et al. Head and neck manifestations of Kawasaki disease. Int J Pediatr Otorhinolaryngol 2000;52(2):123–9.

124. Suddleson EA, Reid B, Woolley MM, et al. Hydrops of the gallbladder associated with Kawasaki syndrome. J Pediatr Surg 1987;22(10):956–9.

125. Benseler SM, McCrindle BW, Silverman ED, et al. Infections and Kawasaki disease: implications for coronary artery outcome. Pediatrics 2005;116(6):e760–6.

126. Jordan-Villegas A, Chang ML, Ramilo O, et al. Concomitant respiratory viral infections in children with Kawasaki disease. Pediatr Infect Dis J 2010;29(8): 770–2.

127. Dajani AS, Taubert KA, Gerber MA, et al. Diagnosis and therapy of Kawasaki disease in children. Circulation 1993;87(5):1776–80.

128. Nakamura Y, Yashiro M, Uehara R, et al. Epidemiologic features of Kawasaki disease in Japan: results of the 2007–2008 nationwide survey. J Epidemiol 2010;20(4):302–7.

129. Durongpisitkul K, Soongswang J, Laohaprasitiporn D, et al. Immunoglobulin failure and retreatment in Kawasaki disease. Pediatr Cardiol 2003;24(2):145–8.

130. Tremoulet AH, Best BM, Song S, et al. Resistance to intravenous immunoglobulin in children with Kawasaki disease. J Pediatr 2008;153(1):117–21.

131. Burns JC, Capparelli EV, Brown JA, et al. Intravenous gamma-globulin treatment and retreatment in Kawasaki disease. US/Canadian Kawasaki Syndrome Study Group. Pediatr Infect Dis J 1998;17(12):1144–8.

132. Caugant DA, Tzanakaki G, Kriz P. Lessons from meningococcal carriage studies. FEMS Microbiol Rev 2007;31(1):52–63.

133. Stephens DS. Uncloaking the meningococcus: dynamics of carriage and disease. Lancet 1999;353(9157):941–2.

134. Kirsch EA, Barton RP, Kitchen L, et al. Pathophysiology, treatment and outcome of meningococcemia: a review and recent experience. Pediatr Infect Dis J 1996; 15(11):967–78.

135. Riedo FX, Plikaytis BD, Broome CV. Epidemiology and prevention of meningococcal disease. Pediatr Infect Dis J 1995;14(8):643–57.

136. Rosenstein NE, Fischer M, Tappero JW. Meningococcal vaccines. Infect Dis Clin North Am 2001;15(1):155–69.

137. Girard MP, Preziosi MP, Aguado MT, et al. A review of vaccine research and development: meningococcal disease. Vaccine 2006;24(22):4692–700.

138. Brigham KS, Sandora TJ. Neisseria meningitidis: epidemiology, treatment and prevention in adolescents. Curr Opin Pediatr 2009;21(4):437–43.

139. van Deuren M, Brandtzaeg P, van der Meer JW. Update on meningococcal disease with emphasis on pathogenesis and clinical management. Clin Microbiol Rev 2000;13(1):144–66.

140. Yung AP, McDonald MI. Early clinical clues to meningococcaemia. Med J Aust 2003;178(3):134–7.

141. Klinkhammer MD, Colletti JE. Pediatric myth: fever and petechiae. CJEM 2008; 10(5):479–82.

142. Wells LC, Smith JC, Weston VC, et al. The child with a non-blanching rash: how likely is meningococcal disease? Arch Dis Child 2001;85(3):218–22.

143. Herrera R, Hobar PC, Ginsburg CM. Surgical intervention for the complications of meningococcal-induced purpura fulminans. Pediatr Infect Dis J 1994;13(8): 734–7.

144. Taha MK, Alonso JM. Molecular epidemiology of infectious diseases: the example of meningococcal disease. Res Microbiol 2008;159(1):62–6.

145. Cummings KC, Louie J, Probert WS, et al. Increased detection of meningococcal infections in California using a polymerase chain reaction assay. Clin Infect Dis 2008;46(7):1124–6.

146. Perkins MD, Mirrett S, Reller LB. Rapid bacterial antigen detection is not clinically useful. J Clin Microbiol 1995;33(6):1486–91.

147. Chanteau S, Dartevelle S, Mahamane AE, et al. New rapid diagnostic tests for *Neisseria meningitidis* serogroups A, W135, C, and Y. PLoS Med 2006;3(9):e337.

148. American Academy of Pediatrics. Meningococcal infections. In: Pickering L, editor. Red Book: 2012 Report of the Committee on Infectious Diseases. Elk Grove Village (IL): American Academy of Pediatrics; 2012. p. 500–9.

149. Visintin C, Mugglestone MA, Fields EJ, et al. Management of bacterial meningitis and meningococcal septicaemia in children and young people: summary of NICE guidance. BMJ 2010;340:c3209.

150. Markovitz BP, Goodman DM, Watson RS, et al. A retrospective cohort study of prognostic factors associated with outcome in pediatric severe sepsis: what is the role of steroids? Pediatr Crit Care Med 2005;6(3):270–4.

151. Zimmerman JJ, Williams MD. Adjunctive corticosteroid therapy in pediatric severe sepsis: observations from the RESOLVE study. Pediatr Crit Care Med 2011;12(1):2–8.

152. Bilukha OO, Rosenstein N, National Center for Infectious Diseases, et al. Prevention and control of meningococcal disease. Recommendations of the Advisory Committee on Immunization Practices (ACIP). MMWR Recomm Rep 2005;54(RR-7):1–21.

153. Leikin SL, Gallagher D, Kinney TR, et al. Mortality in children and adolescents with sickle cell disease. Cooperative Study of Sickle Cell Disease. Pediatrics 1989;84(3):500–8.

154. Halasa NB, Shankar SM, Talbot TR, et al. Incidence of invasive pneumococcal disease among individuals with sickle cell disease before and after the introduction of the pneumococcal conjugate vaccine. Clin Infect Dis 2007;44(11): 1428–33.

155. Vichinsky EP, Styles LA, Colangelo LH, et al. Acute chest syndrome in sickle cell disease: clinical presentation and course. Cooperative Study of Sickle Cell Disease. Blood 1997;89(5):1787–92.

156. Koh A, Pizzo PA. Infectious complications in pediatric cancer patients. In: Pizzo PA, Poplack DG, editors. Principles and practice of pediatric oncology. 6th edition. Philadelphia: Wolters Kluwer/Lippincott Williams & Wilkins; 2011. p. 1190–242.

157. Binz P, Bodmer N, Leibundgut K, et al. Different fever definitions and the rate of fever and neutropenia diagnosed in children with cancer: a retrospective two-center cohort study. Pediatr Blood Cancer 2013;60(5):799–805.

158. Alexander SW, Wade KC, Hibberd PL, et al. Evaluation of risk prediction criteria for episodes of febrile neutropenia in children with cancer. J Pediatr Hematol Oncol 2002;24(1):38–42.

159. Crokaert F. Febrile neutropenia in children. Int J Antimicrob Agents 2000;16(2): 173–6.

160. Lehrnbecher T, Phillips R, Alexander S, et al. Guideline for the management of fever and neutropenia in children with cancer and/or undergoing hematopoietic stem-cell transplantation. J Clin Oncol 2012;30(35):4427–38.

161. Manji A, Beyene J, Dupuis LL, et al. Outpatient and oral antibiotic management of low-risk febrile neutropenia are effective in children–a systematic review of prospective trials. Support Care Cancer 2012;20(6):1135–45.

Heat-Related Illness

Walter F. Atha, MD

KEYWORDS

- Heat emergency • Heat stroke • Environmental heat emergency • Hyperthermia

KEY POINTS

- Evaporation is the most effective cooling mechanism in the emergency department; cooling blankets are less effective.
- Environmental assessment of risk for heat-related illness must include wet bulb global temperature for accurate evaluation of heat stress, including humidity.
- Do not rule out heat stroke based on lack of sweating.
- Definitions of heat-related illnesses are less important than is recognition of the severity of presentation, which drives subsequent evaluation and treatment.
- Elevations in liver function tests may be seen 1 or 2 days after the initial insult.
- Elements of critical care include careful volume replacement and tolerance of mild hypotension.

A heat-related illness is defined as a physiologic insult to the body from exposure to elevated temperature, which can lead to elevation of core body temperature that surpasses the compensatory limits of thermoregulation. Presentations may be acute or delayed. Particularly severe cases can be life threatening. Heat-related illnesses are classically distinguished from "febrile" emergencies in that increased temperature is caused by environmental heat stress, rather than a change in hypothalamic function in the setting of normothermic environmental conditions.[1] Heat-related illness represents a set of syndromes that exist along a continuum from less severe illnesses, such as heat exhaustion, to multiorgan failure with heat stroke. While strict diagnostic criteria remain elusive, common descriptions are generally sufficient to provide working case definitions. For example, the term heat stroke typically implies a core temperature elevated to at least 40°C and the presence of central nervous system (CNS) dysfunction. Working terms to describe various heat-related illness syndromes are also ample, for example, prickly heat, heat edema, and heat cramps.

According to the National Oceanic and Atmospheric Administration (NOAA), 2012 was the hottest year on record for the continental United States, with an average

Disclosures: None.
Department of Emergency Medicine, Howard County General Hospital, 5755 Cedar Lane, Columbia, MD 21044, USA
E-mail address: watha@jhmi.edu

Emerg Med Clin N Am 31 (2013) 1097–1108
http://dx.doi.org/10.1016/j.emc.2013.07.012
0733-8627/13/$ – see front matter © 2013 Elsevier Inc. All rights reserved.

temperature of 55.3°F (12.94°C), 3.2°F higher than the twentieth-century average.[2] If ambient temperatures continue to climb, the incidence of heat-related illnesses is likely to increase, underscoring the importance of better evaluation, diagnosis, and treatment. Epidemiologic data are less robust than they could be if definitions were better standardized; underdiagnosis remains a problem. Even so, high mortality rates have been reported in highly publicized heat waves in the United States and Europe.[3–5] The death of approximately 14,800 individuals was attributed to the heat wave in France during the summer of 2003.[5] The years 2005 to 2009 saw the highest incidence of heat-related sports deaths ever recorded in the United States.

The European heat wave of 2003 emphasized the vulnerability of certain populations to heat-related illnesses, secondary to decreased capacity to dissipate heat and increased likelihood of dehydration. These groups include the elderly, small children (because of their relatively large ratio of skin surface area to body mass), those with medical comorbidities, people with poor access to climate-controlled environments, and those with psychosocial challenges. Occupational and recreational activities requiring strenuous exercise in hot environments may confer significant risk as well (eg, athletes, firefighters, military personnel).

PHYSIOLOGY

Normal human core temperature is maintained at roughly 37°C across all populations. Normal skin temperature is nearly constant at 35°C, creating the temperature gradient necessary to dissipate heat from the core to the periphery. The body's net exothermic metabolism constantly generates heat at a basal rate ofapproximately100 kcal/h.[6]

In addition, the body absorbs heat from and dissipates heat to the environment by 4 basic mechanisms: conduction, convection, evaporation, and radiation (**Table 1**). Conduction is heat transfer via direct contact between surfaces. Convection is heat transfer from a solid or liquid to a moving liquid or ambient air. Both conduction and convection result in net heat loss when the body surface is warmer than the ambient air or surface, and in net heat gain when the ambient air or contact surface is warmer than the body. Radiation is heat transfer via electromagnetic waves. With evaporation of sweat, the water changes from liquid to vapor, with a concomitant reduction in skin temperature of 0.58 kcal per milliliter of sweat.[7] These mechanisms are augmented by therapeutic cooling maneuvers. For example, the use of fans in conjunction with continually wetting the skin increases convection and evaporation-mediated heat transfer. The use of moving water in cold-water immersion systems increases the effectiveness of convective heat transfer. As ambient temperature and relative humidity increase, 2 principal mechanisms of heat dissipation, evaporation and convection, become less effective, thereby diminishing the effectiveness of fans when used alone.[8]

Table 1 Mechanisms of body heat transfer		
	Mechanism	**Dissipation/Absorption**
Conduction	Direct contact between surfaces of divergent temperatures	Both: minimal
Convection	Transfer to a moving liquid or ambient air	Both: moderate
Radiation	Transfer via electromagnetic waves	Both: minimal
Evaporation	Change of state from liquid to vapor or water in sweat	Dissipation only: predominant

Environmental contribution to heat stress must take into account its impact on the body's compensation mechanisms. Relative humidity and temperature must be considered independently in assessing heat stress, because evaporation of sweat is the predominant cooling mechanism in elevated temperatures, and physiologically effective evaporation of sweat ceases when humidity exceeds approximately 75%. Wet bulb global temperature (WBGT) is the best known and most widely used scale of heat stress. WBGT accounts for independent contributions of absolute temperature, humidity, and radiant heat absorption. The calculation is:

WBGT index = [DBT × 0.1] + [WBT × 0.7] + [GT × 0.2]

Dry bulb temperature (DBT) represents true ambient air temperature. Wet bulb temperature (WBT) is measured by covering a thermometer with a white cloth, sometimes called a sock, kept wet by wicking action. Globe temperature (GT) is a measure of the radiant heat effect from the sun and other proximate surfaces producing radiant heat. Analysis of the equation reveals that humidity, via WBT, is the largest contributor to the WBGT index. Complex devices are used to measure the WBGT index, but it can be reasonably approximated using mathematical estimation and allows comparison across regions. For example, WBGT along the east coast of the United States during peak summer months can be very close in range to WBGT in lower-latitude tropical regions and the hottest arid deserts on other continents. At present, the highest WBGT measurements on the planet across all outdoor natural environments are roughly 31°C.[9]

Afferent and efferent apparatuses maintain body thermoregulation. The preoptic nucleus of the anterior hypothalamus (POAH) is the temperature-sensing center in the CNS. The POAH alters the mechanisms for cooling based on temperature relative to its set point. When the hypothalamic set point is elevated, a "febrile" condition exists. A "hyperthermic" condition, on the other hand, is created by an exogenous heat source. When core temperature becomes elevated, the POAH, via sympathetic pathways, signals vasodilatation of the peripheral vasculature and shunting of blood away from splanchnic beds to preferentially perfuse the skin, augmenting heat dissipation. Blood flow to the skin can increase from a baseline of 250 mL/min to 6 to 8 L/min.[10] There is a corresponding increase in cardiac output in response to increased demand.

Increased sweat production, also signaled via the POAH, is another important mechanism of heat dissipation. Eccrine sweat glands cover most of the body, although they are more densely concentrated in the palms and soles, and are cholinergically activated. Apocrine sweat glands found mostly in the axillae are adrenergically activated and play little role in cooling. Evaporation of sweat is an efficient cooling mechanism, but depends on convection of air away from moist skin. Loose-fitting clothing allows air to circulate over moist skin. A core tenet of treatment for elevated body temperature is removal of all clothing, which increases the surface area exposed to convective air currents. Without circulation of air, a thin layer of heated air forms a local insulation barrier, preventing further convective cooling of the skin. High humidity decreases the cooling efficacy of sweating; at 95% relative humidity, sweating becomes essentially ineffective, and for this reason the WBT in the WBGT is weighted more heavily (by a factor of 0.7 vs 0.2 for radiant heat and 0.1 for dry temperature) to determine the effective heat risk.

In the cardiovascular system, increased demand results from decreased peripheral resistance, and shunting of a large portion of the circulating volume to the skin reduces preload. Inotropy is increased, and stroke volume remains the same or increases slightly. The large increase in cardiac demand is mediated primarily by increased heart rate. The increased chronotropy is stimulated by either a direct heat effect on the sinoatrial node, or parasympathetic effects from the baroreflex and sympathetic effects from the heightened adrenergic state in hyperthermia.[11] People with poor baseline cardiac conditioning or decreased cardiac function as a result of myocardial damage or medications that suppress heart rate or cardiac work, such as β-blockers, are less able to increase cardiac output in response to the demand.[12] Hence, they are more likely to have decompensated heat-management mechanisms and rapidly elevate their body temperature. Semenza and colleagues[13] suggested that type 2 diabetics are at increased risk because of decreased peripheral vascular dilatation, presumably neutrally mediated, rather than purely cardiac dysfunction.

Relative dehydration caused by diuretics and other medications leads to the same effects of decreased circulating volume. Sweat production can be decreased by prescription and illicit medications, particularly those with anticholinergic effects. Hyponatremia, caused by increased sodium loss relative to water loss, can develop from increased sweat production. In lower mammals, panting contributes to cooling via convective heat transfer from the pulmonary capillary bed as well as a closed-loop system in the skull, which directly cools the brain; this mechanism is not significant in humans.

PATHOGENESIS AND CLINICAL PRESENTATION

When the cooling mechanisms fail, core temperature rises, leading to pathologic changes in several organ systems. The observed pathologic changes are thought to occur via direct cytotoxicity and a severe systemic inflammatory response (SIRS).[14] The cellular function of any tissue is affected by elevated temperature by denaturation of proteins, release of proinflammatory cellular mediators, including cytokines, and, at very high temperatures, cell death and apoptosis. The critical thermal maximum for humans is 41.6° to 42°C, at which point these cellular changes begin to take place. SIRS is thought to be mediated by direct injury to the vascular endothelium, causing leakage into the interstitial space. Concomitant direct activation by elevated temperature of the coagulation cascade and progression to disseminated intravascular coagulation (DIC) is a common complication of heat stroke.[15]

The 2 tissues most vulnerable to damage by elevated temperatures are the brain, particularly the cerebellum, and the liver. On this basis, the common understanding of the diagnosis of heat stroke requires both CNS changes and evidence of hepatocellular damage, manifested by elevated liver function tests (LFTs). CNS dysfunction can manifest as dizziness, confusion, dysmetria, ataxia, and, eventually, coma. The particular sensitivity of the cerebellum explains the predominance of cerebellar signs and symptoms early in disease progression. Hepatic and renal insult also occurs secondarily to hypoperfusion from CNS-mediated splanchnic and renal blood shunting to the skin, in addition to direct heat damage. Elevations in LFTs might not manifest for more than 12 hours, so normal values should not be used to rule out severe insult in clinically ill patients. Most patients with elevated LFTs will experience complete recovery without hepatic damage, when treated appropriately. However, an interesting case report attributed the death of a normal subject to fulminant hepatic failure that occurred directly after prolonged temperature elevation in a sauna.[16] Abnormalities in the CNS and the hepatic system distinguish heat stroke from heat exhaustion (which is not associated with CNS or liver insult). While many patients with extreme heat illness stop sweating, many continue to sweat profusely. Anhidrosis does not exclude the diagnosis of heat stroke.

Other organ system effects can be severe. Direct cardiomyopathy without evidence of coronary artery disease was attributed to prolonged heat exposure in a case study.[17] The patient described in that report was the first for whom concomitant coronary artery occlusion was excluded by coronary angiography at the time of ST-segment elevation in conjunction with heat stroke. Stress-induced cardiomyopathy caused by heat exposure was the presumed diagnosis. Bowel ischemia from splanchnic shunting can manifest as diarrhea and has been implicated in recent research as contributing to the SIRS-like physiologic response seen in severe heat stroke with multiorgan dysfunction. Direct endothelial damage from heat exposure may also lead to SIRS physiology via the DIC pathway (**Fig. 1**). Using SIRS as a model, novel treatment approaches to severe heat stroke using immune-modulating agents such as recombinant human activated protein C are under consideration.[10]

DIAGNOSIS AND RISK STRATIFICATION

Strict diagnostic criteria for the heat-related illnesses do not exist, except for agreement that the diagnosis of heat stroke should include a temperature of 40°C and CNS dysfunction. Therefore, recognition of the severity and extent of heat exposure as the root cause of the presenting complaint(s) takes precedence. Early recognition of elevated core temperature, knowledge of environmental exposure, careful consideration of the differential diagnosis (**Box 1**), and a search for anything in the medical history that predisposes the patient to heat-related illness are all key. Two reasonably well-defined variants of heat stroke, exertional heat stroke and classic heat stroke, should be understood; they have different causes, but their final pathways are almost identical.

Heat stroke is divided into 2 categories: exertional heat stroke (EHS) and classic heat stroke (CHS). The distinction is important because their pathologic bases are

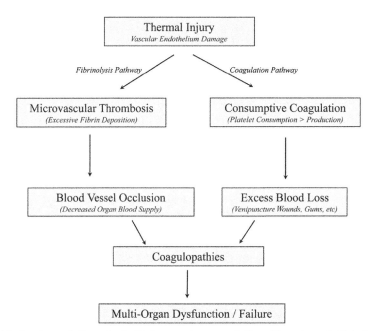

Fig. 1. Mechanisms of disseminated intravascular coagulation. (*From* Leon L, Helwig B. Heat stroke: role of the systemic inflammatory response. J Appl Physiol 2010;109(6):1983; with permission.)

Box 1
Differential diagnosis of hyperpyrexia

Drug associated

  Toxicity

    Anticholinergic

    Stimulant toxicity (phencyclidine, cocaine, amphetamine, ephedrine, MDMA)

    Salicylate toxicity

  Serotonin syndrome

  Neuroleptic malignant syndrome

  Malignant hyperthermia

  Drug withdrawal syndrome: ethanol withdrawal

  Drug-induced fever

Infections

  Generalized infections (eg, bacterial sepsis, malaria, typhoid, tetanus)

  CNS infections: meningitis, encephalitis, brain abscess

Endocrine derangements

  Thyroid storm, pheochromocytoma

Neurologic

  Status epilepticus

  Cerebral hemorrhage

Environmental exposure

  Heat exhaustion

  Heat stroke

Blood clots

  Deep vein thrombosis, pulmonary embolism, deep-seated hematomas

Abbreviation: MDMA, 3,4-methylenedioxymethamphetamine (Ecstasy).
Data from Khoujah D, Hu K, Calvello EJ. The management of the hyperthermic patient. Br J Hosp Med 2011;72:571–5.

different in the populations at risk for them (they can be thought of as "active" [EHS] or "passive" [CHS]). EHS typically occurs in individuals participating in strenuous sports and those whose occupations lead to heat exposure during exertion, such as firefighters and military personnel. Even though these individuals might be in good physical condition, the environment or the use of gear elevates their temperatures beyond the regulatory range of the body's cooling mechanisms. Poor physical conditioning and lack of acclimatization (discussed later in the section on treatment) can contribute to the development of or worsen EHS. The US Army has produced a detailed technical bulletin for the recognition and treatment of heat exhaustion and EHS.[8]

CHS occurs among individuals who have impaired physiologic mechanisms for heat dissipation, stemming from comorbid metabolic or cardiac conditions, or who lack the means to escape a hot environment, for economic, psychiatric, or social reasons, including substance abuse, or because of physical challenges. CHS can be considered a passive process, although it could be exacerbated with even minimal exertion in vulnerable populations. Decreased cardiac function limits the significantly increased cardiac output demands created by blood flow to the skin vasculature. Cardiac function can be decreased by structural heart disease and by medications used to treat heart disease. Diabetes can dampen the skin vascular vasodilatation response itself. The poor and homeless often do not have access to air conditioning, leading to group-cooling solutions that many cities adopt during hot summer months. Chronic behavioral/psychiatric challenges can prevent affected individuals from seeking appropriate environments during periods of elevated temperatures.

In the patient with undifferentiated altered mental status, heat illness may be overlooked unless core temperature is measured during the initial assessment. Patients at increased risk for CHS are also at increased risk for myriad other causes of depressed CNS status, so the diagnostic workup should not cease with the recognition of elevated core temperature. Other life-threatening causes to be considered include infection, endocrine derangements, neurologic issues, and drug-induced syndromes (**Table 2**).

The clear consensus for assessment of core temperature is rectal measurement. Oral, axillary, skin sensing, and tympanic membrane methods have all been shown to be inferior to rectal measurement.[18] Rectal temperature assessment is recommended by sports medicine organizations as the preferred methodology, although poor acceptance and impracticality are cited as impediments.[19] Although there is no absolute criterion for core temperature, most literature cites a core temperature of 40°C for the diagnosis of heat stroke.

The term heat-related illness encompasses any pathologic process caused by an acute increase in core temperature resulting from exertion, passive environmental exposure, or both. Heat exhaustion is at the less extreme end of the spectrum and can present with fatigue, rapid pulse, profuse sweating, vomiting, and weakness,

Table 2
Heat-related illness syndromes

Elevated body temperature at presentation	Heat exhaustion	Systemic symptoms: tachycardia, weakness, nausea/vomiting, profuse diaphoresis	Temperature may be normal in heat exhaustion, although presentation uniformly follows very recent exposure to high temperature
	Heat stroke	Temperature >40°C Central nervous system symptoms	Progresses to multiorgan system failure
		Exertional heat stroke	"Active": found in athletes, military personnel, firefighters
		Classic heat stroke	"Passive": found in elderly, many comorbidities, socially/environmentally limited
Normal body temperature at presentation	Prickly heat	Rash caused by chronic heat exposure	
	Heat edema	Dependent edema in poorly heat-acclimated elderly	
	Heat cramps	Severe leg cramps seen some time after cessation of vigorous exercise	

but without CNS symptoms not attributable to orthostasis. Most cases of heat exhaustion are a mixture of sodium and water depletion and are rarely pure presentations of either.

The heat-related illnesses typically seen in normothermic patients after ongoing low-grade heat exposure are prickly heat, heat edema, and heat cramps. Prickly heat, also called lichen tropicus, is a dermatologic condition presenting as a rash caused by the plugging of sweat ducts with material from the stratum corneum produced by excess sweating. As sweat production continues behind the plugged sweat duct, the resulting pressure causes the duct to rupture, leading to an inflammatory vesicular reaction. With repeated cycles of rupture and replugging of the duct with desquamated material a deeper chronic pruritic dermatitis develops, known as miliaria profunda.[20] Treatment is symptomatic for pruritus, unless secondary infection occurs (*Staphylococcus aureus* is the most common pathogen).

Heat edema is lower extremity–dependent edema seen after heat exposure, attributed to microvascular transudate of fluid with prolonged peripheral vasodilatation. It can also present in the hands. This type of edema is not associated with volume overload, and is commonly seen in elderly patients with relative hypovolemia caused by inadequate replacement of volume losses in hot environments. Heat edema is commonly found immediately following abrupt transition from a cold to a hotter climate. Elevation and compression stockings are the preferred treatment; diuretics have no role.

Heat cramps, most often experienced in the lower extremities, occur after cooling has occurred. These cramps are thought to be caused by hyponatremia, can be quite painful, and can be treated with balanced electrolyte oral solutions. The hyponatremia in heat cramps is associated with volume loss due to sweating, which should be replaced by hypotonic oral solutions rather than balanced electrolyte-containing solutions.

Heat syncope can occur in response to skin vasodilatation, resulting in functional orthostasis after exposure to heat. An elevated core temperature is not required to make the diagnosis. In a young, otherwise healthy patient who experiences only brief syncope clearly associated with orthostasis and returns to completely normal function, the diagnosis is minor heat-related illness. However, if syncope occurs in the same population at risk for CHS, a more aggressive evaluation is warranted.

Regardless of cause, the hyperthermic patient should undergo diagnostic testing proportionate to the severity of presentation. The diagnostic workup should not be guided strictly by meeting clinical definitions of discrete syndromes, but rather by clinical suspicion for morbidity based on the patient's medical history and presentation, and an understanding of the effects of severe heat stress. Laboratory evaluation might include basic chemistries to assess sodium levels and renal function, creatine kinase levels for consideration of rhabdomyolysis, and coagulation parameters for assessment of DIC/SIRS. In the obtunded patient, a chest film, electrocardiogram, computed tomography scan of the head, and, possibly, lumbar puncture are appropriate means to look for other causes of, and direct disorders arising from, elevated temperature.

TREATMENT

Because heat-related illness includes a wide spectrum of severity, the therapeutic options range from simple cooling measures and oral hydration to intensive care services. Young, healthy adults with normal examination results, other than mildly elevated core temperature, may be observed in a cool environment and provided oral hydration with cooled, slightly hypotonic solutions. Solutions with high osmolality slow gastric emptying, delaying transition of cooled fluids to the small intestine and leading to improvement in core cooling. Most clothing should be removed to expose as much skin surface as possible to the cooler environment; wet clothing, even of light weight, significantly impairs the efficacy of evaporation of sweat in cooling.

The cornerstone of treatment in more severe heat illness is rapid reduction of core temperature and supportive care. Most elements of treatment are empiric, starting with an ABC (airway/breathing/circulation) approach. Obtunded or hemodynamically compromised patients may require endotracheal intubation. Core cooling methods should be started immediately. Almost all patients with a heat illness at any point along the spectrum will be hypovolemic, so volume replacement should occur early in the course of treatment. The preferred solution for volume replacement is normal saline, given the high likelihood of some degree of hyponatremia after sweating profusely. These measures should all be instigated by field personnel, with a focus on rapid cooling. Heled and colleagues[21] proposed that the traditional emergency medicine "golden hour" should be thought of as the "golden half-hour" in the case of heat emergency; morbidity is reduced dramatically if cooling measures, usually in the field, begin within 30 minutes after recognition.

Because studies of cooling methodologies tend to involve small numbers of patients, it is difficult to control for the many variables involved; therefore, most recommendations regarding treatment are experiential, and based on empiric understanding of the pathophysiology of heat stress and the body's response. Based on experience with young healthy athletes with EHS cited in the sports medicine literature, complete immersion of the patient below the neck in cold water seems to be the most efficient cooling method, when appropriate and available.[19] There is no such body of evidence for immersion therapy in CHS patients. The high thermal conductivity of water eliminates the local insulating effect of heated air immediately adjacent to the skin; however, circulating water is presumed to improve cooling via convection. Concerns about peripheral vasoconstriction induced by cold water, leading to decreased efficacy of cooling, as well as shivering induced by cold water, serving to continue the increase in temperature, are outweighed by the therapeutic benefit.[16] Some sports trainers advocate vigorous massage of the extremities to overcome the vasoconstriction effect and promote blood flow to the extremities. If severe shivering causes the patient significant discomfort or impedes resuscitative efforts, benzodiazepines can be used to reduce it. Phenothiazines should be avoided, as should any medication with anticholinergic properties that could reduce sweating. Immersion in ice water (2°–3°C) is more effective than immersion in cold water (10°–20°C) for rapid reduction of core temperature.[18]

Cold-water immersion is often not practical. Equipment used to resuscitate sicker patients (eg, cardiac monitoring leads, intravenous equipment, endotracheal tubes) as well as agitation, poor patient tolerance, and vomiting and diarrhea make immersion in cold water challenging. Most emergency departments do not have the facilities necessary for cold-water immersion. The most common and effective cooling method in the emergency department is a combination of spraying the skin with tepid water and running a fan to augment evaporation and convection. Although this method does not provide cooling at a rate comparable with that of immersion, it is better tolerated, practical, and associated with a low mortality rate.[19]

In theory, when immersion is not available, placing ice as close as possible to the great vessels provides high-volume exposure to the cold. Application of ice packs to the neck, groin, and axilla is another commonly used cooling method. Military units and emergency medical service organizations have used the downdraft from a stationary helicopter to cool overheated personnel and patients.[22]

Administration of cold intravenous fluids is typically not recommended. A recent case study, however, described a severely hyperthermic patient suffering EHS (multiorgan system failure, including coma, seizures, and DIC parameters) who was placed on the therapeutic hypothermia protocol used for cardiac-arrest patients. The patient made a full recovery, pointing out the need for further study of this approach.[23] Wilson and Crandall[12] suggested consideration of this method, because (1) therapeutic hypothermia has clearly demonstrated efficacy in preserving brain function after insult resulting from cardiac arrest, (2) no research-based lower-limit temperature goal has been established, and (3) a broad body of literature has established the relative safety of hypothermia-inducing methods, including infusion of cold intravenous fluids. Other internal cooling measures, such as cold-water gastric lavage, peritoneal lavage, and rectal or bladder lavage, are poorly studied in humans and can result in water intoxication. Cooling blankets are not effective.

In general, cooling measures are often stopped before the patient becomes normothermic, so as to avoid "overshooting" and causing hypothermia. Dantrolene, an inhibitor of muscle contraction via decrease of calcium released from the sarcoplasmic reticulum, has not been shown to have benefit in hyperthermia.[24]

Hypotension should be treated as distributive shock, caused by shunting of a large proportion of the circulating volume to the periphery via vasodilatation, although hypovolemia must also be considered. Initial permissive hypotension during the cooling phase allows gradual peripheral vasoconstriction and redistribution of the circulating volume centrally. Overly aggressive volume expansion during the initial phases of management can result in pulmonary vascular congestion. Because of this concern, it is reasonable to provide isotonic intravenous fluids in 500-mL aliquots with frequent clinical assessments, including measurements of central venous pressure in critical care management. If vasopressors are needed to manage severe refractory hypotension, agents with predominant α-adrenergic effects, such as norepinephrine, should be avoided because of the theoretical concern about peripheral vasoconstriction leading to decreased core cooling. Use of vasopressor agents is associated with poor outcomes.[12]

Prevention is also particularly important. Acclimatization is an important and highly effective preventive measure, especially for people at risk for EHS, namely those who cannot completely avoid heat stress for occupational or other reasons. Although there is overlap in the physiologic effects of acclimatization and conditioning, good physical conditioning does not confer the full protective effects of acclimatization. Acclimatization requires daily exposure to high temperatures over a 1- to 2-week period. Prolonged exposure causes predictable adaptation of the body via increased plasma volume, onset of sweating at lower temperatures, increased sweat volume with lower electrolyte concentration in the sweat, lower heart rate in response to exercise, and increased stroke volume.[20]

Other preventive measures include ensuring adequate oral hydration, frequent and systematic assessment of those at risk for EHS, and avoidance of strenuous athletic activity during temperature extremes. It is critical to not leave the elderly or young children unattended in vehicles, even for a short time with partially open windows. In response to concerns about the increasing frequency of high-temperature weather emergencies, 12 European countries have set up heat-wave early warning systems.[25] Many of these systems specifically address populations at risk by arranging monitoring of socially isolated and disadvantaged individuals during a heat wave.

SUMMARY

Heat-related illnesses can be avoided or minimized by using proper preventive measures, such as correct evaluation of the environment and acclimatization or, when a high-temperature environment is unavoidable, reducing activities that create heat stress. Recognition of a primary heat-related illness, while considering the complete differential diagnosis of hyperpyrexia, is key to appropriate treatment. Current research indicates that the most effective means of reducing core temperature is cold-water immersion, when feasible, or evaporative techniques, which are more widely accessible in the setting of an emergency department. Any CNS manifestation of heat-related illness is an ominous finding and indicates higher severity of impact, warranting more aggressive evaluation and treatment.

REFERENCES

1. Simon HB. Current concepts: Hyperthermia. N Engl J Med 1993;329(7):483–7.
2. National Climatic Data Center, National Oceanic and Atmospheric Administration. State of the climate. Available at: www.ncdc.noaa.gov/sotc. Accessed March 12, 2013.
3. Jones TS, Liang AP, Kilbourne EM, et al. Morbidity and mortality associated with the July 1980 heat wave in St. Louis and Kansas City, MO. JAMA 1982;247: 3327–31.
4. Dematte JE, O'Mara K, Buescher J, et al. Near-fatal heat stroke during the 1995 heat wave in Chicago. Ann Intern Med 1998;129(3):173–81.
5. Argaud L, Ferry T, Le QH, et al. Short- and long-term outcomes of heatstroke following the 2003 heat wave in Lyon, France. Arch Intern Med 2007;167: 2177–83.
6. Webb P. The physiology of heat regulation. Am J Physiol 1995;268:R838–50.
7. Platt M, Vicario S. Heat illness. In: Marx JA, editor. Rosen's emergency medicine. 7th edition. Elsevier; 2009. p. 1882–92.
8. Wyndham CH, Strydom NB, Cooke HM, et al. Methods of cooling subjects with hyperpyrexia. J Appl Physiol 1959;14(5):771–6.
9. Sherwood SC, Huber M. An adaptability limit to climate change due to heat stress. Proc Natl Acad Sci 2010;107(21):9552–5.
10. Leon L, Helwig B. Heat stroke: role of the systemic inflammatory response. J Appl Physiol 2010;109:1980–8.
11. Charkoudian N. Skin blood flow in adult human thermoregulation: how it works, when it does not, and why. Mayo Clin Proc 2003;78:603–12.
12. Wilson T, Crandall C. Effect of thermal stress on cardiac function. Exerc Sport Sci Rev 2011;39(1):12–7.
13. Semenza J, McCullough J, Flanders W, et al. Excess hospital admissions during the July 1995 heat wave in Chicago. Am J Prev Med 1999;16:269–77.
14. Lugo-Amador N, Rothenhause T, Moyer P. Heat-related Illness. Emerg Med Clin North Am 2004;22:315–27.
15. Gader AM, al-Mashhadani SA, al-Harthy SS. Direct activation of platelets by heat is the possible trigger of the coagulopathy of heat stroke. Br J Haematol 1990;74: 86–92.
16. Erarslan E, Yüksel Í, Haznedaroglu S. Acute liver failure due to non-exertional heatstroke after sauna. Ann Hepatol 2012;11(1):138–42.
17. Chen WT, Lin CH, Hsieh MH, et al. Stress-induced cardiomyopathy caused by heat stroke. Ann Emerg Med 2012;60:63–6.
18. Smith JE. Cooling methods used in the treatment of exertional heat illness. Br J Sports Med 2005;39(8):503–7.
19. Bouchama A, Dehbi M, Chaves-Carballo E. Cooling and hemodynamic management in heatstroke: practical recommendations. Crit Care 2007;11(3):R54.

20. Bouchama A, Knochel J. Heat stroke. N Engl J Med 2002;346(25):1978–88.
21. Heled Y, Rav-Acha M, Shani Y, et al. The "golden hour" for heatstroke treatment. Mil Med 2004;169(3):184–6.
22. Poulton TJ, Walker RA. Helicopter cooling of heatstroke victims. Aviat Space Environ Med 1987;58(4):358–61.
23. Hong J, Lai Y, Chang C, et al. Successful treatment of severe heatstroke with therapeutic hypothermia by a noninvasive external cooling system. Ann Emerg Med 2012;59:491–3.
24. Hadad E, Cohen-Sivan Y, Heled Y, et al. Clinical review: treatment of heatstroke: should dantrolene be considered? Crit Care 2005;9(1):86–91.
25. Lowe D, Ebi K, Forsberg B. Heatwave early warning systems and adaptation advice to reduce human health consequences of heatwaves. Int J Environ Res Public Health 2011;8:4623–48.

Index

Note: Page numbers of article titles are in **boldface** type.

Emerg Med Clin N Am 31 (2013) 1109–1116
http://dx.doi.org/10.1016/S0733-8627(13)00102-8
0733-8627/13/$ – see front matter © 2013 Elsevier Inc. All rights reserved.

emed.theclinics.com

United States Postal Service

Statement of Ownership, Management, and Circulation
(All Periodicals Publications Except Requestor Publications)

1. Publication Title	2. Publication Number	3. Filing Date
Emergency Medicine Clinics of North America	0 0 0 - 7 1 4	9/14/13

4. Issue Frequency	5. Number of Issues Published Annually	6. Annual Subscription Price
Feb, May, Aug, Nov	4	$298.00

7. Complete Mailing Address of Known Office of Publication (Not printer) (Street, city, county, state, and ZIP+4®)

Elsevier Inc.
360 Park Avenue South
New York, NY 10010-1710

Contact Person
Stephen R. Bushing

Telephone (Include area code)
215-239-3688

8. Complete Mailing Address of Headquarters or General Business Office of Publisher (Not printer)

Elsevier Inc., 360 Park Avenue South, New York, NY 10010-1710

9. Full Names and Complete Mailing Addresses of Publisher, Editor, and Managing Editor (Do not leave blank)

Publisher (Name and complete mailing address)

Linda Belfus, Elsevier, Inc., 1600 John F. Kennedy Blvd. Suite 1800, Philadelphia, PA 19103-2899

Editor (Name and complete mailing address)

Patrick Manley, Elsevier, Inc., 1600 John F. Kennedy Blvd. Suite 1800, Philadelphia, PA 19103-2899

Managing Editor (Name and complete mailing address)

Barbara Cohen - Kligerman, Elsevier, Inc., 1600 John F. Kennedy Blvd. Suite 1800, Philadelphia, PA 19103-2899

10. Owner (Do not leave blank. If the publication is owned by a corporation, give the name and address of the corporation immediately followed by the names and addresses of all stockholders owning or holding 1 percent or more of the total amount of stock. If not owned by a corporation, give the names and addresses of the individual owners. If owned by a partnership or other unincorporated firm, give its name and address as well as those of each individual owner. If the publication is published by a nonprofit organization, give its name and address.)

Full Name	Complete Mailing Address
Wholly owned subsidiary of	1600 John F. Kennedy Blvd., Ste. 1800
Reed/Elsevier, US holdings	Philadelphia, PA 19103-2899

11. Known Bondholders, Mortgagees, and Other Security Holders Owning or Holding 1 Percent or More of Total Amount of Bonds, Mortgages, or Other Securities. If none, check box ☐ None

Full Name	Complete Mailing Address
N/A	

12. Tax Status (For completion by nonprofit organizations authorized to mail at nonprofit rates) (Check one)
The purpose, function, and nonprofit status of this organization and the exempt status for federal income tax purposes:
☐ Has Not Changed During Preceding 12 Months
☐ Has Changed During Preceding 12 Months (Publisher must submit explanation of change with this statement)

PS Form 3526, September 2007 (Page 1 of 3 (Instructions Page 3)) PSN 7530-01-000-9931 PRIVACY NOTICE: See our Privacy policy in www.usps.com

---

13. Publication Title	14. Issue Date for Circulation Data Below
Emergency Medicine Clinics of North America	August 2013

15. Extent and Nature of Circulation		Average No. Copies Each Issue During Preceding 12 Months	No. Copies of Single Issue Published Nearest to Filing Date
a. Total Number of Copies (Net press run)		902	819
b. Paid Circulation (By Mail and Outside the Mail)	(1) Mailed Outside-County Paid Subscriptions Stated on PS Form 3541. (Include paid distribution above nominal rate, advertiser's proof copies, and exchange copies)	546	500
	(2) Mailed In-County Paid Subscriptions Stated on PS Form 3541 (Include paid distribution above nominal rate, advertiser's proof copies, and exchange copies)		
	(3) Paid Distribution Outside the Mails Including Sales Through Dealers and Carriers, Street Vendors, Counter Sales, and Other Paid Distribution Outside USPS®	151	148
	(4) Paid Distribution by Other Classes Mailed Through the USPS (e.g. First-Class Mail®)		
c. Total Paid Distribution (Sum of 15b (1), (2), (3), and (4))	▲	697	648
d. Free or Nominal Rate Distribution (By Mail and Outside the Mail)	(1) Free or Nominal Rate Outside-County Copies Included on PS Form 3541	74	71
	(2) Free or Nominal Rate In-County Copies Included on PS Form 3541		
	(3) Free or Nominal Rate Copies Mailed at Other Classes Through the USPS (e.g. First-Class Mail)		
	(4) Free or Nominal Rate Distribution Outside the Mail (Carriers or other means)		
e. Total Free or Nominal Rate Distribution (Sum of 15d (1), (2), (3) and (4))	▲	74	71
f. Total Distribution (Sum of 15c and 15e)	▲	771	719
g. Copies not Distributed (See instructions to publishers #4 (page #3))	▲	131	100
h. Total (Sum of 15f and g)	▲	902	819
i. Percent Paid (15c divided by 15f times 100)		90.40%	90.13%

16. Publication of Statement of Ownership

☐ If the publication is a general publication, publication of this statement is required. Will be printed in the November 2013 issue of this publication.   ☐ Publication not required

17. Signature and Title of Editor, Publisher, Business Manager, or Owner	Date
Stephen R. Bushing Stephen R. Bushing – Inventory Distribution Coordinator	September 14, 2013

I certify that all information furnished on this form is true and complete. I understand that anyone who furnishes false or misleading information on this form or who omits material or information requested on the form may be subject to criminal sanctions (including fines and imprisonment) and/or civil sanctions (including civil penalties).

PS Form 3526, September 2007 (Page 2 of 3)

mergencyMed **Advance**~

ll the latest emergency medicine news and research you need, all in one place

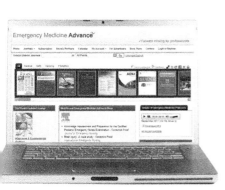

EmergencyMedAdvance.com is a new essential online resource offering valued high-quality content and news for the global community of Emergency Medicine professionals to save time and stay current—from physicians and nurses to EMTs.

ay current
Emergency Medicine news

ve time
Access relevant articles in press from 16 participating journals

nd more...
ournals' profiles
Personalized search results
Emergency Medicine bookstore

- Upcoming meetings and events

- Search across 500+ health sciences journals
- Learn how to submit a manuscript

- Sign up for free e-Alerts
- Emergency Medicine jobs

**ookmark us today at
mergencyMedAdvance.com**

ELSEVIER

Printed and bound by CPI Group (UK) Ltd, Croydon, CR0 4YY

03/10/2024

01040478-0001